THE GROWTH OF
BUREAUCRATIC
MEDICINE

HEALTH, MEDICINE, AND SOCIETY:
A WILEY-INTERSCIENCE SERIES

DAVID MECHANIC, Editor

THE GROWTH OF BUREAUCRATIC MEDICINE

An Inquiry into the Dynamics of Patient Behavior and the Organization of Medical Care

DAVID MECHANIC
University of Wisconsin-Madison

WITH THE COLLABORATION OF

Linda H. Aiken, Robert Wood Johnson Foundation
James R. Greenley, University of Wisconsin-Madison
Doris P. Slesinger, University of Wisconsin-Madison
Bonnie L. Svarstad, University of Wisconsin-Madison
Richard Tessler, University of Massachusetts-Amherst

A WILEY-INTERSCIENCE PUBLICATION

JOHN WILEY & SONS, New York • London • Syndey • Toronto

Library of Congress Cataloging in Publication Data:
Mechanic, David, 1936–
    The growth of bureaucratic medicine.

    (Health, medicine, and society)
    "A Wiley-Interscience publication."
    Includes bibliographical references and index.
    1. Social medicine.   2. Medical care.   3. Health
attitudes.   4. Medical care—United States.
I. Title.   [DNLM: 1. Delivery of health care—U.S.
2. United States. W84 AA1 M48g]

RA418.M33   362.1   75-29347
ISBN 0-471-59021-5

Printed in the United States of America

10 9 8 7 6 5 4 3 2 1

FOR ROBERT

Preface

This book examines central aspects of the organization of medical care, and particularly primary medical care, from the perspective of patients, health professionals, and policymakers. It contains analytic essays by me on medical organization and the problems of effectively designing human services, and empirical studies of patients, health professionals, and policymakers carried out by me and some of my colleagues and students in the past few years. Some of these studies deal with patients, others with doctors; some with the attitudes and behavior of healthy people in the population, others with patients with serious medical problems such as myocardial infarction; some with special populations such as black mothers, troubled adolescents, or poverty populations, others with more representative cross sections of the population. Most frequently we focus on physicians as providers of service, but occasionally we examine their roles in medical politics, in research, and in educational activities.

We are concerned here with illness in its various manifestations—physical, psychological, and behavioral. Our program of research is based on the belief that effective understanding of the functioning of the health care delivery system requires a broad perspective and an examination of the aspirations, problems, and constraints affecting its various participants. Only by viewing the system from different vantage points can we begin to appreciate the complex synthesis that results from the interaction of the varying participants involved. Doctor and patient, administrator and policymaker, each comes to view care in terms of how he or she relates to the system of care; each constitutes part of the reality, but not the entire reality. By examining the fit that evolves at the point of service delivery, we obtain a better picture of how to make the needs of patients and the delivery of services more congruent.

Although the studies reported here are varied, they all relate to a general theme involving the following questions. When we examine the problems and needs of patients, and the constraints operating on health professionals, how do we design systems that bring them into a better congruence? How do policymakers at the federal, state, or delivery system level, who design programs to improve access to care, quality, or efficiency, remedy obvious deficiencies in medical care in an effective and humane manner? What are the important needs that patients have that are not being dealt with, and how might the health care system be mobilized to do better?

The program of studies described in this book has been supported by grants from the Robert Wood Johnson Foundation, the National Institute of Mental Health, the National Center for Health Services Research, and the Milbank Memorial Fund. I conceived the book and did much of the writing as a Fellow at the Center for Advanced Study in the Behavioral Sciences at Stanford, and I very much appreciated the hospitality and stimulation so evident there. The University of Wisconsin Graduate School Research Committee was generous in providing part of my support during this year. I am grateful to many of my colleagues who have read the manuscript or parts of it and have made helpful comments: Jacob Fine, Burton Fisher, Eliot Freidson, Lawrence Friedman, Robert Haggerty, William Parson, Herman Stein, and Aaron Wildavsky.

Four of the collaborators in this book were doctoral and postdoctoral students of mine at Wisconsin. The fifth, James Greenley, has been a member of the Wisconsin faculty. They have been stimulating and cordial colleagues, and I am particularly pleased to present some of our joint efforts here.

I am grateful for the very able assistance of my secretary Lorraine Borsuk who typed the manuscript and assisted with a variety of other details. I also thank Christine Valentine for her excellent copy editing and Ann Wallace for her proofreading and indexing.

DAVID MECHANIC

Center for Advanced Study
in the Behavioral Sciences
Stanford, California
July 1975

Acknowledgments

Some of the chapters appearing in the book are adapted from work published elsewhere, and I am grateful for permission from the publishers to use these materials in this volume. Chapter 1 is adapted from a paper entitled "Health and Illness in Technological Societies," published by the *Hastings Center Studies*, **1**:7–18 (1973). Chapter 2 is adapted from a review reprinted, with permission, from *Annual Review of Sociology*, Volume 1, 1975, copyright by Annual Reviews, Inc. All rights reserved. Chapter 6 is based on a paper appearing in the *Ethics of Health Care*, published by the Institute of Medicine, National Academy of Sciences, 1974. Chapter 7 is based on two papers previously appearing in the *Journal of Health and Social Behavior*, **16**:95–113, (1975) and in *Health and Society*, **53**:149–172 (1975). Finally, Chapter 15 is adapted from a paper on evaluation appearing in Jack Zusman and Cecil Wurster, eds., *Evaluation of Alcohol, Drug Abuse, and Mental Health Service Programs,* published by Lexington Books, 1975.

I am also grateful to the various publishers who granted permission to quote copyrighted materials: Holt, Rinehart and Winston, Inc. (excerpts from A. Bandura, *Principles of Behavior Modification,* 1969, pp. 9, 111–112); *Politics and Society* (excerpt from R. Alford, "The Political Economy of Health Care," **2**:164, 1971); Random House, Inc. (excerpt from William Nolen, *A Surgeon's World,* © 1970, pp. 211–212); The Williams & Wilkins Co., Baltimore (excerpt from C. Hofling et al., "An Experimental Study in Nurse Physician Relationships," *Journal of Nervous and Mental Disease,* **43**:173, 178, 1966); University of California Press (excerpt from J. Pressman and A. Wildavsky, *Implementation,* 1973, pp. 93–94, originally published by the University of

California Press, reprinted by permission of The Regents of the University of California); Russell Sage Foundation (excerpt from Edward A. Suchman, Ph.D., *Evaluation Research: Principles and Practice in Public Service and Social Action Programs,* © 1967 by Russell Sage Foundation, pp. 7–8); The Minneapolis Medical Research Foundation, Inc. (excerpt from S. Mushkin, "Evaluations: Use with Caution," *Evaluation,* 1:30–35, reprinted by permission of the copyright holder. Copyright © 1973, The Minneapolis Medical Research Foundation, Inc.); Baywood Publishing Co., Inc. © (excerpt from R. Logan, "National Health Planning." *International Journal of Health Services,* 1:11–12, 1971); Basic Books, Inc. (excerpts from Chapter 6, "Paying for Medical Care," from Victor Fuchs, *Who Shall Live?: Health, Economics, and Social Choice,* © 1974 by Basic Books, Inc., Publishers, New York); *Yale Journal of Biology and Medicine* (excerpts from Paul Beeson, "Moral Issues in Clinical Research," 36:465, 1964); and the American Medical Association (excerpts from Henry Beecher, "Consent in Clinical Experimentation," *Journal of the American Medical Association,* 195:124, © 1966, American Medical Association).

D. M.

Contents

PART III ILLNESS, ILLNESS BEHAVIOR, AND HELP-SEEKING:
          IMPLICATIONS FOR THE DESIGN OF HEALTH SERVICES

PART IV   TRENDS IN HEALTH POLICY, SOCIAL REGULATION,
          AND IN THE EVALUATION OF HEALTH PROGRAMS

THE GROWTH OF
BUREAUCRATIC
MEDICINE

Introduction

There is an unmistakable trend toward the growing bureaucratization of medical care in the United States and other highly developed nations. This trend receives its momentum from growing knowledge and the technological development of medicine, the increased involvement of government in the financing and regulation of health care, and the search for mechanisms that increase efficiency and accountability of providers of medical service. The increased organizational elaboration of medical settings is an inevitable consequence of the growing complexity of medical tasks. At issue is the type of organizational approaches appropriate to the varying character of medical technology and to the special human problems of medical care. While the concept of bureaucracy is not used here pejoratively, it is abundantly clear that the future organization of medicine requires organizational approaches that are very much at variance with traditional models of formal organization. As government plays a larger role in medical care, it tends to impose bureaucratic forms with which it is particularly familiar, without special sensitivity to the unique aspects of delivering sensitive personal services. Although I argue for the advantages of greater organizational coherence in the planning and practice of medicine, my thesis is that to graft organizational concepts developed in more traditional areas of governmental activity—particularly the traditional bureaucratic model—would be inappropriate for the effective and humane performance of medicine.

Although I find little cause for optimism about future developments, a sensitivity to the special needs of human services organizations exists. And although discussions of approaches better fitted to important personal aspects of care are increasing, organizational theory in sociology has been slow to break from traditional concepts of bureaucracy and to see new organizational possibilities. Today we depend more and more on the conscious design of complex systems to achieve our objectives. Bureaucrats who develop plans, legislators who design bills, and administrators who devise guidelines all approach their tasks with some conception, either explicit or implicit, of the motivations, values, and life concerns of those who will be affected. The legislation and the guidelines contain incentives and disincentives that have as their purpose the shaping of human behavior.

In many respects, the static design of administrative systems is not well fitted to the transactional quality of human interaction. As with the stimulus-response experimental design, the designer of human organizations can provide certain incentives, but has no opportunity to control the complex transactions that might result from those incentives. Just as the traditional experimenter could only observe what happened in response to the experimental stimulus, and therefore could not capture the way in which subjects in a more open system might manipulate or subvert the stimulus to their own advantage, the architect of human systems designs incentives and hopes for the best. The failures to achieve desired effects are notorious.

The inherently difficult task of designing effective incentives is made even more problematic by the fact that those who design such systems are often one-dimensional in their thinking and lack understanding of various human factors or social forces that affect the behavior and adaptive strategies of participants. Human beings are more than pawns to be moved at the will of high-level bu-reaucrats; they actively monitor and adapt to their environments. People in-terpret the various manipulations designed to affect them, and manage situa-tions in terms of their own goals and values and the constraints to which they are exposed.

To the extent that we deal with organizations that produce clearly definable and measurable products or services, organizational designs are more easily ap-plied, although even in these circumstances participants may be unwilling partners who divert, delay, and manipulate efforts to increase productivity. But as we move into areas where organizational objectives are more ambiguous and intangible, there is greater opportunity for the actors involved to exercise coun-tercontrol, to shape the system in their own images and on the basis of their own concerns. The human services field is particularly vulnerable to miscal-culation by those who attempt to impose "rational" incentives to achieve valued objectives. As frequently as not, such incentives produce effects quite dif-ferent from those intended.

This book deals with one type of human services organization—the medical care bureaucracies. Although medical care is only one part of a larger pattern of helping institutions in an organizational society, consideration of this limited sphere permits close examination of the enormous difficulties and possibilities of the planning process, whether it be embodied in legislative intent or in the translation of such intent by administrative agencies and personnel. The lessons we learn from this close examination will, I hope, have wider implications for understanding how more effectively to release the potentialities of human beings.

THE PLAN OF THIS BOOK

One view that emerges from the perspective developed in this book and the results reported from our research is that organizational behavior is enormously complex. Participants' responses vary, and are difficult to anticipate or to direct. The sociological approach that examines behavior from the viewpoint of each of the relevant participants, and that attempts to understand their behavior in terms of opportunities and constraints in their interactions with others, provides a level of explanation often lacking in ordinary commentary on human affairs. But this is hardly enough; it is too easy to "understand" why people behave as they do, why they fail to conform to more lofty designs. The danger in such explanations is that we become content to account for what is, and fail to seek a definition of something better toward which we must strive.

Although we may be criticized for failure to suggest, in some chapters, clear blueprints for creating new organizational environments, our basic premises are clear throughout. First, our bureaucratic organizations, ostensibly organized to serve people more efficiently, too frequently come to serve those who control them and who treat their clients in an impersonal and dehumanizing fashion. Second, under the guise of science, efficiency, and effectiveness, we often degrade the human qualities of helping institutions. Third, our society desperately needs experiments in new forms of social organization that provide renewed bases for personal commitment, that contribute to the deprofessionalization of the expert, and that encourage a higher level of caring. And, finally, medicine as a social institution is as important in its functions as a source of human sustenance and support as it is in its technical interventions. Medicine without caring is technics run wild.

Yet the problems are extraordinarily difficult. They are embedded in our complex economic and sociocultural environment, and pose their own special dilemmas as well. Much of the advocacy on medical affairs is facile or so out of tune with current realities as to make its relevance very limited. Readers who want panaceas or clear blueprints for the future had better seek them elsewhere; I offer no obvious, grand solutions. The chapters that follow offer a statement of values about what we would like medicine to offer as a social institution, and an exploration of existing barriers in achieving the appropriate behaviors of health professionals, managers, and patients. This book takes a stand on many issues. It argues that medicine must be structured to give more emphasis to the psychological and behavioral aspects of health and disease; that the necessary decision on how to ration services should be made by inducing providers to economize rather than by placing barriers on the initial access of consumers to care; that, despite many difficulties, a national health care system that provides universal access to care as a right, and that introduces limits on economic allocations through prospective national budgeting, offers the greatest potential for a sane and equitable system of health care services in the United States.

Some readers will be impatient with the qualifications that accompany my commitments and recommendations. Why, they will ask, can you not advocate what you stand for unequivocally, without hedging? Although I believe that planning is better than no planning, my research has made me increasingly skeptical of grand solutions, of well worked out designs, of simple answers to complex issues. More and more I believe that we require a combination of planning and muddling through. This stance offers direction but also flexibility, and supposes a willingness to experiment with alternatives and to concede failure when failure is evident.

The book begins with a general and comparative survey that traces the dramatic organizational changes mandated by the growth of knowledge and technology. These changes, which are evident throughout the developed world and in some underdeveloped countries, require that we consider new organizational frameworks for medical care, new roles for health professionals, and the social and ethical implications of technological advances. Chapter 1 provides a general description of these trends; Chapter 2 provides a comparative framework, reviewing from a sociological perspective the limited existing research on comparative health care systems; and Chapter 3 briefly reviews some of the emerging conflicts in the roles of physicians who work in more complex organizational settings. Chapter 4, on the design of human services systems, sets the stage for much of the research and analyses that follow. It deals with varying concepts of organizational management and with disputes about the forces that either give organizations their impetus or impede their effective performance. Although the discussion deals with general issues, it focuses primarily on medical care and provides a framework for the specific studies that follow.

Parts II and III report on studies of the performance of varying health care delivery programs and of the perceptions and reactions of patients. Part II focuses on the prepaid group practice model, the most frequently advocated solution for dealing with many current problems in medical care. We examine the diversity of entities included within this rubric, and compare the ways in which patients and physicians respond to various types of practices. A major issue is how to organize prepaid practice to assure that the reality more closely fits the idealistic claims made for it. In Part II we do not explore problems by enumerating them; we let the difficulties and dilemmas become apparent as we examine how patients and doctors perceive and respond to one another, how physicians organize their work in varying settings, and how strategies of practice affect patient care.

Part III is more specifically focused on patients, and how their sociocultural background, social situation, and special problems affect their views of illness and their reactions to life difficulties. In our view, it is absurd to consider organizational design without giving substantial attention to the special inclinations, needs, and typical reactions of the individuals the system is designed to serve. Thus, we also consider how medical services can be responsive, given the variability and complexity of patient reactions. In a formal sense, research on patients is tangential to the consideration of bureaucratic organization. But in our view it is central; human services bureaucracies must have the capacity to respond flexibly, not only to the technical contingencies of medical tasks, but also to the wide range of problems and behaviors and social situations of patients. Chapter 8 poses the general issues, and is followed by four research studies, each focusing on a specific aspect. Chapter 9 examines alternative sources of help for similar problems, and explores the factors that lead people into varying networks of care. Chapter 10 examines the barriers to using preventive services, and suggests some ways of overcoming them. Chapter 11 examines doctor-patient communication, and particularly the difficulties in achieving conformity with medical advice. Chapter 12 illustrates the psychosocial complexity of the treatment of myocardial infarction, one of the most common of the serious conditions physicians must deal with, and considers how treatment might be organized to respond not only to medical factors but also to psychosocial adaptations that may facilitate or retard the effects of medical care.

The final part of the book explores issues of health policy and evaluation, and the role of social science research in these matters. The chapter on informed consent illustrates some of the difficulties in balancing the needs of the individual patient or subject against the needs of the larger society. By exploring social psychological dimensions of informed consent, it becomes clear why some of the formal regulatory mechanisms developed in recent years have had only limited success. I then consider how social scientists might be more useful in policy formulation and evaluation, and particularly how their location in the network of policy considerations is likely to affect their influence. This is followed by more specific consideration of evaluation research in health care, which is one of the areas where social scientists, particularly if they understand the policy formulation process, can make a special contribution.

I complete the book by considering alternative approaches to national health insurance and some of the potentials, but also cautions, in choosing to go in either one or another direction. The considerations are of a general kind and are likely to be relevant in understanding future developments, regardless of whatever legislation may pass in the next year or two. Although I favor an approach based on a prospective budgetary allocation and the organization of services within restraints set by a budgetary allowance, I also examine some of the difficulties we should anticipate in attempting to implement such an approach. In short, I offer no simple or utopian solutions. I anticipate that, whatever course we take, we will face the need for continuing reconsideration and readjustments. Equity and quality will come only by continuing pressure on the system of care, by monitoring and reassessment, and by a willingness to experiment with alternative approaches and alternative incentive systems. Our success will depend on our willingness to modify programs on the basis of experience and assessment, abandoning those concepts that turn out more elegant in theory than in reality.

I
THE GROWTH OF
BUREAUCRATIC
MEDICINE:
A COMPARATIVE
PERSPECTIVE

Chapter 1

Health and Illness in
Technological Societies

Cultural attitudes and behavior relevant to health and Illness vary widely depending on social conditions, levels of education and socioeconomic status, and stages of technological development. In the more highly developed technological societies, the biomedical sciences and medical practice are well developed, and there is a growing congruence between medical and lay conceptions of them. But in much of the world, highly sophisticated and scientifically oriented attitudes and behavior exist alongside elaborate folk beliefs, and social position and education are predictive of health orientations. The privileged experience low rates of infant mortality and considerable longevity, and die primarily of heart disease, cancer, strokes, and accidents. The impoverished suffer a high rate of infant loss, consume diets often deficient in calories, protein, and vitamins; and experience a wide range of preventable disorders including gastroenteritis, tuberculosis, trachoma, and a variety of other water-borne and infectious diseases. The low level of nutrition results in general vulnerability to diseases and problems of growth and development.

Although education is highly correlated with health status and health practices, the close correspondence between education and other living conditions sometimes leads public officials to place undue emphasis on acquisition of knowledge by itself. The improved state of health in highly technological societies probably results more from a nutritious diet, better immunization practices, and improved sanitation and water supply than it does from acquisition of correct information. Well-organized public health programs and improved standards of living are the core of efforts to raise the levels of health. At any given living standard, education and knowledge are important in facilitating the maximum use of available resources, but the emphasis on knowledge in the absence of other efforts becomes a rationalization to excuse existing inequalities.

Many of the folk practices characteristic of underdeveloped rural communities and urban slums help in coping with the anomic and disorganized social conditions that prevail. They constitute part of a pattern that holds groups together under conditions of social strain and uncertainty. The few patterns of folk tradition and culture that remain are often the rural peasant's or the migrant's only insulation against the worst consequences of industrialization and urbanization. Understanding the functional utility of traditional belief systems assists us in introducing change in the least disruptive fashion and in a manner that makes the population more receptive to the adoption of health innovations.

Folk beliefs persist in even the most modern nations, but they are very much submerged in countries with highly developed, scientific systems of medical practice. As medical science and technology have developed in modern nations, there has been a growing convergence in health attitudes and provision of medical care. This is true not only within nations but also among nations with great differences in ideology, historical and social background, and economic organization, and reflects common adaptations to the demands of new knowledge, the elaboration of medical technology, the demonstration of efficacy in various spheres, and growing expectations of populations who now experience a relatively high living standard.

The growth of technology and the scientific base of medicine have mandated an elaborate and specialized technical system that is extremely expensive. At the same time, conditions in the society at large create enormous demand for health services and growing expectations about the achievements of medical care. As a result, health care absorbs an increasing proportion of gross national products and societal resources, and the natural possibilities for continuing expansion seem at this time to be unlimited. Therefore, all developed nations are seeking solutions that allow them to be responsive to expectations and also to protect budgetary processes from being overwhelmed by health expenditures.

Although health systems in developed countries are enormously complex and involve an elaborate technology, medicine continues to play the sustaining role it has in more simple and underdeveloped societies. Indeed, as society itself becomes increasingly bureaucratized and impersonal, and as populations become more geographically mobile—disrupting kinship relations, traditional helping patterns, and opportunities for expressing intimacy—problems that were dealt with informally are increasingly part of professional work in the health sector. Epidemiological investigations of the occurrence of illness and seeking of medical care suggest that much of the motivation for contact with the health care system results from environmental stress and life problems; and physicians who man the front lines of the health care system increasingly complain of the trivial and inappropriate complaints of their patients. Thus, there is an indication that the technological structure, which characterizes modern medicine, is viewed somewhat differently by the professional and the client, and is a good deal less than perfectly responsive to the forces bringing patients into the health care system.

Traditionally, the institution of medicine developed to provide sustenance to those facing uncertainty, anxiety, and distress. Patients sought out physicians before physicians had much technical ability to provide help. Throughout much of the world today, people still seek help for their ills from diviners, witch doctors, and other healers—often at the same time that they use the facilities of modern medicine. For centuries the major function of medicine was to ameliorate distress and to provide support and relief from pain and discomfort. It is ironic that now that medicine has developed the capacity to be helpful in a variety of ways, it has lost much of its capacity to communicate compassion, so central to the healing process. Indeed, even from a purely technical perspective, the effectiveness of medical care depends on the patient's cooperation. The patient must be able and willing to provide information, to conform with medical advice, to return to the physician, to take medication properly, and to carry out numerous other tasks. Failures in communication and empathy not only harm a vital function of medical care, but also diminish the opportunities for technical quality and effectiveness.

The question of why persons who have access to excellent technical facilities use healers, folk remedies, and other nonrational approaches attunes us to important issues about the character of health institutions. The common answer heard in medical settings is that such persons are superstitious and ignorant, and that progress is possible only through education.

Ignorance can be attributed so smugly to those who use nonscientific therapists and practices because in developed technological societies we have come to take for granted the medical perspective, and there is a relatively close correspondence between lay perspectives and scientific-medical points of view. In part, this reflects the diminution of the authority of religious views of bodily functions and a growing dependence on a medical view of physical experience. The National Fertility Study in the United States documents this growing trend among, for example, Catholics who reject church dogma on contraception despite religious adherence in other respects. One of the most impressive characteristics of modern technological nations is the extent to which outlooks previously shaped by moral standards and religion have been increasingly influenced by technical developments, and the authority of traditional institutions in molding these perspectives has been very much diminished. Correspondence between lay concepts and scientific-medical views is much greater than in underdeveloped countries; but despite the more limited nature of client referral networks and lay healing systems in modern society, great strains still persist between medical practices and lay perceptions. This is particularly evident in the United States, for example, among American Indians and Spanish-speaking Americans.

Correspondence between medical and lay perspectives develops to the extent that a secular value system exists, and also depends on demonstrated effectiveness of established medical knowledge. Where medical technology is effective, as in contraceptives, immunization, or antibacterial drugs, there is an absence of competing perspectives. Competing conceptions are more likely to thrive in areas where medical intervention is itself uncertain—for example, in the psychiatric area and in the behavior disorders, where there are strong competing nonmedical interpretations, and in such areas as cancer, the common cold, and arthritis and rheumatism. In modern nations, once physicians demonstrate effective intervention, competing theories appear to weaken dramatically.

Although we take it for granted, the extent to which medical concepts have come to dominate other concepts in many realms of life is truly a remarkable phenomenon. The growing domain of medicine has served effectively to sustain social patterns in a manner consistent with a modern industrial society. As medicine has developed, it has increasingly taken over the functions of care provided by family and close associates and has facilitated the smooth persistence of social activities despite sickness and social disability among some family members. Hospitals, in particular, have facilitated social life by assuming responsibility for the mentally ill, the aged, the retarded, and those with a variety of other problems in functioning; and the standardized technology of medicine and its general availability, in contrast to community helping patterns and kinship networks, has facilitated geographic mobility and a pattern of family organization consistent with the demands of industrial organization. With new technologies, such as psychoactive drugs and home dialysis units, and changing concepts of care, the medical system is increasingly attempting to develop ways of managing patients in the community without total dependence on hospitals, which are expensive and not always the most effective way of providing care. But such efforts require new community facilities, such as support systems and day and night hospitals, that limit the responsibilities placed on the family which in modern society usually lacks the resources to take on these functions in any extensive way.

As the domain of medicine has extended to all aspects of behavior and society, it has frequently gone well beyond its technical competence. As society develops a less intimate pattern of social intercourse, persons in difficulty increasingly look to the physician as a source of sustenance and care. Such behavioral patterns as drug abuse, alcoholism, and sexual behavior—previously viewed as largely under the control of individual volition and socioenvironmental influences—are increasingly accepted as medical problems to be dealt with within the context of the medical model. As medicine has moved rapidly into these more controversial and more poorly defined areas, it has met opposition from traditional institutions, but the direction of the drift is clear. Medicine as an institution has developed great potentialities for facilitating social control of the population, and these potentialities are very much increased by the growing centralization and bureaucratization of medical practice. The momentum of this tendency in modern societies makes it necessary to consider both the character of scientific-medical orientations and the manner in which medical institutions in society are integrated with other social institutions and the roles they perform.

MEDICAL CONCEPTIONS OF HEALTH AND ILLNESS

Medical conceptions of disease are derived from a model that attempts to identify clusters of symptoms causally related in some fashion and to establish the etiology, course, and treatment of the particular entity. Within the more traditional domain of medicine, such entities may be well understood (as in the case of pernicious anemia), partially understood (as in the case of diabetes or coronary heart disease), or highly uncertain (as in the case of sarcoidosis and schizophrenia). The approach, however, proceeds on the assumption that disease states are definable, and much effort is devoted to more reliably identifying new disease states and searching out their various characteristics and appropriate treatments.[1]

Most complaints brought to the physician by a patient are characterized by pain, distress, and disrupted functioning. Increasingly, such complaints result from the failure of individuals to meet certain established social and behavioral norms: complaints such as obesity, alcoholism, sexual problems, mental illness, child misbehavior, and the like. Faced with such problems, the traditional medical approach seeks to identify an underlying disorder in the organism that explains the apparent deviant manifestations, and these behavioral syndromes are increasingly identified as diseases. Such definitions, like all definitions of disease, are arbitrary. The only justification for depending so substantially on the medical model is its assumed utility. But as the characteristic morbidity pattern of modern nations is defined increasingly by chronic and recurrent illness, accidents, and psychological disorders, the utility of the traditional disease model for understanding many important health problems is unclear.

A contrasting model usually advocated by nonphysicians but also by some physicians is particularly obvious in the evaluation of deviant behavior. This model seeks to understand the problems within social, cultural, legal, and moral paradigms. The deviant behavior is seen not as disease, but as a reflection of life style, social adaptation, or philosophical or political struggles. In dealing with most deviant behavior, the utility of the medical model is usually uncertain, and the viewpoints of physicians often reflect their own biases and social viewpoints. Yet physicians' authority and decision-making powers in society permit them frequently to act on unconfirmed theories, and such actions have great societal consequences.

Similarly, there is a competing perspective among some medical scientists to the predominant medical one, a perspective that views disease not as discrete clusters but as adaptations to life environments. It emphasizes an epidemiological approach that considers the interrelations between host, agents, and the larger socioenvironmental context. It seeks to elucidate the environmental conditions conducive to disease processes and to examine what differentiates those who become sick from those who do not, why they are vulnerable to attack in certain bodily systems, and why illness becomes apparent at certain times and not at others.

In short, modern societies are characterized by medical conceptions that are varied and in flux. As the preventable diseases and those that can be brought under control with existing interventions are alleviated, the modern medical system faces a residue of other conditions to which the predominant causal models do not easily apply. However, the biomedical basis of medical practice continues to develop and has encouraged an elaborate technology—and related task specialization—which has had spectacular categorical successes but has failed to come to terms with the profound moral and social issues in the practice of medicine and its role in society. Both the difficulty of these issues and the momentum of technology have contributed to the view that medical practice is what medical advances make possible. Modern health systems have forged ahead, following the technological imperative—physicians must do everything possible for their patients—while neglecting the question of patients' rights and wishes, the impact of biomedical advances on society, and the allocation of resources in society among competing sectors. As a result, we see growing attempts to gain control over medical technology and to direct its impact on society.

MEDICINE AND THE STATE

The same forces that stimulate the state to exert greater control over medical practice pose dilemmas for the role of medicine in society more generally. As the domain of medicine grows, so does its potential influence over the lives and activities of the average citizen; and as its technology becomes more effective, medical care holds a more central and important place in the perceptions of the public. Traditionally we have come to view the physician as an agent of the patient. In most cases, the relationship between patient and physician was entered voluntarily, and ethics required the physician to give the patient's interests highest priority. If the reality departed from the ideal, at least the nature of the contractual relationship between healer and client depended on the continued willingness of the patient to define the practitioner as his or her agent and to continue to provide the necessary remuneration. In these circumstances, the uncertainties of medical assessments and the ambiguities of the ethical context were less central since the situation was based on the premise that the patient's best interest would be supreme. Whether the healer was to exorcise the spirits, lower a fever, or remove an inflamed appendix, the direction of the therapy originated from the patient's initial definition of his or her problem.

As medical technology developed and new forms of medical organization emerged, the institution of medicine itself became a more powerful interest in the relationship between patient and practitioner. In the major medical centers, the patient's interests were no longer supreme. Teaching, research, and the maintenance of a routinized and effective system of operation also played important roles. At the community level, industrialization brought physicians an increased responsibility in work certification, disability determinations, legal and insurance assessments, and similar areas. In these circumstances, the auspices of the physician probably affect the outcomes for patients in subtle ways.

With new forms of organization emerging to encompass recent developments in medical technology and to provide more accessible and more equitable care, there is a trend toward a change in the auspices of medical care. Increasingly, the physician and other health workers are employees of a bureaucratic organization, resulting in a shift in their loyalties from the individual patient providing the fee to the organization, the profession, or the physicians' sponsors. Although the character of such shifts needs more careful study, indications are that the technical quality of care is enhanced, but that patients are dealt with more impersonally. Patients are more likely to feel that physicians are inflexible, less interested in them, and less willing to take time to listen to them. There is a tendency in such organizations to give relatively less attention to the patients' concerns and relatively more attention to the problems of organization and work demands.

The extent to which medicine as an institution can exercise social control is seen in the military uses of medicine or in the organization of health care in totalitarian regimes. Medicine can be used to assure adequate industrial manpower, or to justify release from work for employees who hate their jobs. Which course it is more likely to take will depend as much on who controls medical institutions as on the nature of medical knowledge and technology. In military situations the physician is an agent of the armed forces and not of the patient and, unless a dissenter from within, the pressures are to pursue a course consistent with the interests of the organization, which may vary from the interests of patients. The outcome of employment medical examinations similarly may depend on whether the physician works for the patient or for industry. In legal contests, the physician's stand is often predictable, depending on which side is paying him. Many medical decisions of interest to society in its daily affairs are discretionary, and the character of decisions is likely to be influenced by who it is the physician represents.

ETHICAL ISSUES AND SOCIAL CONTROL

As biomedical knowledge and technology continue to confront society with new dilemmas, the decision-making processes that direct events must be improved. Thus far, it has been enormously difficult to control new technologies or to shape their implications for society, and we have followed developments more than we have directed them. We have attempted to devise rules on an ad hoc basis. For example, when transplant technology confronted us with the issue of obtaining viable organs, we began to reconsider the biological meaning of death and to ponder the legal questions of organ acquisition and disposal. Such ad hoc processes help avoid societal confrontations, but provide little time for planning and tend to be reactive.

The difficult ethical issues raised by many biomedical advances bring into sharp contrast existing cultural and moral differences in society. Rigid, normative prescriptions governing the physician's traditional obligation to preserve life, and the ideology of doing whatever one could, contributed to stability in society even if the gap between theory and reality was considerable. For in acclaiming the shared value of the sanctity of life, the existing deviations appeared idiosyncratic rather than systematic or based on public policy. Because decisions were less visible they were more acceptable. Attempts to translate informal behavior into public policy—as was attempted in an English hospital when age guidelines for resuscitation were made explicit in a written order—result in mass public outcries. But informal practices, however valuable in minimizing conflict, tend to be inequitable. They favor the rich and the conventional over the poor and the deviant. While they facilitate bootlegging humanistic solutions to difficult personal dilemmas—as occurred in informal medical procedures for obtaining abortions—these solutions were not equally distributed to those in need. There is no question that open confrontation, such as has occurred over the legalization of abortion, exacerbates social conflict and acrimony among religious and social groups, but it also exposes the issues and helps clarify them. Open discussion creates new possibilities for the development of social movements and agitation for social change.

It is not at all clear whether modern societies are as yet prepared to confront openly the dilemmas of biomedical advances. While informal practices have a certain expediency and solve difficult problems for the society, the statement of principles has a cementing quality and is difficult to reverse. It is one thing to experiment with transplantation and other spectacular techniques; it is quite another to make a societal commitment to provide the technology for all of those in need. Each of these ethical issues is for some an abstract question and for others the stark reality. Do those who only ponder the issue as a matter of philosophy have equal say to those who confront the reality? In the case of advances affecting small numbers of people, do we have the capacity to communicate to the public the contingencies and implications of following one or another course? In making informal decisions a wide variety of factors come into play—the situation of the patient and the family, their social circumstances, the quality of living at stake, and the moral and social attitudes of the decision makers. Bringing such considerations into the public arena in a constructive way is one of the difficult challenges we face. For it is not clear that we know how to consider or make such decisions.

It is almost trite to reflect on the enormity of the ethical and moral issues that future developments in the biomedical sciences suggest. How we shall deal with them is unclear, but it is apparent that the informal solutions that have been so prevalent in the past are less likely to prevail in the future because of the changes taking place in medicine itself. Traditionally, we have seen many of the dilemmas as problems to be worked out by patients and their individual physicians in their continuing relationship, which was viewed as confidential and intimate. But medicine is now more complex; physician services are more specialized, stratified, and segmented, and a wide variety of nonmedical personnel plays an important role in the delivery of patient care. Moreover, the nature of the information system is very much altered; decisions are more widely known by a variety of others. Furthermore, the organizational auspices of care—and particularly payment arrangements and the implementation of Professional Standards Review Organizations—are likely to have tremendous bearing on what is attempted and what is done. The inclusion of particular technologies, such as transplantation, within any kind of insurance scheme is likely to have important consequences for the financing of the health care system as a whole and the allocation of resources between health care and other sectors.

The complexities of a changing technology encourage bureaucratic solutions. But, at the same time, people in modern societies are seeking greater autonomy over decisions affecting their own lives. How individual rights to use one's own body as one wishes are balanced against larger organizational needs is likely to depend on the impact of any particular practice on societal functioning. Although such practices as abortion are very much involved with religious and social ideologies, the drift of events is clearly related to views on population policy as a whole. In all likelihood the right to abortion would be viewed very differently in a context where individual decisions markedly interfered with societal purposes. In the chapter on informed consent (Chapter 13) some of the conflicts between protection of individuals and social needs are explored, as are the difficulties in developing effective regulatory policies.

LAY CONCEPTIONS AND THE SCIENCE OF MEDICINE

In general scientific practitioners proceed from a theoretical perspective that is far removed from the conceptions of those who seek their assistance. To the extent that medical practitioners have given convincing demonstrations that they can treat illness, persons may come seeking help; but they share little of the information and scientific understanding available to the physicians. Rather, they construct their world on an experiential and empirical basis modified by prior assumptions, cultural learning, and world views. Western physicians often feel frustrated with such patients because they are frequently uncooperative in adhering to medical advice. They follow practices that are clearly detrimental to their health, and they fluctuate back and forth between scientific and traditional healers. The difficulties that modern practitioners have with such patients reflect the fact that the patients, although users of medical facilities, are not converts to modern medical conceptions. They may accept the authority of the physician in only a limited sphere and may leave the relationship or ignore medical advice when their cultural conceptions of cause or therapy are violated.

Although similar problems exist in modern nations, they are more submerged and have lesser overall impact. Those in underdeveloped countries have influential and culturally supported systems of belief in conflict with modern medicine, while persons in modern nations find less social support for competing points of view, except in some ethnic enclaves. Thus, although folk beliefs—particularly those consistent with experience—may continue to persist and may affect the provision of care, they do not usually constitute competing systems of belief. Recently developed countries, such as China, continue to retain strong traditional beliefs—particularly in rural areas—and Chinese medicine constitutes an interesting attempt to merge traditional and modern medical practices.

Increased levels of education and the influence of mass media have contributed importantly to the growing convergence of patients' and practitioners' concepts of disease. Health is a popular public theme, and the public's interest in biomedical developments is impressive. As the public has become more conversant with medical concepts, physicians are more frequently confronted with requests for new drugs, therapies, and devices, and with searching questions concerning their professional advice. Indeed, the sophisti-cated consumer is increasingly straining the traditional doctor-patient relation-ship and challenging the authority of the physician in a fashion that many phy-sicians find uncomfortable. As the momentum for consumer input grows, as support for encouraging informed and articulate patients develops, and as the public increasingly becomes more sophisticated about medical science and medical practice, the character of traditional physician-patient relationships will change significantly.

All our experience to date suggests that we will continue to welcome new ad-vances in medical science and technology. The current crisis in modern nations is not with medical technology, but rather with its costs and the difficulty of meeting rising expectations and demands for equity of access, concerns that result in part because of the successes of medicine. While decision makers seek an optimal balance, the sick and their loved ones usually seek whatever relief and assistance science can offer. While at the margins the extension of life raises difficult issues in active societies dominated by a practical scientific ethic, few will accept less than what science makes possible.

PATIENT BEHAVIOR AND MEDICAL PRACTICE SYSTEMS

In focusing on new developments in the biomedical sciences, we risk neglecting the fact that most medical care is a relatively mundane matter. The overwhelm-ing majority of the population seeking medical care comes to physicians' offices complaining of routine symptoms and illnesses. In general, medical care has a limited impact on morbidity and longevity in society. As modern science has af-fected physicians' views about the nature of their work, the discrepancy between those views and the patient's motivation in seeking care is enlarged.

Various surveys in modern nations indicate that only a small proportion of patients with symptoms seek the assistance of a physician. Although severity of symptoms and the extent to which they disrupt ordinary activities are im-portant factors, there is enormous overlap between presenting complaints and untreated symptoms. Physicians throughout the world report that patients come for trivial and inappropriate reasons, but doctors themselves do not agree on what is trivial and inappropriate; and in the aggregate, physicians' percep-tions of both trivial symptoms and those worthy of care may be different from the conceptions of their patients. Patients come to emphasize symptoms that are discomforting, frightening, or disrupt usual activities; physicians are likely to think in terms of symptoms for which their techniques of practice apply. This fundamental difference in perspective contributes to a lack of congruence between the motivation for seeking care and what physicians wish to do.

The view of the physician has been shaped, in large part, by biomedical advances. Increasingly, doctors have been trained to depend on sophisticated, diagnostic tools and complex approaches. In this light, many patient complaints appear trivial and inappropriate. Although various studies suggest that life problems are important factors in medical utilization, the science base of medicine has had little behavioral science content. Behavioral technologies, however limited, might be useful in orienting physicians to more appropriate management of many patients.

THE GROWTH OF THE BIOMEDICAL SCIENCES IN MODERN NATIONS

Modern nations have experienced the rise of highly developed social institutions to support the growing scope of biomedical science activity. Research and development constitute essential aspects of the health sector, and it is widely believed that science and technology will provide new solutions that will cure disease, increase longevity, and improve the quality of life. These expectations have been consistently reinforced by the enormous progress that has characterized medical care in recent decades. But as René Dubos has repeatedly emphasized, each social environment creates new health problems in its own image, reflecting its goals, priorities, and concepts of progress. Disease problems often reflect the consequences of how people have chosen to live, and even the impressive advances of the biomedical sciences have created new health problems of major dimensions. The ability to support life, longevity, and functioning among persons with genetic vulnerabilities to serious disease increases the birthrate among such persons and thus the need for continuing care. For example, it is commonly believed that the proportion of diabetics in populations has increased; and under community care programs made possible by biomedical advances, schizophrenic women have higher birth rates. Anyone familiar with such programs as renal dialysis appreciates not only the enormous advantage of these technologies, but the profound and continuing problems that such patients and their families face, not only in relation to their treatment but also in respect to work, family life, and the quality of living in general.[2]

In considering future investments in biomedical research and development, we must realize that varying technologies have very different consequences for society. Some, such as polio immunization, are oriented toward early prevention and reduce the need for medical care and specialized personnel in the health system. Others, such as transplantation, result in large increased costs and expenditures and in highly developed and specialized health personnel. Some developments allow persons whose lives would have been hopeless in the not-too-distant past to lead full and vigorous lives, while others create horrendous problems of coping with a life that will never retain functional viability, but will involve complex and agonizing decisions for health professionals and the families of patients. With all the existing uncertainties and the difficulty of predicting the nature of biomedical advances in the future, establishing priorities is an enormously difficult task. But the alternative is to let events take us where they will, and inaction may involve graver consequences than difficult and uncertain decisions.

The biomedical sciences have become an establishment in their own right seeking funding, autonomy, and a free lease on taking discovery wherever it may lead. The advocates of the establishment repeatedly emphasize the gains through biomedical developments—the antibiotics, polio immunization, renal transplants—maintaining that inquiry is likely to reap greater gains in the future. Legislators and their constituencies, concerned about particular disease threats, usually express categorical priorities, but funding has been sufficiently diffuse in the past to support an extensive basic science infrastructure necessary for science advancement generally. Although the emphasis on targeted approaches threatens the infrastructure, in all likelihood administrative definitions will be sufficiently flexible to sustain the core of basic studies necessary to the future advance of biomedical science activities.

As medicine has been institutionalized as a dominant profession and one of high prestige, it has become increasingly independent of its clients. The value of medical services is not significantly questioned in modern societies except perhaps by a few social scientists, and the patient is assumed to value the services available. Thus, physicians have felt no great need to proselytize or to offer their services in a form responsive to cultural subgroups more skeptical of medical care and influenced by competing belief systems.

Everywhere in the world the groups least educated, most needy, and suffering from the greatest morbidity are most likely to have frames of reference discordant with the assumptions dominant in everyday medical practice. Too frequently, physicians are contemptuous of what they see as superstitious and ignorant attitudes and behavior. Yet medical practice can be conveyed in a fashion consistent with subcultural values and beliefs. Care can be provided so that it is less likely to violate subcultural expectations and norms. The failure to concern itself with the conditions for establishing relationships, inducing cooperation, achieving conformity with suggested regimen, or managing effective follow-up and continuance in care, is a major failure of medicine.

Similarly, the low levels of penetration of immunization and other preventive practices in subgroups of the population are indicative of the incapacities of medical organization. For in the final analysis, the success of medical care must be measured by what is achieved in the aggregate rather than by its scientific elegance or its more miraculous achievements. Medical care is as much a form of organization as a set of technical tasks. Without an effective plan to translate knowledge into action, it becomes elitist in orientation and ineffectual in maintaining community health. With appropriate organization and societal direction as to goals and priorities, medical science provides the means to vastly enhance life and reduce suffering. But, unless encased in a context defining social goals and individual rights, biomedical advance can contribute to the further alienation and dehumanization of man as a social and a moral actor.

NOTES

1. D. Mechanic (1968), *Medical Sociology: A Selective View* (New York: Free Press).
2. R. Fox and J. Swazey (1974), *The Courage to Fail* (Chicago: University of Chicago Press).

Chapter 2

The Comparative Study
of Health Care
Delivery Systems

O nly recently has significant effort been made to examine comparatively the organization and performance of health care delivery systems. But since even recent efforts have been largely developed within a health services framework, they have lacked significant theoretical perspectives. The existing data describe particular locations and periods of time, and thus are limited for testing sociological hypotheses. As with comparative research in other areas, the definition and measurement of comparable units within varying sociocultural and historical circumstances are difficult, and samples of complex entities, such as delivery systems, are only obtained with considerable effort and cost.

One possible level of sociological analysis involves examining the character of the health care delivery system in relation to the structure of society. Glaser,[1] for example, on the basis of visits to various countries and through interviews and written material available on health care delivery in those countries, posed a number of hypotheses concerning the relationships between the religious, familial, and economic aspects of social organization and the character of hospital organization, including such matters as recruitment into hospital occupations and the development and uses of technology. Careful, empirical investigation of these hypotheses would be a task of major proportions. While it is interesting to know, for example, to what extent the strength of a religious mandate to help strangers affects motives for employment, the priority of hospital work, and the length of working hours, such propositions do not tell us a great deal about varying dimensions of performance among health care systems within modern industrial societies. However, Glaser's approach is useful in bringing to our attention the extent to which variabilities in the structure and performance of modern health care systems have been narrowed by industrialization, urbanization, secularization, and the growth of technology; and his hypotheses provide useful concepts from which to examine the differences in medical care in developed and underdeveloped nations.

Health care delivery systems have broad social functions not only in treating disease and disability, but also in alleviating tensions and distress and in sustaining persons in the performance of social roles.[2] The health care delivery system frequently deals with conflicts and dilemmas resulting from larger societal demands, and may be either an instrument of social control, a means of social support, a context in which difficult social disputes can be informally managed, or all of these.

The intangible consequences of many health services and their varying social functions make comparative study difficult. Even within more narrow conceptual limits, there is a lack of specification of outputs reasonably expected to be affected by the types of inputs characteristic of medical organization.[3] Levels of investment in health services and variations in organization—so far as we can presently ascertain—have had limited impact on the most readily available output measures, such as infant and adult mortality.[4] More subtle indicators are underdeveloped, and it is only recently that greater effort is being devoted to developing more appropriate measures.[5] Thus, sociological researchers have concentrated almost all of their effort on inputs and processes of care in contrast to performance measures. Across nations, such inputs and processes reflect different traditions, cultures, and political and economic processes.

THEORETICAL CONSIDERATIONS

It is commonly agreed at a more general level that the organization and priorities of health care organization reflect the political and economic priorities of its sponsors, and that each health care system has developed within its own historical and sociocultural contexts, which lead to many of its more unique qualities. However, such observations are confirmed more by case studies of individual systems than by comparative studies of the economic and political bases of medical care in diverse settings.

At the macro level, the most sustained and fertile analysis derives from Parsons'[6] conceptualization of the functional role of health services within the larger social system. At the individual level illness serves as an accepted excuse for relief from ordinary obligations and responsibilities, and may be used to justify behaviors and interventions not ordinarily tolerated by the social system without significant sanctions. At the societal level the definition of illness may be used more or less as a mechanism of social control to contain deviance, to remove misfits from particular social roles, or to encourage continued social functioning and productive activity. Thus, from a sociological standpoint, the locus of control for medical decision-making is a key variable in examining the implications of medical care for social life more generally. For the most part, sociologists have not carefully examined varying approaches to regulation, the extent to which physicians in different countries have power and responsibilities extending beyond ordinary medical work, and the resulting implications for society. But with the growing bureaucratization of medicine and increased regulation, sociologists will inevitably direct more of their attention to such issues in the future.[7]

Given the diversity of political contexts among nations, the extent to which most medical care delivery systems have resisted intrusion of larger political interests is remarkable, and reflects in part the immense worldwide status and autonomy of the medical profession.[8] The growth of medical knowledge and technology has so pervasively influenced the shaping of health delivery systems that nations with very different ideological preferences have similar forms of medical care systems and face common problems and dilemmas.[9, 10] Although government sponsorship and control of medical care have in some contexts resulted in radical alterations in the distribution of services,[11-14] forms of service delivery and professional organization are less varied than might be anticipated on the basis of ideological, political, or economic differences among nations.

One consequence of increasing knowledge and technological potential is the growth of specialization and fragmentation in the delivery of services in all modern medical care systems. Although it is difficult to meet ordinary primary care needs with increasing reliance on specialized technologies and an elaborate division of labor, new organizational models for meeting these basic functions have been slow to develop. The slow adaptiveness of social organization to emerging technologies reflects both the economic and political strength of the health professions throughout much of the world, and the extraordinary difficulties in developing an adequate accommodation between a rapidly growing knowledge base and sophisticated technology and the expectations, understandings, and preferences of populations.[15]

A major difficulty in the sociological investigation of comparative medical organization is the inadequacy of traditional concepts describing emerging structural arrangements and ongoing organizational processes. The conceptual approaches that fit centralized, bureaucratized organizations are poorly adapted for studying intraorganizational programming and cooperation, coordination among agencies, and organizational networks. In the American context, for example, we have no adequate sociological paradigm that facilitates the classification and study of such organizational entities as health sciences centers, prepaid group practices, comprehensive medical foundations, hospital mergers, and the like. An examination of any of these organizational devices suggests a wide range of dimensions on which entities having similar designations may differ, but we have yet to develop an adequate set of generic concepts that are meaningful in understanding prevailing forms of organization within single countries, much less on a crossnational level. Most research depends on commonly understood designations such as hospitals, clinics, medical schools, and so forth.

Because of the meager development of comparative sociological study of national systems of medical care, I focus on several types of comparative studies both between and within national systems. The appropriate boundaries of medical care systems are frequently unclear since medical work may be more or less closely related to the delivery of social welfare services. In this chapter I emphasize the health care sector as compared with broader social welfare functions in varying societies. From the point of view of clients, however, varying delivery systems are often alternatives for dealing with similar problems.

After a brief examination of the world system of medical care, a tentative paradigm describing the operation of national health systems is suggested, followed by more specific models of various components of health delivery systems and their comparative effects on health outcomes. All of these models are exploratory; they help define issues for research and help organize disparate efforts in the area. But since available comparative data are both limited and frequently flawed, these suggested models primarily direct attention to issues requiring more focused research.

THE INTERNATIONAL KNOWLEDGE, TECHNOLOGY, AND MANPOWER MARKETPLACE

Science and technology transcend national boundaries. With the facility of rapid transmission of information in modern societies, new knowledge or technological innovations may rapidly diffuse throughout the world. The character of medical care is dependent on the degree of established knowledge and technological development at any given time. Education for medical science and practice derives from the existing base of science and technology. Medicine, in particular, is characterized by intricate and rapid communication networks involving innumerable scientific journals—many of an international character—and abstracting, indexing, and translating services. Moreover, drugs and medical products are produced by industries of considerable size that aggressively market their technologies on a worldwide basis.

Even in less developed countries there is a strong trend toward approaches to medicine characteristic of modern nations, despite the fact that such development may be ill-suited to major population needs or to the economic ability of the country. This results—except for some of the socialized countries—in a highly stratified system of medical care, where a well-developed medical capacity characteristic of modern Western nations caters to a tiny minority of the population. The limited affluence of many of these countries and their priorities for development make it unlikely that such services will be offered to a significant proportion of the population.

Medical schools throughout the world tend to emulate those characteristic of modern nations and are part of the worldwide medical community. Medical education thus encourages a pattern of practice that these countries can ill afford to implement widely. This results in limited economic and scientific opportunities for medical practice, and encourages an international migratory pattern of medical and scientific manpower for both education and employment. This migratory pattern is supported by greater available opportunities in modern nations (including more prestige, income, and autonomy), and by political factors. The ability to migrate is influenced by the need for physicians in receiving areas, immigration and licensing requirements, cultural and language similarities, and political orientations consistent with the prevailing medical system in the receiving country. The migratory pattern is one from the less to the more affluent countries that can offer better facilities and social opportunities to practice scientific medicine. The United States is a major recipient of physicians from other countries, and foreign-trained physicians constitute a significant proportion of doctors licensed in any year. During the past decade England and Wales lost a significant number of physicians through immigration to the United States, Canada, New Zealand, and Australia, but replaced them with doctors from India and Pakistan.[16] It may be that models describing the flow of populations from areas of lesser to greater opportunities through stages can successfully describe physician migration, but only fragmentary data are available, and most of the existing studies have been carried out from an American or British perspective.

PATTERNS OF MORTALITY AND MORBIDITY AND NATIONAL DEVELOPMENT[17]

In this century, patterns of mortality and morbidity in developed nations have shifted significantly from a preponderance of infectious disease problems to a variety of chronic degenerative diseases, accidents, and psychological and behavior problems.[18,19] Underdeveloped countries continue to show the characteristic pattern of malnutrition, abundant deaths from diarrhea and dysentery, tuberculosis, and a variety of other infectious, intestinal, and respiratory diseases.[20] The pattern of disease has a devastating effect on the population, and interacts with malnutrition to produce substantial disability and mortality in the population.

Patterns of disease and disability in underdeveloped countries clearly take an enormous toll on the capacities of those afflicted. The actual interaction between the health status of the population and national development, however, is far less clear. Most of the data available cannot clearly differentiate such relevant factors as the capacity of workers, underemployment related to economic forces, the effects of increased education, and other changes that often accompany improvements in health status, and the consequences of increased fertility. Measures of health status and economic development vary from one analysis to another and may be an important factor in conflicting data and conclusions. Health, for example, may be defined in terms of mortality rates from specific diseases, life-expectancy rates, man-years of labor available, infant mortality rates, and levels of health expenditure.

Much of the literature on health and national development is speculative and is written more to convince the reader about the economic value of health investments than to unravel the complex dynamics underlying the relationship. Most empirical efforts have been carried out by economists interested in human capital and those from the public health field.[21-26] These studies have illustrated some of the intervening processes that make it difficult to come to any simple conclusions about the effects of improved health. The studies examine such varied outcomes as the productive capacities of individual workers, of entire farms, or of regional areas using such measures as per capita gross national product, per capita energy consumption, total acreage under cultivation, production levels of specific crops or products, and per capita agricultural output. Some public health programs, such as malarial eradication, have beneficial effects on human health and also allow land to be reclaimed for agricultural development, but long-term effects are complicated by changes in fertility.[27, 28]

Although specific impacts of the delivery of health services on national development are difficult to measure, it is clear that in underdeveloped nations preventive health programs, such as those concerned with improved nutrition, sanitation, pure water sources, family planning, and the like, bring far greater benefits than those associated with curative medicine as practiced in modern nations.[29] The application of relatively simple public health measures has an enormous capacity to reduce mortality and increase longevity. From the perspective of national development, however, control of fertility is essential. The translation of medical techniques characteristic of modern nations to underdeveloped countries has relatively little impact in contrast to investments in broader public health measures.

The elaboration of the health care delivery system usually accompanies national development and interacts with improved economic and social conditions. However, the premature application of highly specialized curative medical care often captures for the few resources that could potentially reap greater benefits for the larger population. Countries with centralized control over the expenditure of medical resources are developing priorities along these lines; those more closely allied with a capitalistic ethic tend to develop a curative medical care system that serves the affluent.[30-32] Although inappropriate approaches to medical education may be developed in undeveloped countries for reasons of prestige, politics, and the desire to develop highly trained manpower for the country as a whole, economic ideologies appear to play a major role in explaining different orientations to the training of health manpower.

HEALTH CARE DELIVERY
SYSTEMS IN MODERN NATIONS

Health care delivery systems are shaped by the historical context in which they are embedded. Such factors as economic organization, ideological forces, the available technology, and pre-existing professional organization affect access to medical care, the distribution of health care services and ultimately the quality of health care. Figure 2.1 depicts a variety of gross categorizations that can serve as a framework for organizing various studies and helps make apparent how few of the possible areas of investigation concerning national systems have been explored. Beyond an occasional case study almost no data exist on the influence of ideology, economic organization, and the level and character of technology and its relationship to variables describing either the social structure of the country or the organization of health care delivery. There are attempts to link economic investment in medical care to health care outcomes, as in Abel-Smith's study,[33] and ideology to the organization of the health occupations,[34-36] but such analyses are infrequent.

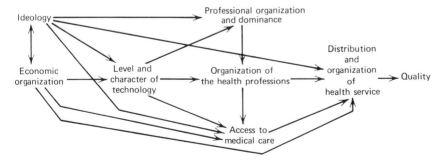

Figure 2.1.   System determinants of the distribution and quality of health services.

Almost all of the research efforts by sociologists have dealt with the organization of the health professions and occupations and with access to and distribution of medical care. Most influential is the work of Freidson[37, 38] on medical dominance of physicians over the work of other health professions and his study of professional controls. Physicians throughout the world have been able to control substantially their conditions of work as well as those of other health occupations. Research on access to medical care has focused on economic and sociocultural barriers to utilization[39, 40] and only indirectly speaks to larger issues of social organization. The great mass of studies deals with client perceptions, conflicts among health workers, factors affecting demand for medical care, differential reactions to services, and the like.[41, 42] Thus, for the most part, sociological inquiry in medicine, as well as work in the health services area, contributes relatively little to understanding health care at the institutional level.[43]

National ideology, as it pertains to medical care, may be defined in terms of government involvement in the financing, administration, and regulation of the health sector. Government participation may vary in terms of the proportion of medical costs assumed by the public sector, the extent of government intrusion and control over various types of decisions, and the extent to which government itself owns and operates the health care delivery system. Although various historical studies suggest the danger of attempting to understand contemporary developments outside the context in which professional patterns and relationships have developed,[44–46] it is possible to order national systems on various criteria describing the relationship between government and the medical sector. Anderson[47] makes an ambitious attempt to examine inputs and outputs in the United States, England, and Sweden, and to relate this to the larger sociopolitical and historical context. He reaches certain conclusions about equity and the propensity toward innovation in these three countries, but it is not clear on what particular indicators these conclusions rest and whether there is a clear basis for the assessment. Anderson's study and the comparative studies by Stevens[48] on the United States and England both suggest the complexity of the issues, the intangibility of the criteria, and how difficult it is to unravel organizational features from the unique historical forces that have come to shape the evolution of each system of care.

In general, it appears that in nations in which government assumes the highest proportion of total medical care costs, greater emphasis is given to public health, preventive medicine, and ambulatory medical care. Moreover, in these countries government is more willing to intrude on the professional dominance of medicine in establishing medical care priorities, although they tend not to intrude on clinical professional work. An important intervening factor is the degree of bureaucratic organization of medicine, which appears to be related to both government investment and the extent of regulation.

Most of the literature on medical care systems deals with costs and various aspects of administering medical care services. As government investment increases, there are greater incentives to impose various cost controls. Throughout most of the world, government agencies or insurance funds must negotiate with physician groups on payment and service-related matters. An enormous array of devices has been developed around the world to establish appropriate remuneration schedules for different types of health manpower.[49] Among Western nations, medical groups retain considerable influence in these negotiations and generally have sufficient political support to determine the mechanism by which they are paid.[50, 51]

In sum, sociological contributions to understanding the medical care sector are highly limited. Much of the problem involves the failure to specify the aspects of the health care sector of greatest significance to sociology, in contrast to health economics or health administration. Moreover, few sociologists have directed themselves to the role of medicine relative to other social institutions and to the larger social and cultural significance of health care institutions. We now turn to such issues.

THE SOCIAL FUNCTIONS OF HEALTH CARE

Although much of social science inquiry is oriented toward analyzing failures in medical care relationships—failure or delay in seeking medical care, the client's use of marginal healers, noncompliance with the physician's advice—the remarkable fact is that the authority of the physician extends as widely as it does. In fact, we take it so for granted that seeking medical care is the rational and natural thing to do when ill that we are frankly surprised at the persistence of folk and religious concepts in what we view as the legitimate province of medicine. As Parsons and Fox[52] noted, with industrialization, medicine increasingly took over the functions of family care and thus facilitated the smooth flow of social activities despite sickness and social disability among family members.

Henry Sigerist[53] and Talcott Parsons[54] alerted sociologists to the importance of health care as a means of relieving social tensions produced by other social institutions, such as the factory or the home, or as a mechanism to control deviance in the society. In an illuminating monograph, Field[55] illustrated how illness could be manipulated by both clients and the state, each to achieve its own particular goals. The most direct attempt to attack this issue empirically is a study by Shuval[56] in which she develops measures of different levels of social need among Jews of varying ethnic origins, and relates these to measures of reported utilization of Kupat Holim, the largest health service program in Israel. She found that higher levels of need for catharsis, legitimation of failure, and resolution of the magic-science conflict is associated with higher levels of utilization. Although this study is provocative, Shuval unfortunately had no data from medical records that could validate utilization reports and add depth to the study. Another study in Israel by Mann and his colleagues[57] found that latent social need was influential in the long-term pattern of use of health services. Persons who had been in concentration camps showed far higher levels of utilization over a period of years than could be accounted for solely on the basis of existing measurable morbidity. Cole and Lejeune,[58] in a study of welfare mothers, build a persuasive empirical case to support the contention that reported illness behavior is used to legitimate failure. And many studies have found a relationship between life change, psychological distress, and help-seeking behavior.[59, 60]

Antonovsky[61] suggests an epidemiological model that attempts to explain variations in physician utilization among populations comparable in morbidity. Host characteristics include latent need, intolerance of ambiguity of symptoms, and an orientation toward the use of professionals. Characteristics describing medical institutions include availability of facilities, the ability to be responsive to various latent functions, and the degree of receptivity of physicians to patients. Characteristics of the larger sociocultural environment include organizational facilitation in using medical services, absence of stigma for such use, cultural pressures to have problems diagnosed, and the degree of availability of functional alternatives. In contrast, Andersen[62-64] presents a less theoretical approach that has been useful in regression models of medical utilization. He views utilization as a consequence of predisposing, enabling, and illness variables. Predisposing variables include demographic variables (age, sex, and marital status, for example), social structural variables (race, education, religion, and ethnicity, among others), and beliefs and knowledge about health and medical care. Enabling factors include family income, availability of health insurance, source of care, and access to regular source of care, as well as the availability of health services, price of health services, and other community characteristics. Illness variables include disability, symptoms, diagnoses, and the like. Also, various social psychological models have been suggested to describe how persons come to perceive and react to illness or to decide to engage in preventive health behavior.[65-67]

The social psychological models and those suggested by Antonovsky and Shuval are most interesting theoretically, but thus far they have not been particularly powerful in explaining aggregate utilization data. In contrast, the Andersen model appears to account for greater variation, but lacks a theoretical conception of the dynamics of the behavior at issue. Antonovsky's suggested model provides a basis for developing a clearer understanding of variabilities in physician utilization among different national systems. Such variation in visiting physicians is substantial among developed nations. Countries such as the Soviet Union and Israel have a per capita utilization of 9 to 12 visits; the

United States and England average 4 to 6 visits; and such countries as Sweden fall within the 2 to 3 visit range. These differences reflect cultural variations, availability and accessibility of services, and social ideologies as well as other factors. The only empirical study with comparative data on physician utilization in varying countries is the International Collaborative Study.[68] Bice and colleagues[69] have examined various predicted relationships in each of 12 study areas in seven countries, using a path model including age, education, income, skepticism of medical care, and the reported tendency to use services, and have found some to be relatively consistent in predicting physician use. Skepticism of medical care significantly predicted lower utilization in 11 of the 12 areas; tendency to adopt the sick role predicted correctly to high utilization in 10 areas, but only 7 of the relationships reached statistical significance. Sociodemographic variables such as age, education, and income yielded inconsistent relationships or patterns contrary to those predicted.

Although these various approaches raise questions of sociological interest, they face conceptual problems. Social need and psychological distress affect not only medical utilization but also morbidity states. Thus, it is not clear to what extent social and psychological factors influence utilization by modifying morbidity, and the extent to which they trigger help-seeking behavior.[70] Current data suggest that social and psychological stresses can affect utilization directly as well as modify illness states. The role of different types of social stress on illness has received much attention.[71–73] There is considerable controversy as to whether social change itself contributes to illness, irrespective of its positive or negative features, or whether illness and utilization follow only adverse life changes. This issue is further complicated by the specific physical or behavioral dysfunctions under consideration.[74, 75]

In sum, why people seek help and where they choose to bring their problems are issues to which sociologists can make a distinctive contribution. Illness is not only an event that happens to people, but also an important explanation that can be used to sustain one's social identity and social functioning. Although medical utilization is a common source of help-seeking, it is only one of many alternatives. The processes through which persons come to see themselves as having a problem, the way they come to define the problem as one that calls for seeking particular types of assistance, and how they present the problem are all aspects that can help us understand the larger significance of medical care and social services for life activities more generally.[76, 77] We now turn to this issue.

POPULATION SELECTION AND HEALTH CARE

In any population at risk, only some persons with symptoms and illness will enter the available health care services system. Indeed, the formal helping system in the community may be only part of a far more elaborate system of formal and informal help made available by religious agencies, self-help groups, and kinship networks. The nature of the selection process will depend in part on the sociocultural and psychological characteristics of the population and in part on the availability and character of the formal health services system, its various components, and the broader system of helping services in the community at large. Assuming that individuals perceive a problem and define the problem as worthy of assistance—processes which themselves require sociological illumination—an assessment must be made also of the nature of the problem and to which of various alternative sources to bring it. Decision-making is influenced by the processes of definition and evaluation of symptoms and their cause, but depends as well on the scope of helping facilities available, their compatibility with cultural beliefs and behavior patterns, ease of access and barriers to use, and the larger network of helping patterns in the community, particularly as they relate to the formal helping system.

The process of help-receiving is dependent on the character of the first-contact service and how it is linked with other components of the helping system. While the initial arrival of a person to a first-contact service depends on sociocultural and personal contingencies, decisions concerning further care are more substantially influenced by the organization and interlinking of various components of the help-giving system. First-contact care may be isolated from a larger system of helping services if the person in need of assistance first contacts a religious healer or a chiropractor. If the patient begins the search for care from a rural general practitioner or from a small community hospital, the possibilities for referral and further services suggested by the helper are far greater but considerably less expansive than those characterized by major teaching centers that offer a wide array of technological possibilities and specialized consultants. The data on performance show that the more elaborate facilities generate greater cost and more services, in part reflecting a different case load typical of such institutions but also indicative of the institution's potential. That such services are more than just a costly addition is reflected in a variety of studies that show teaching institutions to have generally higher levels of performance.[78]

Thus, each part of the helping system—whether a physician, a medical group, or a facility such as a community hospital—tends to be related to a larger organizational field which influences the options possible and the types of decisions made. The organizational fields are characterized by varying technological and manpower capacities, different levels of demand for services and the ability to respond to them, and varying propensities to generate certain types of services. Crossnational studies, as well as those concerned with variations within single countries or regions, suggest no clear rational basis for large fluctuations in rates of services generated relative to the likely patterns of morbidity in the community. For example, fluctuations of rates of hospitalization, length of stay, and rates of surgical procedures from one setting to another suggest that the availability of hospital resources is the best single predictor of gross rates, although it is far more difficult to demonstrate that excess capacity results in "unnecessary use."[79–82] Existing literature suggests that such services can be significantly reduced as a matter of policy without obvious adverse consequences. The use of hospital beds or any other resource within an organizational service field will in part be a product of the organization of resources, the culture of the practicing professions, the types of regulation, and the incentives characteristic of the system. The outputs of these systems are often intangible, difficult to measure precisely, and highly responsive to explicit and implicit incentives which may be more or less consistent with "ideal practice."

In theory, the organization of delivery systems has an implicit logic. Such systems, as one moves from the points of first contact to secondary and tertiary facilities, are organized to deal with more complex and specialized problems, and it is assumed that the sequence of referral reflects increasing severity or the life threatening nature of the illness, the complexity of the clinical picture, and the need for more specialized care. Although such factors generally determine the flow of work, much of the variance remains unexplained by such objective variables. However, if one examines each of the components of the delivery system as a minisocial system, it is evident that the flow of patients and decision-making in each results in part from sociocultural and psychosocial factors unrelated to the severity of the conditions treated or the objective needs of the patients.[83] These include the wishes and manipulations of patients to receive certain kinds of treatments irrespective of their objective value, the incentives and nonmedical needs that influence how physicians work, the actual resources available, and the pressures on varying components of the system. In addition, the fact that many hospitals and clinics are multipurpose institutions involving patient care, education, and research requires that they construct their populations not only on the basis of patient care needs but also in terms of the institution's other goals.

THE COMPARATIVE EFFECTS OF
HEALTH CARE DELIVERY SYSTEMS

Although the effects of medical care on global indices of health and mortality have received much attention in recent years, the rationale of such analysis is frequently defective. Values on the dependent variables used are determined by a wide range of influences related to social technology, levels and styles of living, nutrition and public health, and it is not apparent that medical care should have a particularly large positive effect. Indeed, to the extent that medical care identifies more illness, sustains life among chronically ill persons, and allows the survival of persons with congenital and other defects, it contributes to higher levels of recognized morbidity and disability in the population. Moreover, global indicators such as mortality are summary measures affected by numerous factors, no single one of which—however important—can reasonably be expected to have a major impact on the gross indicator under conditions existing in modern nations.[84]

A more appropriate means for evaluating the effectiveness of a particular delivery procedure or set of procedures is through controlled clinical trials. Although drug and other medical interventions are commonly evaluated through randomized controlled trials, similar methodology has only recently been applied to health service patterns. Cochrane[85] reviews both the logic and some of the successful applications of randomized controlled trials, but in most situations randomization remains impractical or extremely difficult, and we continue to depend on multivariate statistical approaches to judge the effectiveness of health services. All that is possible here is to offer some important examples of the possibilities and problems of such evaluation.

One reason for recent criticisms of our health services stems from evidence of large disparities in infant mortality and the fact that on this score the United States, despite its affluence and large investment in health services, is in an unfavorable position relative to other developed nations. Implicit in much of the criticism is that the large white-nonwhite differential is a product of lack of access to medical services; the overall high American rate relative to other countries is seen in part, if not totally, as a product of the ineffective organization of health care in the United States.

Although there is a profound belief that effective maternal and child health care prevents infant mortality and other injuries and defects in the child, there is no clear evidence that this is the case. Birth weight is the single best predictor of infant mortality, and when introduced into a multiple regression analysis, other variables fail to explain any appreciable additional variance. Both infant mortality and birth weight, however, are related to socioeconomic status, color, education of the mother, less than optimal age, high parity, illegitimacy of the child, and so on.[86] These variables, however, are all intercorrelated. While age and parity reflect certain biological risks, the other variables are largely viewed as proxies for such variables as social living conditions, nutrition, mothering skills, and access to medical care. We know that the introduction of medical services into an underserved area results in a reduction in the rate of infant mortality, but there has been little direct evidence that in areas with medical resources, the use of adequate prenatal and postnatal care results in lower infant mortality. A study of infant mortality[87] in New York City for 1968, using matched birth and death records, examined infant death in relationship to socioeconomic and ethnic differences, medical and social risk, and the use of adequate medical care as indexed by time of first prenatal visit, number of prenatal visits, and whether the baby was delivered in a public or private service. The last component was used on the assumption that those whose babies were delivered in public services in New York City had poor continuity of care. The results of the study show that for almost every ethnic, social, and medical risk and socioeconomic subcategory, mothers who had adequate care were less likely to lose their infants than those who received lesser care.

As with most other studies that do not include random allocation, the conclusion that medical care affects infant deaths is open to alternative explanations. Given the fact that postneonatal deaths are more responsive to socioeconomic factors than they are to biomedical factors, it would have been expected that good prenatal care should have had a greater effect on neonatal than postneonatal rates, but the study found no such differential effect. The design leaves open the possibility that the relationship between good care and lower mortality is a result of social selection, and not of the influence of medical care. Certainly it is plausible to suspect that a black woman with low education, or a member of any other subgroup with social risk and low education, who obtains adequate prenatal care may be different from others in the subgroup who do not receive comparable care. The lack of information in the study on other characteristics of the women makes it difficult to interpret clearly the findings. More recently, Slesinger,[88] in analyzing data from a sample of black women and their children in Washington, D.C. concerning utilization of prenatal and child care, found that a significant amount of variance in preventive medical care—controlling for socioeconomic status—is attributable to household composition and various attitudes toward health. Mothers who were more isolated from informal relationships with associates or formal community groups had lower utilization of preventive medical care (see Chapter 10).

Similar selection possibilities exist in various studies of the effects of prepaid group practice relative to more conventional services on such outcomes as infant prematurity and mortality among the aged. Careful studies examining outcomes among recipients of services from the Health Insurance Plan of New York in contrast to nonsubscribers with similar sociodemographic characteristics show some advantage in rates of prematurity and mortality for prepaid practice recipients.[89–92] These findings have been widely cited as demonstrating the medical advantages of prepayment, and have been used by policymakers to support the enlargement of prepayment programs.[93] However, even when socioeconomic and other controls are applied, the alternative remains that the better outcomes observed in the prepaid contexts are attributable to social selection. Persons with greater health consciousness and interest in maintaining health, when given a choice, may have been more likely to select prepaid practice. However, Mechanic and Tessler,[94] studying health selection into a prepaid practice program in Milwaukee, Wisconsin could find little evidence of significant selection on the basis of health consciousness or preventive health patterns (see Chapter 7).

Even if we assume that the health outcomes observed can be attributed to prepaid group practice rather than to social selection, the extent to which we can generalize such findings to various other settings remains uncertain. Although much has been written in recent years on prepayment, we cannot be certain that these studies deal with the same types of social organization and service patterns. Prepaid group practices are usually discussed as if they are a common form of practice organization; and to the extent that they offer prepaid services from a group practice setting, they have a distinctive similarity. The fact, however, is that these limited criteria are not adequately descriptive. Very few groups are exclusively based on prepayment, and the degree of prepayment from one group to another varies widely. Most prepaid groups are small, but some are very large. Although some are general practice groups, others are primarily multispecialty groups. The groups also may differ substantially in economic organization and how the physician is paid, the use of ancillary manpower, task allocation and delegation, ownership and other relationships to hospitals, scope of services, and availability of specialized services.[95] Moreover, in the United States, legislation pertains to the more global entity, "Health Maintenance Organization," which refers both to prepaid groups and to medical foundations. Thus, generalization on the basis of case studies is hazardous; but no investigator has yet made a serious effort to define the population of prepaid practices and to sample systematically from them in order to evaluate outcomes in relation to competing practices. This, of course, would be a costly and difficult task.

Comparability and generalizability are salient issues in almost all comparative research on health care systems, and characterize comparative research in general. A national system of care, or a health delivery system such as a prepaid practice, constitutes a single case. Very few studies involve a large number of units of whatever kind. When such studies have been undertaken, they usually involve relatively superficial analyses or assess organizational variables on the basis of averaging individual interviews with organizational respondents. Studies that relate to quality of medical care or responsiveness of health personnel tend to involve individual institutions (for some exceptions, see Georgopoulos and Mann; Heydebrand; Roemer and Friedman[96–98]). It becomes extremely difficult, therefore, to separate effects that are due to organizational characteristics shared in common by other organizations, characteristics idiosyncratic to the structure of the particular organization not shared by similar units, or even idiosyncratic traits of professionals who work in that particular organization. Much research is written up as if professional and other health personnel are randomly distributed among varying organizations. The more realistic assumption, of course, is that each type of organization recruits participants who either select themselves or have been selected on the basis of certain characteristics. The same case can be made for clients of professionals and organizations. Often they have gone through a search in which they have selected certain helpers and facilities that complement their own needs.[99] Few studies of delivery systems delve sufficiently deep to assess such selective tendencies and what role they might have in explaining observed outcomes.

COMPARATIVE STUDY OF PREPAYMENT AND CAPITATION SYSTEMS

The difficulty we encounter in specifying appropriate criteria for defining organizational units such as prepaid group practices is exacerbated when we try to define comparable units within different national organizational structures. Whether experience with particular payment mechanisms or devices to ration medical services can be generalized from one setting to another, or whether they are so confounded by the sociocultural context to make generalization impossible, must await repeated studies in different social contexts. Most conclusions from such research, therefore, must remain tentative.

In the United States considerable evidence exists that prepaid practices have lower rates of hospital admissions, lower rates of surgical intervention, and thus lower overall costs per capita.[100, 101] These differences persist even when taking into account the composition of patient populations they treat and correcting for the purchase of additional services outside the plan. Generally, the cost advantage of the HMO has been attributed to the removal of the incentive to the physician to provide unnecessary services and the possible addition of a financial incentive to avoid hospitalization. Although it has been argued that such savings are the result of an incentive to keep patients healthy to avoid later costs for the health care plan, there is little evidence to support such contentions, and even the theory of the health maintenance function is somewhat tenuous. A plausible alternative explanation for cost savings of prepaid group practices is simply the limited specialty personnel and hospital beds available to the enrolled group. Most of the major prepaid groups depend on a lower proportion of specialists and hospital beds relative to competing facilities in the community, and international variations in rates of admission to hospital and surgical intervention are consistent with the hypothesis that the availability of resources affects the rate of utilization.[102-104] In all probability, the rather consistent observed differences between prepaid and other contexts is a product of a variety of influences including patient composition, physician incentive, and the different availability of treatment resources.

A continuing concern in the comparative health literature is the manner in which payment incentives affect the motivation and behavior of physicians and the quality of care they provide. After the most comprehensive review of the effects of remuneration in varying countries around the world, Glaser concludes that "once the procedures and levels of pay suffice, and if the nonpecuniary rewards are protected, doctors will adjust to any system of compensation. In practice, the most familiar system usually arouses the least protest."[105] This conforms with more general findings on job satisfaction, which suggest that although perceived adequate remuneration is an important condition for satisfaction, once a certain level of remuneration is reached, attention focuses on nonremunerative aspects of work satisfaction such as conditions of work, personal autonomy, and opportunities for self-improvement and actualization.[106] Mechanic and Faich,[107] in studying a remuneration dispute between general practitioners and the English government, concluded that other dissatisfactions and status insecurities were expressed through conflicts over remuneration since payment issues were the regularized means for dealing with doctor grievances.

From the policy point of view, Glaser's conclusion is inadequate since it does not provide a basis for understanding how to shift from a familiar remuneration system to one less familiar without undermining the motivation and performance of doctors. Increasingly, for example, the United States is considering types of medical organization that propose to shift physician payment from the predominant fee-for-service format to one based on capitation, which the majority of physicians oppose. Although little systematic sociological study of such questions is available, Colombotos'[108] study of doctors' attitudes prior to and following Medicare is helpful in understanding the larger context. Although prior to the Medicare program physicians were very much opposed, following its implementation physicians became more favorable and overwhelmingly participated in the program. Thus, prior attitudes and responses were not predictive of later behavior following implementation. Medicare, of course, basically maintained the structure of the existing payment system, and thus the program was an economic asset from the physician's point of view. In contrast, Medicaid, a federal-state matching program that more seriously regulates physicians' fees and conditions of reimbursement, had more difficulty achieving physician cooperation. It seems reasonably clear from the American and other contexts that cooperation can be achieved in moving from one structure and system of remuneration to another if the terms are generous, but not if the new conditions threaten the economic position of the profession.

The difficulty with attempting to shape physician behavior using payment incentives is that physicians are in a position to modify easily their pattern of work to subvert the incentive system when they are unsympathetic with it. As Glaser[109] points out, when the payment system remunerates definable units of work, physicians then manipulate their patterns of work to generate more payable units. This might be achieved through the procedures used to diagnose and treat illness or through the extent to which physicians encourage patients to return for follow-up care. Medical activity is highly discretionary and very much under the control of the physician.[110] Carelessly developed incentives can induce a variety of undesirable and unintended behaviors on the part of the physician. Both consumer studies and studies of physicians in the American system report that doctors on capitation arrangements appear to be less oriented to satisfying the patient's psychosocial needs, are more inflexible, and are more likely to respond to patients' problems as if they are trivial.[111] It is not fully clear to what extent this is a product of the capitation system itself or the fact that physicians on capitation are more likely to limit their hours of work and thus expose themselves to a more concentrated and demanding case load. The perceived lack of responsiveness of physicians on capitation is probably due to the fact that they work under heavy time pressure, while fee-for-service physicians are more likely to expand their hours of work to deal with increased patient demand and to feel rewarded for this additional effort.

PROFESSIONALISM IN MEDICINE AND THE ORGANIZATION OF ROLES

Throughout the world there has been growing bureaucratization of medical practice, and as physicians more commonly work in organized settings they are increasingly subjected to conflicting demands and incentives. Physicians tend to have an elaborate role-set involving not only patients and colleagues but increasingly managers and administrators, third parties who pay and regulate the services provided, and personnel involved in training and research. Physicians in institutional settings frequently face conflicts between service, research, training, and economic and administrative needs.

A few efforts have been made to describe how conflicts between professional and managerial needs are dealt with in varying contexts. Goss,[112] for example, has dealt with the conflicts between hospital administration and medical decision-making, and suggests a pattern of advisory bureaucracy in which accommodation is attempted through tactful suggestion and negotiation rather than bureaucratic authority. The growing literature on service bureaucracies describes the greater autonomy and flexibility of roles, the extent of role development and institutionalization, and the difficulty of developing bureaucratic standards to control a multipurpose organization with intangible goals.[113-116] Similarly, a literature is emerging to deal with intraorganizational negotiation and cooperation, which is an important aspect of the service sector.[117, 118] However, little of this organizational theory is adequate for effectively conceptualizing the increasingly complex service sector, and particularly medical practice.

One of the most important and persistent problems in the provision of medical care involves the most effective and economical division of labor among physicians, and between physicians and other health workers. Although a small minority of all health personnel, physicians dominate the organization and control of health work in most if not all societies. Although many of the poorer countries face a great scarcity of health personnel, and thus must develop ancillary personnel if they are to have basic services, the medical profession in most countries has attempted to maintain a monopoly over the organization of medical work. Historically—and at present—the development of specialization and subspecialization follows economic and status needs of the dominant profession as much as the requirements of technology and knowledge or the need for effective performance.[119]

This is not to say that medical technology has not significantly advanced in a fashion requiring a more specialized division of labor. But an examination of the substance of specialties and how they developed, and how they relate to the organization of work more generally, would show that their shape is as much a product of the pursuit of self-interest as it is of the scientific elaboration of medicine. In any case, with a more specialized division of labor and a greatly expanded technology, the needs for coordination and integration are more acutely felt in all developed medical systems. Thus, all developed systems of care appear to be struggling with the common problem of how to make use of the growing sophistication of medical knowledge and still retain basic services for the common needs that people have and the ordinary problems they bring to doctors.

CONVERGENCE OF HEALTH CARE DELIVERY SYSTEMS IN POSTINDUSTRIAL SOCIETY

An examination of the available descriptive materials on health care delivery systems in various countries suggests that the demands of medical technology and the growth of the science base of medical activity produce pressures toward common organizational solutions despite strong ideological differences.[120, 121] One difficulty with this hypothesis is the lack of specification of criteria for convergence and the extent to which they have been met in various national contexts. Recent developments in Chinese medicine, for example, can be viewed as supporting or contradicting the convergence hypothesis depending on which of various features of Chinese developments are emphasized.

Most countries of the world have developed modern medical practices to some degree, if for no other reason than national pride, to serve an elite, or for political expedience. In many poorer countries, a developed scientific structure exists for the rich, and only very limited services are available for the poor. As populations increasingly demand medical care, there is growing concern among nations to provide a minimal level of service to all and to decrease obvious inequalities in care. To use available technology and knowledge efficiently and effectively, certain organizational options are most desirable. Thus one finds that there is a general tendency throughout the world to link existing services to defined population groups, to develop new and more economic ways to provide primary services to the population without an overelaboration of technological efforts, to integrate services increasingly fragmented by specialization or a more elaborate division of labor, and to seek ways to improve the output of the delivery system with fixed inputs. Although these concerns to some extent characterize national planning in underdeveloped countries, they particularly describe tendencies among developed nations as they attempt to control the enormous costs of available technologies.[122] Throughout the world there is increasing movement away from medicine as a solitary entrepreneurial activity and more emphasis on the effective development of health delivery systems.

The hypothesis of convergence does not imply that medical systems, which develop out of the particular historical and cultural background of a nation and its dominant ethos, will not continue to have distinct characteristics reflecting the ideological orientations and the sociocultural context of a country. But the basic pattern of practice in modern society is increasingly dominated by the imperatives of the emerging technology, the objective pattern of morbidity in the population, and the worldwide phenomenon of growing public expectations.

NOTES

1. W. A. Glaser (1970a), *Social Settings and Medical Organization: A Cross-National Study of the Hospital* (New York: Atherton).

2. D. Mechanic (1968), *Medical Sociology: A Selective View* (New York: Free Press).

3. A. Donabedian (1973), *Aspects of Medical Care Administration: Specifying Requirements for Health Care* (Cambridge: Harvard University Press).

4. B. Abel-Smith (1967), *An International Study of Health Expenditure and Its Relevance for Health Planning* (Geneva: World Health Organization), Public Health Paper Number 32.

5. J. Elinson (1973), "Toward Sociomedical Health Indicators," paper presented at the International Conference of Medical Sociology, Warsaw, Poland.

6. T. Parsons (1951), *The Social System* (New York: Free Press).

7. M. Goss et al. (1973), "Professional Organization and Control," report presented at the annual meetings of the American Sociological Association, New York City.

8. The current debate concerning the uses of psychiatry in the Soviet Union reflects international sensitivities to the political uses of medical institutions.

9. D. Mechanic (1974b), *Politics, Medicine, and Social Science* (New York: Wiley-Interscience).

10. M. Field (1973), "The Concept of the 'Health System' at the Macro-Sociological Level," *Social Science and Medicine,* 7:763–785.

11. I. Douglas-Wilson and G. McLachlan, eds. (1973), *Health Service Prospects: An International Survey* (Boston: Little, Brown).

12. J. Horn (1969), *Away With All Pests* (New York: Monthly Review Press).

13. V. Sidel (1971), "Medicine in the People's Republic of China," *Proceedings of First Annual Meeting of the Institute of Medicine* (Washington, D.C.: National Academy of Sciences).

14. Z. Stein and M. Susser (1972), "The Cuban Health System: A Trial of a Comprehensive Service in a Poor Country," *International Journal of Health Services,* 2:551–566.

15. D. Mechanic (1972a). *Public Expectations and Health Care* (New York: Wiley-Interscience).

16. B. Abel-Smith and K. Gales (1964), *British Doctors at Home and Abroad* (London: Bell).

17. I am indebted to Bruce Turetsky for his assistance in reviewing the literature on the role of health in national development.

18. D. Mechanic (1968), op. cit.

19. T. McKeown (1965), *Medicine in Modern Society: Medical Planning Based on Evaluation of Medical Achievement* (London: Allen and Unwin), pp. 21–74.

20. J. Bryant (1969), *Health and the Developing World* (Ithaca: Cornell University Press).

21. R. Baldwin and B. Weisbrod (1974), "Disease and Labor Productivity," *Economic Development and Cultural Change,* 22:414–435.

22. R. Barlow (1967). "The Economic Effects of Malarial Eradication," *American Economic Review,* 57:130–148.

23. W. Malenbaum (1970), "Health and Productivity in Poor Areas," in H. E. Klarman, ed., *Empirical Studies in Health Economics* (Baltimore: Johns Hopkins), pp. 31–54.

24. W. Scott (1971), "Cross-National Studies of the Impact of Levels of Living on Economic Growth: An Example," *International Journal of Health Services,* 1:225–232.

25. C. E. Taylor and M. Hall (1967), "Health, Population and Economic Development," *Science,* 157:651–657.

26. B. Weisbrod, R. Andreano, R. Baldwin, E. Epstein, and A. Kelley (1973), *Disease and Economic Development: The Impact of Parasitic Diseases in St. Lucia* (Madison: University of Wisconsin Press).

27. H. Frederikson (1962), "Economic and Demographic Consequences of Malaria Control in Ceylon," *Indian Journal of Malariology,* 16:379–391.

28. R. Barlow (1967), op. cit.

29. B. Benjamin (1965), *Social and Economic Factors Affecting Mortality* (The Hague: Mouton).

30. E. F. Weinerman (1969), *Social Medicine in Eastern Europe: The Organization of Health Services and the Education of Medical Personnel in Czechoslovakia, Hungary, and Poland* (Cambridge: Harvard University Press).

31. I. Douglas-Wilson and G. McLachlan, eds. (1973), op. cit.

32. D. Mechanic (1974b), op. cit.

33. B. Abel-Smith (1967), op. cit.

34. O. Anderson (1972). *Health Care: Can There Be Equity? The United States, Sweden, and England* (New York: Wiley-Interscience).

35. R. Alford (1975). *Health Care Politics: Ideological and Interest Group Barriers to Reform* (Chicago: University of Chicago Press).

36. M. Field (1967), *Soviet Socialized Medicine* (New York: Free Press).

37. E. Freidson (1970a), *Profession of Medicine: A Study in the Sociology of Applied Knowledge* (New York: Dodd, Mead).

38. E. Freidson (1970b). *Professional Dominance: The Social Structure of Medical Care* (New York: Atherton).

39. J. B. McKinlay (1972), "Some Approaches and Problems in the Study of the Use of Services—An Overview," *Journal of Health and Social Behavior*, **13:**115–152.

40. L. A. Aday (1972), *The Utilization of Health Services: Indices and Correlates* (Washington, D.C.: National Center for Health Services Research and Development), DHEW Pub. No. HSM 73-3003.

41. H. E. Freeman, S. Levine, and L. G. Reeder, eds. (1972), *Handbook of Medical Sociology*, 2d ed. (Englewood Cliffs, N.J.: Prentice-Hall).

42. A. Donabedian (1973), op. cit.

43. R. Alford (1972), "The Political Economy of Health Care: Dynamics Without Change," *Politics and Society*, **2:**127–164.

44. B. Abel-Smith (1964), *The Hospitals, 1800–1948: A Study in Social Administration in England and Wales* (London: Heinemann).

45. R. Stevens (1966), *Medical Practice in Modern England: The Impact of Specialization and State Medicine* (New Haven: Yale University Press).

46. H. Eckstein (1964). *The English Health Service: Its Origins, Structure, and Achievements* (Cambridge: Harvard University Press).

47. O. Anderson (1972), op. cit.

48. R. Stevens (1971), *American Medicine and the Public Interest* (New Haven: Yale University Press).

49. W. A. Glaser (1970b), *Paying the Doctor: Systems of Remuneration and Their Effects* (Baltimore: Johns Hopkins Press).

50. H. Eckstein (1960), *Pressure Group Politics: The Case of the British Medical Association* (Stanford: Stanford University Press).

51. T. Marmor and D. Thomas (1971), "The Politics of Paying Physicians: The Determinants of Government Payment Methods in England, Sweden, and the United States," *International Journal of Health Services*, **1:**71–78.

52. T. Parsons and R. Fox (1952), "Illness, Therapy and the Modern Urban American Family," *Journal of Social Issues*, **8:**31–44.

53. H. E. Sigerist (1960), "The Special Position of the Sick," in M. I. Roemer, ed., *Henry E. Sigerist on the Sociology of Medicine* (New York: MD Publications).

54. T. Parsons (1951), op. cit.

55. M. Field (1957), *Doctor and Patient in Soviet Russia* (Cambridge: Harvard University Press).

56. J. Shuval (1970), *Social Functions of Medical Practice* (San Francisco: Jossey-Bass).

57. K. J. Mann, J. H. Medalie, E. Lieber, J. J. Groen, and L. Guttman (1970), *Visits to Doctors* (Jerusalem: Jerusalem Academic Press).

58. S. Cole and R. Lejeune (1972), "Illness and the Legitimation of Failure," *American Sociological Review*, **37:**347–356.

59. D. Mechanic (1972), "Social Psychologic Factors Affecting the Presentation of Bodily Complaints," *New England Journal of Medicine*, **286**:1132–1139.

60. B. Dohrenwend and B. Dohrenwend (1974), *Life Events: Their Nature and Effects* (New York: Wiley-Interscience).

61. A. Antonovsky (1972), "A Model to Explain Visits to the Doctor: With Specific Reference to the Case of Israel," *Journal of Health and Social Behavior*, **13**:446–454.

62. R. Andersen (1968), *A Behavioral Model of Families' Use of Health Services* (Chicago: Center for Health Administration Studies), Research Series 25.

63. R. Andersen, B. Smedby, and O. Anderson (1970), *Medical Care Use in Sweden and the United States: A Comparative Analysis of Systems and Behavior* (Chicago: Center for Health Administration Studies), Research Series 27.

64. R. Andersen and J. F. Newman (1973), "Societal and Individual Determinants of Medical Care Utilization in the United States," *Milbank Memorial Fund Quarterly*, **51**:95–124.

65. D. Mechanic (1968), op. cit.

66. I. M. Rosenstock (1969), "Prevention of Illness and Maintenance of Health," in J. Kosa, A. Antonovsky, and I. K. Zola, eds., *Poverty and Health: A Sociological Analysis* (Cambridge: Harvard University Press), pp. 168–190.

67. I. K. Zola (1964), "Illness Behavior of the Working Class," in A. Shostak and W. Gomberg, eds., *Blue-Collar World: Studies of the American Worker* (Englewood Cliffs, N.J.: Prentice-Hall).

68. D. Rabin, ed. (1972), "International Comparisons of Medical Care," *Milbank Memorial Fund Quarterly*, **50**:Part II.

69. T. Bice et al. (1972), "International Comparisons of Medical Care: Behavioral Results," *Milbank Memorial Fund Quarterly*, **50**: 57–63.

70. D. Mechanic (1974c), "Discussion of Research Programs on Relations Between Stressful Life Events and Episodes of Physical Illness," in B. Dohrenwend and B. Dohrenwend, eds., op. cit.

71. B. Dohrenwend and B. Dohrenwend (1974), op. cit.

72. G. E. Moss (1973), *Illness, Immunity, and Social Interaction: The Dynamics of Biosocial Resonation* (New York: Wiley-Interscience).

73. S. Levine and N. Scotch (1970), *Social Stress* (Chicago: Aldine).

74. G. Brown and J. L. P. Birely (1968), "Social Change and the Onset of Schizophrenia," *Journal of Health and Social Behavior*, 3:203–214.

75. G. Brown, M. Bhrolcháin, and T. Harris (1975), "Social Class and Psychiatric Disturbance Among Women in an Urban Population," *Sociology*, **9**:225–254.

76. C. Kadushin (1969), *Why People Go to Psychiatrists* (New York: Atherton).

77. J. Shuval (1970), op. cit.

78. M. Goss (1970), "Organizational Goals and Quality of Medical Care: Evidence from Comparative Research on Hospitals," *Journal of Health and Social Behavior*, **11**:255–268.

79. A. Donabedian (1973), op. cit.

80. J. Wennberg and A. Gittelsohn (1973), "Small Area Variations in Health Care Delivery," *Science*, **182**:1102–1108.

81. J. Bunker (1970), "Surgical Manpower: A Comparison of Operations and Surgeons in the United States and England and Wales," *New England Journal of Medicine*, **282**:135–144.

82. H. Klarman (1965), *The Economics of Health* (New York: Columbia University Press), pp. 139–141.

83. D. Mechanic (1974d), "Patient Behavior and the Organization of Medical Care," in Institute of Medicine, *Ethics of Health Care* (Washington, D.C.: National Academy of Sciences), pp. 67–85.

84. S. Mushkin (1973), "Evaluations: Use With Caution," *Evaluation*, **1**:30–35.

85. A. L. Cochrane (1972), *Effectiveness and Efficiency: Random Reflections on Health Services* (London: Nuffield Provincial Hospitals Trust).

86. D. Mechanic (1968), op. cit.

87. Institute of Medicine (1973), *Infant Death: An Analysis by Maternal Risk and Health Care* (Washington, D.C.: National Academy of Sciences).

88. D. Slesinger (1973), "The Utilization of Preventive Medical Services by Urban Black Mothers: A Socio-Cultural Approach," Ph.D. dissertation, University of Wisconsin, Madison.

89. S. Shapiro et al. (1967), "Patterns of Medical Use by the Indigent Aged under Two Systems of Medical Care," *American Journal of Public Health*, **57**:784–790.

90. S. Shapiro, S. L. Weiner, and P. M. Densen (1958), "Comparison of Prematurity and Perinatal Mortality in a General Population and in the Population of a Prepaid Group Practice Medical Care Plan," *American Journal of Public Health*, **48**:170–187.

91. S. Shapiro, H. Jacobziner, P. M. Densen, and L. Weiner (1960), "Further Observations on Prematurity and Perinatal Mortality in a General Population and in the Population of a Prepaid Group Practice Medical Care Plan," *American Journal of Public Health*, **50**:1304–1317.

92. S. Shapiro (1967), "End Result Measurements of Quality Medical Care," *Milbank Memorial Fund Quarterly*, **45**:7–30.

93. Department of Health, Education, and Welfare (1971), *Toward a Comprehensive Health Policy for the 1970's: A White Paper* (Washington, D.C.: Government Printing Office).

94. D. Mechanic and R. Tessler (1974), "Comparison of Consumer Response to Prepaid Group Practice and Alternative Insurance Plans in Milwaukee County," *Research and Analytic Report Series*, 5-73, Center for Medical Sociology and Health Services Research, University of Wisconsin, Madison.

95. D. Mechanic (1972a), op. cit.

96. B. S. Georgopoulos and F. C. Mann (1962), *The Community General Hospital* (New York: Macmillan).

97. W. V. Heydebrand (1973), *Hospital Bureaucracy: A Comparative Study of Organizations* (New York: Dunellen).

98. M. I. Roemer and J. W. Friedman (1971), *Doctors in Hospitals: Medical Staff Organization and Hospital Performance* (Baltimore: Johns Hopkins University Press).

99. C. Kadushin (1962), "Social Distance Between Client and Professional," *American Journal of Sociology*, **67**:517–531.

100. A. Donabedian (1969), "An Evaluation of Prepaid Group Practice," *Inquiry*, **6**:3–27.

101. Department of Health, Education, and Welfare (1971), op. cit.

102. J. Bunker (1970), op. cit.

103. A. Donabedian (1973), op. cit.

104. J. Wennberg and A. Gittelsohn (1973), op. cit.

105. W. A. Glaser (1970b), op. cit., p. 289.

106. R. Faich (1969), "Social and Structural Factors Affecting Work Satisfaction: A Case Study

of General Practitioners in the English Health Service," Ph.D. dissertation, University of Wisconsin, Madison.

107. D. Mechanic and R. Faich (1970), "Doctors in Revolt: The Crisis in the English National Health Service," *Medical Care,* **8:**442–455.

108. J. Colombotos (1969), "Physicians and Medicare: A Before-After Study of the Effects of Legislation on Attitudes," *American Sociological Review,* **34:**318–334.

109. W. A. Glaser (1970b), op. cit.

110. V. R. Fuchs and M. J. Kramer (1972), *Determinants of Expenditures: For Physicians' Services in the United States 1948–1968* (Washington, D.C.: National Center for Health Services Research and Development), DHEW Pub. No. HSM 73-3013.

111. D. Mechanic (1974d), op. cit.

112. M. Goss (1963), "Patterns of Bureaucracy Among Hospital Staff Physicians," in E. Freidson, ed., *The Hospital in Modern Society* (New York: Free Press).

113. W. Rushing (1964), *The Psychiatric Professions: Power, Conflict, and Adaptation in a Psychiatric Hospital Staff* (Chapel Hill: University of North Carolina Press).

114. R. Bucher and J. Stelling (1969), "Characteristics of Professional Organizations," *Journal of Health and Social Behavior,* **10:**3–15.

115. D. Mechanic (1974c), op. cit.

116. B. S. Georgopoulos (1972), *Organization Research on Health Institutions* (Ann Arbor, Mich.: Institute for Social Research).

117. S. Levine and P. E. White (1972), "The Community of Health Organizations," in H. Freeman et al., op. cit., pp. 359–385.

118. M. Aiken and J. Hage (1968), "Organizational Interdependence and Intra-Organizational Structure," *American Sociological Review,* **33:**912–930.

119. R. Stevens (1971), op. cit.

120. M. Field (1971), "Stability and Change in the Medical System: Medicine in the Industrial Society," in B. Barber and A. Inkeles, eds., *Stability and Social Change* (Boston: Little, Brown), pp. 30–60.

121. D. Mechanic (1974b), op. cit.

122. Ibid.

Chapter 3

Conflicts in the Roles
of Bureaucratic Physicians

With the growing bureaucratization of medical practice, physicians and other health professionals face complex and competing demands that pose new social and ethical dilemmas for them. Although we presently conceive of the physician as largely autonomous, the fact is that the modern physician is increasingly an organizational man.[1] In the United States, approximately 8 per cent of physicians work for the federal government, mostly in hospital-based practice but also in administrative, research, and teaching roles. Many of these physicians serve the armed forces and their dependents in one of the largest systems of organized, socialized care in the world. Seven per cent of nonfederal physicians work in teaching, research, and administration. Of the more than 90 per cent of physicians in the nonfederal sector, approximately one-fourth are in hospital-based practice and most of the others have some hospital attachment. Even those primarily in office-based practice are dependent on their hospital affiliations to pursue their work, and increasingly face restrictions under the rules of the hospital as a social and legal entity.

Increasing numbers of physicians are employed by drug firms, medical industries, insurance companies, and public agencies. Doctors, more than ever before, participate in the courts, in quasi-judicial determinations on disability compensation and other matters, in industrial health settings, and in the schools. In short, the roles of physicians in defining the social consequences of illness and disability, and the special privileges or limitations to be placed on

49

those affected, are far-reaching and have important implications for the exercise of individual rights and the adjudication of claims for special consideration.

Although public employment, or salary as a source of payment, may tell us little about the organization of physicians' roles and how they actually function, the employment of physicians by complex organizations involves certain changes in the auspices of medical care that depart in significant ways from traditional concepts. In the existing model of medical ethics, and the legal structure that supports it, the primary responsibility of physicians is to their patients. Patients consent to the implicit contract with the physician on the assumption that the doctor acts as their agent, and on their behalf. Obviously there are constraints stemming from the limits of the physician's knowledge and understanding, and the legal and other ethical requirements of the role. To the extent that the physician violates the patient's trust either by carrying out procedures without the patient's consent, or divulging information harmful to the patient, the patient has access to redress through malpractice litigation.

The traditional concept of private physicians acting as agents on behalf of their patients is of course an oversimplification, for in reality the dependence and limited knowledge of patients set up a variety of opportunities for physicians to focus on competing interests in addition to those of the patients. Such activities may be carried out in good faith, reflecting certain incentives operating in a fee-for-service context, ethical and social dilemmas in the society at large, or the particular sociopolitical orientations of the physician. Thus the distinction between the private, and autonomous, practice of medicine and bureaucratic practice is not as obvious as it might appear. But the growing bureaucratization of medicine complicates the physician's role, the various persons involved in patient care, and the operation of incentives affecting how the physician works.

The increased potentialities for conflict of interest in bureaucratic settings reflect the fact that such settings are more likely to be defined by multiple interests. In addition, the provision of patient care is shared by a larger number of physicians and other health workers, which to some extent diffuses responsibility, and privileged information about patients and their conditions is more widely accessible, and therefore less private. The organizational setting, which requires greater cooperation and reciprocity among workers, puts the physician under pressure to sacrifice certain interests of the patient to satisfy organizational needs or to help maintain working relationships within the organization. These points can be brought out more clearly by contrasting the simple traditional model with its elaboration in bureaucratic settings.

In the private setting in which there is a simple dyadic relationship between doctor and patient, and in which some competition for patients exists among doctors, patients exercise certain countercontrols on doctors' behavior. As Freidson[2] has noted, physicians may be required to make certain concessions to patients to retain their patronage, concessions that may require deviations from a preferred pattern of work and medical judgment. In communities where they are attempting to build a practice, physicians are especially likely to respond to patients' requests for quasi-medical services, for house calls, and for amenities of service that might be less available when patients are more abundant. As the doctor's practice grows, the time given to any patient relative to the rest must be weighed. The fee-for-service context may encourage the physician in marginal situations to carry out "unnecessary services" or to have the patient return "too frequently" in the opinion of an outside medical observer with no personal interests at stake. Where the physician is not sufficiently busy, there may be an implicit conflict between the physician's economic self-interest and the patient's optimal interests, although I do not mean to suggest that the typical physician consciously takes advantage of the patient.

Certainly, physicians encounter requests, demands, and other circumstances in conflict with their social and ethical views. Doctors often take moralistic stances toward patient behavior. They may express reluctance to prescribe contraceptives,[3] provide little assistance in obtaining an abortion, refuse the patient certain prescription drugs about which they hold strong moral views, or steer away from issues they consider embarrassing such as sex and family conflict. In the medical encounter, physicians are limited by their own psychological and social needs and capacities.

Much of medical decision-making involves social and ethical considerations in which the therapist finds it difficult to be neutral. Physicians may relieve their own anxiety and uncertainty by conceptualizing moral choices as medical problems. Take, for example, the mundane and typical instance in which a patient with a sore throat requests antibacterial treatment. The well-trained physician has been taught to ascertain the character of the infection prior to issuing such a prescription, and sees the indiscriminate use of antibiotics as poor medicine. Some physicians will meet patient requests for such drugs on the basis that the patient would be dissatisfied if the demand was not met and might obtain the drug elsewhere. But if we more carefully dissect the character of the medical problem, it is clear that it has components that are both medical and social.

A patient with a sore throat has a given probability of having a bacterial infection. Ascertaining whether this is the case, and knowing the appropriate use of antibiotics and their value and adverse effects, are clearly aspects of medical expertise. Ordinarily, this leads to the decision-rule that because of the possible adverse effects, antibiotics should not be used until the bacterial basis of the infection has been demonstrated. But the rule also has exceptions, as in medical situations where a bacterial infection would pose special dangers to the patient, and under these circumstances prophylactic antibacterials may be medically justified. The decision to use or not to use antibiotics without further investigation is made by weighing different probabilities: the probability of danger from a possible bacterial infection against the probability of danger from the drug. However, some patients, for social reasons, are willing to assume the dangers of using a drug unnecessarily in order to gain the added protection of decreasing the probability or length of morbidity. Take, for example, people who feel they are at a stage in their business or professional life where they "can't afford" to become sick. These patients may be willing to incur a greater and perhaps medically unjustifiable risk for a higher probability of protection. The decision then becomes a social decision, not a medical one, since the medical determination does not take into account the social costs of an increased probability of morbidity or inconvenience. One could argue that in these cases physicians should give patients the benefit of medical advice, which the patients can then weigh against the contingencies of their life situation. This example appears from a superficial perspective to be purely a medical determination. As one moves into consideration of psychoactive drugs, contraception, radical versus conservative techniques of managing certain illnesses, and the like, the social aspects of the decision loom very large indeed.

The opportunities for nonmedical influences on medical activities are extensive even in routine situations. In the physical examination, for example, the rectal exam is one of the procedures most frequently neglected, and this in all probability reflects the inconvenience of performing the procedure in a busy outpatient practice, the physician's expectation that the patient may be reluctant to have the procedure performed, and the aesthetic aversion that physicians may feel about the procedure despite their medical socialization. The doctor-patient interaction, like any other human association, may activate unconscious tendencies of the physician, such as attitudes toward certain ethnic and minority groups, toward men or women, or whatever. Thus, physicians in even the most simple private relationships with patients carry out their practice within a social and ethical context in which their attitudes, personalities, and the constraints of the practice situation play a role in the decisions made. Moreover, the same doctor who serves members of a family will occasionally face conflicts in resolving the competing or conflicting interests of members. Should the physician prescribe contraceptives for a teen-age girl, aware of the fact that her parents disapprove, but also aware of the fact that she is vulnerable to pregnancy without such a prescription? Should a physician divulge to one member of a family information obtained from another without that person's consent, even if the physician believes that to do so is in the interests of the family as a whole? What should the physician's attitude be toward pain, toward using drugs as "crutches" to deal with family and employment conflict, and toward certifying illness and disability, even when doubts exist that they are really incapacitating? To the extent that these decisions are treated as medical determinations, and they usually are, the intrusion of other social and ethical interests against those of the patient may be considerable. Although the simplicity of the dyad may insulate the interaction from other pressures to be discussed shortly, there are abundant forces remaining in this context to dilute the interests of the patients as he might see them.

Physicians who work in bureaucratic settings usually continue to regard themselves as autonomous professionals, and they resist many of the demands that would alter their role as agent of the patient. But despite such resistance, the requirements of many of the physicians' roles in organizations create strong incentives and pressures that may be inconsistent with the individual patient's interests. Some of these pressures result from the growing complexity of the organization and the degree to which the bureaucratic physician can be more independent of client control than the autonomous community practitioner. But in the bureaucratic context, the influences from organizational requirements, and other professionals involved in the patient's care, have greater force. Indeed, the definition of the physician's employment, under some circumstances, transforms the definition of who the client is.

In many circumstances—military psychiatry, prison medicine, institutional psychiatry, industrial medicine, and research and teaching, to name some—clear and apparent conflicts develop between the best interests of the patient and other competing interests that are perceived as legitimate. Similarly, there are circumstances such as those evolving in prepaid practices and medical foundations, school health services, and the courts where the physician faces conflicting loyalties and demands from various constituencies—the patient, the administration of the plan, colleague standards, other patients, the research and teaching program, and the like. Moreover, as specialties develop that define their responsibilities not to a single patient, but to a family, a community, or an enrolled population, the possibilities for conflicts between the varying interests among members of these collectivities mount.

There is an old aphorism that he who pays the piper calls the tune; and following this logic there is reason to anticipate that physicians paid by employers rather than employees, by school administrations rather than by students, the military rather than soldiers, and the court rather than adversaries to a proceeding, may have a tendency to resolve conflicts and dilemmas in favor of the organization that gives them their remuneration and controls their advancement. When industrial physicians consider policies concerning safety requirements that deal with uncertain risks for workers and economic costs for employers, the fact that they are employed by the company may affect their judgment. School physicians often find it difficult to resist divulging information concerning a student. The process is subtle. Students come and go, but the physician tends to have a regularized relationship with the school and, indeed, depends on the school for employment. Close and friendly relationships are often developed with the administration, and the doctor's self-image may be that of an agent of the school community rather than of the student under consideration. No conspiracy theory is required to explain deviations from privileged communication under such circumstances. Similarly, the military psychiatrist must treat patients who may be in an adversarial relationship with the military organization that employs the psychiatrist, and the auspices of this employment is no trivial factor in how the psychiatrist contributes to the resolution of the situation. Physicians obviously have retained a strong professional base so that even in these organizational contexts they can usually do what they feel is in the interests of particular patients, but it is prudent for us to assume that where there is stress, there is some give.

In the cases described above, the conflicts are sufficiently obvious that both patient and professional are likely to recognize them. Students are suspicious of student health services, as perhaps they should be. For some problems they are more likely to seek out their peer group or free clinics than recognized sources of care. Employees, and the unions that represent them, are aware that industrial physicians may not act in their interests, and they often use their own medical consultants to challenge industrial conditions they believe to be conducive to ill health. Similarly, lawyers sense that health professionals working for the court are not always to be trusted, and that they may be influenced by their own special relationship to the court system and the judge.[4] But even where there is awareness of potential conflicts of interest and values, the failure to clarify roles leads to a general suspiciousness that erodes the potential of the medical role.

Perhaps of greater concern are those instances that are more ambiguous, more pervasive, and where the role of the physician appears more innocent. In such cases as the HMO, the teaching hospital, or the research ward, the conflicts in the physicians' role are more submerged and the various interests are less adversarial in their nature. In the case of HMOs, for example, there are increasing attempts to develop incentives that encourage physicians to avoid providing unnecessary services. But since the concept of "necessary" is itself vague, the determination is likely to reflect the balance of pressures on the physician. As the personal incentive increases to economize on the provision of services, as may occur especially in profit HMOs, pressures may exist to withhold various expensive services—some of which may be of a lifesaving nature. It is difficult to anticipate the effect of a system in which patients come to believe that physicians are withholding service because it is in their economic interest to do so, but it seems reasonably obvious that such beliefs, if they became widespread, would erode the effectiveness and quality of medical service.

The bureaucratization of medicine also has the effect of diluting the personal responsibility of the provider, making it more likely that interests other than those of the patient will prevail. By segmenting responsibility for patient care, the medical bureaucracy relieves the physician of direct continuing responsibility. If the patient cannot reach a physician at night or on weekends, obtain responsive care, have inquiries answered, or whatever, the problem is no longer focused on the failure of an individual physician, but on the failures of the organization. It is far easier for patients to locate and deal with individual failures where responsibility is clear, than to confront a diffuse organizational structure where responsibility is often hazy and the buck is easily passed. To the extent that a physician knows that a patient is his or her charge, the physician feels a certain responsibility to protect the patient's interests against organizational roadblocks and requests that may not be fully appropriate. But when responsibility is less clear it is easier to make decisions in the name of other interests such as research, teaching, or demonstration.

The teaching hospital that brings together a variety of legitimate interests in service, teaching, and research presents conflicts in weighing priorities. Although, in name, the interests of the patient are supreme, there are strong pressures to insure the continuance of the teaching and research programs. The psychological comfort and integrity of the patient's family may be important, but so is the need for organs for transplant, permission to obtain an autopsy, and a variety of other matters that contribute to the institution. Individuals of integrity no doubt become victims of the structures within which they find themselves, and they are "forced" to engage in behaviors they may basically disapprove of. When a physician in an HMO is pressured by its administration to withhold what the administration defines as an unnecessary service, he must choose to yield or to stand up to the administration, knowing full well that the person who stands on principle often pays a price. Does a physician-researcher, committed to an important research project, withhold certain information on risks, or at least dampen the threatening information, to insure that the necessary formal consent is obtained? How much is it proper to badger relatives to obtain autopsy permission, or how much pressure is justified to obtain organs for transplant? If the organization encourages, however subtly, deceptive and unethical behaviors to cope with competing demands and needs, what options are available to the physician who disapproves?

Needless to say, conflicts exist in all complex organizations. That they also exist in medical institutions is neither surprising nor cause for alarm. But unlike many other participants in complex organizations, the physician has greater autonomy and a more profound mystique, and patients tend to be both more dependent and trustful. Thus, it is especially important that mechanisms be developed that allow for recognition of existing conflicts and ways of adjudicating them so as to allow the work of the institution to go on while also protecting patients' rights. Even though some hold great hopes for peer review as a means of recognizing and checking abuses, we have little evidence that self-policing is effective in dealing with such problems.[5–7]

Still another danger of the bureaucratization of medicine is the growing extent to which sensitive information about patients is shared by a wide variety of persons, and the threat of access to this information by unauthorized persons. Although much of this fear is directed to the computerization of medical records, in some ways the dangers that presently exist may be greater. Computerization and the concerns it arouses at least direct the attention of organizational personnel to the issues involved. But as clinics and institutions get larger, the archaic means of storing confidential records provide little security, and records are easily accessible to large numbers of people. It is difficult to know how frequently such reports are violated, but in all probability the problem is greater than generally recognized.

With the growth of third-party insurers and increasing auditing of medical records, data on patients are accessible not only to a wider range of health personnel, but to others involved in managerial functions. Unlike physicians, these persons are not indoctrinated in issues of medical confidentiality, and to the extent that such training is important in preventing abuse, the range of access should raise concern. Records will have to be available not only for medical communication but also for review and managerial functions, but as the access is increased so must be efforts to protect against improper disclosure.

Physicians are practical and active individuals who do not easily buckle to bureaucratic pressures. While this may create problems in an organizational society concerned with efficiency and accountability, it also provides certain protections against the overzealous manager who knows more about efficiency and systems theory than about patient care. Physicians have been quite successful in thwarting attempts to impose a traditional bureaucratic structure on them, and for the most part the administration of health institutions has remained relatively weak. Even in the military, where the authority structure is strong, physicians and psychiatrists have often been able to protect their professional discretion to a considerable extent. The growing organizational basis of medicine and its associated technologies make possible programs of care that could not be provided under other auspices. As we evolve new organizations, we obviously require mechanisms of control to insure that we make use of knowledge and technological potential without sacrificing patient rights or responsive care.

NOTES

1. S. G. Vahovich, ed. (1973), *Profile of Medical Practice* (Chicago: Center for Health Services Research and Development, American Medical Association), pp. 4, 13.
2. E. Freidson (1970), *Profession of Medicine: A Study in the Sociology of Applied Knowledge* (New York: Dodd, Mead).
3. M. J. Cornish et al. (1963), *Doctors and Family Planning* (New York: National Committee on Maternal Health), Publ. 19.

4. A. Blumberg (1967), *Criminal Justice* (Chicago: Quadrangle).

5. E. Freidson (1976), *Doctoring Together* (New York: Elsevier).

6. B. Gray (1975), *Human Subjects in Medical Experimentation: A Sociological Study of the Conduct and Regulation of Clinical Research* (New York: Wiley-Interscience).

7. B. Barber et al. (1973), *Research on Human Subjects: Problems of Social Control of Medical Experimentation* (New York: Russell Sage Foundation).

Chapter 4

The Design of Human Services Systems: Implications from Organizational Theory

The conceptions that legislators, administrators, and managers have about how people function affect the types of organizational designs and incentives they advocate. As Herbert Simon points out, organizations refer to "the complex pattern of communications and other relations in a group of human beings. The pattern provides to each member of the group much of the information, assumptions, goals, and attitudes that enter into his decisions, and provides him also with a set of stable and comprehensible expectations as to what the other members of the group are doing and how they will react to what he says and does."[1] The pattern of incentives and how they are communicated also affect how people go about doing their jobs and how they relate to others in the organization.

Most writings on organizations deal with industrial or business settings. Such organizations tend to have a well-defined technology and a limited and clearly defined set of goals. They produce a product and compete in the marketplace with companies selling similar products. The design of the organization depends on the type of technology necessary in the production and distribution processes and on the needs to be efficient. Since the goals of the organization are reasonably clear, supervision of work is not difficult. In contrast, organizations providing helping services to clients have less clearly defined goals, have more uncertain technologies for achieving desired effects, and depend to a larger extent on professionals and paraprofessionals. Thus, work patterns in such organizations involve greater discretion and less direct supervision. Even in highly supervised industrial situations workers manage to assert their individuality or control over their work through informal practices developed on the job or through small work groups. In human services organizations, where it is more difficult to measure production and its effects, such adaptations are a much larger part of everyday activity.

Much of our thinking on bureaucracies in government and the service sector has been influenced by traditional concepts of bureaucratic organization. The civil service bureaucracy, which has a clearly hierarchical structure and defined channels of communication and decision-making, is our typical model. When such organizations have as their main object delivering personal services to clients—for example, welfare agencies—they often appear inflexible, unresponsive, and self-protective. These organizations not only give clients inferior, and sometimes degrading, treatment, but they also often have a deadening effect on their employees, offering limited opportunity for personal growth or for increased satisfaction through improved performance. Work often becomes routine and dull, and employees' satisfaction tends to come from interactions on the job, not from the main work of the organization.

This chapter focuses on the management of bureaucracies that provide personal services to clients as a major aspect of their work. It explores, in a very preliminary way, how the delivery of personal services can be designed to provide more effective and responsive service as well as higher levels of performance and self-fulfillment among employees. Since my concern in this book is with medicine, I dwell on examples in the health area, but the implications of the discussion extend to a wide range of organizations that focus on providing personal services to clients.

This chapter establishes the framework for those that follow. While I flesh out the main arguments and considerations that govern my thinking about human services bureaucracies here, the chapters that follow illustrate one or another aspect of the problem by examining some facet of medical care—how it is organized, how it is viewed by providers and consumers, and the problems of assessment and implementation. One way of approaching the problem is to examine the reasons currently offered for failure or poor performance in service bureaucracies. Analyses have been made at two levels, institutional and organizational. After examining these conceptions, I discuss more explicitly the concepts of personality and human functioning that are most appropriate in thinking about the design of administrative guidelines or other types of organizational incentives. I illustrate the problem by contrasting the concepts of organization of Herbert Simon and Chris Argyris, and then by suggesting a conception of personality that builds on both. Throughout this chapter I focus on one major question: How can delivery be organized so that human services meet people's needs in a personal and effective way, but also in a way that is efficient? All organizations must operate within limits of resources—time, money, personnel. Our task is not to define a utopian model that has no reasonable relationship to the world in which we live, but rather to understand better how we can make most effective use of the resources that are likely to be available.

SOME INSTITUTIONAL CONCEPTIONS OF
THE DELIVERY OF HUMAN SERVICES

A commonly held view of the failure of human services bureaucracies is that they are organized to enhance the interests of particular groups—for example, those who provide the services—and thus do not place highest priority on meeting the needs of clients.[2] This perspective can be traced to the power elite conception associated with the work of C. Wright Mills and his followers.[3] In brief, the argument is that important decisions in health care, as in other sectors, are controlled by a relatively few persons who are interlinked and who exercise power in their own interest and in the interests of their group. Although this theory does not assume that the group in power will always dominate decision-making, exceptions are explained as insignificant concessions required to avoid conflict and to exercise power smoothly. Many who hold this view believe that significant change is impossible because those who hold power will not allow their interests to be threatened. It follows, therefore, that incremental change is unimportant, since serious redistributions of power do not take place.

Since this theory suffers from circular thinking, it is difficult to test its basic assumptions and hypotheses. It is obvious that certain persons and groups in society exercise disproportionate influence and power in certain sectors; it is equally obvious that the views and interests of certain groups and individuals are not represented when decisions are made. However, these facts do not constitute a basis for maintaining that there is a power elite that has control over the sector in question and has the ability to thwart all significant change.

A contrasting view, associated with the pluralists, accepts that power in any sphere may be disproportionately concentrated, but treats the processes of social participation, decision-making, and influence as problematic.[4] Some people have varying access to power and decision-making; others may even be disenfranchised because of the lack of skills or inability to organize effectively. But control over institutions is seen as the outcome of a political process in which varying interests clash, negotiate, and often compromise.

To see how the debate over power and control in institutional spheres relates to medical care, we can turn to Alford's essay on the political economy of health.[5] Alford maintains that we fail to correct problems in the delivery of care to clients because organizational change in medical care is orchestrated to serve the interests of professionals and bureaucrats who manage the health delivery system. He notes that

> the "crisis" of health care is *not* a result of the necessary competition of diverse interests, groups, and providers in a pluralistic and competitive health economy, nor a result of bureaucratic inefficiencies to be corrected by yet more layers of administration established by government policy. Rather, the conflicts between the professional monopolists—seeking to erect barriers to protect their control over research, teaching and care—and the corporate rationalizers—seeking to extend their control over the organization of services—account for many of the aspects of health care. . . . These conflicts stem, in turn, from a fundamental contradiction in modern health care between the character of technology of health care and the private appropriation of the power and resources involved. The integration of all aspects of the health care system . . . would require the defeat or consolidation of the social power that has been appropriated by various discrete interest groups and that preserve existing allocations of social values and resources. . . . Change is not likely without the presence of a social and political movement which rejects the legitimacy of the economic and social base of pluralist politics.[6]

Alford's utopian analysis of health services contrasts the existing system with an ideal system, and thus fails to offer any clear criteria for evaluating the delivery of health care. Nor does Alford establish any clear guidelines by which we can evaluate the extent and meaningfulness of change. Thus, his argument is made to appear true by definition, in contrast to the presentation of standards and data indicating how well or poorly we met them. Moreover, he leaves us with the inference that anything less than rejection of "the legitimacy of the economic and social base of pluralist politics" would constitute merely a symbolic deflection of the needs and demands of less powerful groups in the society. Given the nature of his analysis any change, no matter how extensive—National Health Insurance, Medicare and Medicaid, HMOs, Regional Health Planning—is passed off as having little substance. Nevertheless, we find no statement of criteria that would allow us to assess the changes either in terms of the prior situation or in terms of a clear set of ideal standards.

It is certainly true that the health sector, like any other, reflects the social and political forces dominant in the society at large. However, it is incorrect to assume that modifications of health organization do not have important substantive consequences. Medical care has been undergoing continuing adaptations from a variety of interventions aimed at dealing with access, cost, and quality. Certainly we are far from an ideal system, but we must recognize that the one that has evolved has been shaped by many compromises among competing groups. Neither physicians, health administrators, executives of health industries, nor patients presently feel that the current system of care is optimal from their point of view. Indeed, part of the current problem is that in the process of negotiation and compromise the system of care becomes distorted in numerous ways, and comes to have a variety of irrational features.

The imperfections of our present system of providing medical care are discussed later in this book. To recognize difficult problems is not the same as asserting that interventions in the medical field are merely "dynamics without change," or merely symbolic gestures that protect the power of professional monopolists and corporate rationalizers. In recent years we have seen important changes in the delivery of medical care. Medicare, despite its imperfections, brought many new services to the elderly, and the traditional obverse relationship between socioeconomic status and physician visits has been eliminated.[7] Group practice, HMOs, and health care regulation have grown considerably. Powerful influences who have an important role in deciding the form in which programs are implemented certainly exist in the health field, but these forces cannot take their power for granted, nor do they always prevail. Improvement of health care delivery is not consistent with our aspirations for a variety of reasons: the interventions may be weak and diluted because of the necessary compromises in legislating new programs, the goals may be poorly defined and there may be significant disagreements as to priorities, the solutions themselves may be poorly formulated and ineffective, and the processes of implementation may be complex and may require agreements and cooperation that are difficult to obtain.

As the discussion of comparative health care systems in previous chapters noted, medical systems varying substantially in organization, centralization, and degree of government involvement face many of the same problems that Alford describes as characteristic of the American political economy, thus leading us to question his attributions of causality. Further, his analysis begs the more serious questions of how to define our health care goals more clearly, how to assess the efficacy of varying alternatives, and how to cope with the numerous problems of implementation. In Part II of this volume, problems of rationing and allocating services are discussed in the context of varying forms of medical practice. As we illustrate in these analyses, each way of organizing health care services and dealing with clients has distinct advantages, but also special problems. Since the best of all possible worlds necessarily eludes us, we must seek the best possible trade offs and an overall solution that is satisfactory to both clients and providers. There are, of course, disagreements on what the best trade offs are and whether certain possibilities can work in practice. Since there is growing discussion on the uncertainties of planned social change, let us examine this area in somewhat greater detail.

Associated with the disillusionment of those who advocated major social programs in the 1960s only to see these programs fail is the view that our difficulties in many social areas result not from the power of special interests, but simply from the lack of individual and organizational know-how to design solutions adequate to deal with competing objectives. In medical care, for example, we want access and quality, but we also want to control the costs of care. We wish to enhance our capacities in primary medical care and in prevention, but we also want protections against incapacitating and catastrophic illness and facilities to cope with them. We want doctors to be technically proficient and on the cutting edge of medical advance, but also to have interest in our minor complaints and life problems. As Alice Rivlin has argued,

> we are failing to solve social problems because we do not know how to do it—the problems are genuinely hard. The difficulties do not primarily involve conflicts among different groups of people, although these exist. Rather, current social problems are difficult because they involve conflicts among objectives that almost everyone holds. These conflicts create technical or design difficulties that override the political ones.[8]

Rivlin poses the problem here as conceptual—one where it is difficult to define the most effective allocation of resources among competing goals. Even within a single sector, such as medical care, it is difficult to make allocative decisions. But if one also seeks to define trade offs in enhancing health between investments in other programs and medical care, the problems become even more troublesome. The issues are not only technical, but also involve people's expectations and the political process more generally. Thus, it requires considerable ingenuity to devise solutions that "work" and that also create minimal conflicts among interested persons and in relation to dominant values. Because of the need to overcome political as well as technical obstacles, the route to implementation often must be circuitous. And such routes, because they are so indirect and because they involve cooperation from so many individuals and groups, are frequently ineffectual. For example, in this country for several decades there has been concern with the poor distribution of physicians relative to need in the population. The many government programs that have been instituted to achieve improved distribution have tried to do so without coercive measures and have failed. Pressman and Wildavsky, in a study of the implementation of a federal program at the local level, note the complex chains of cooperation that are required to meet desired objectives.

> What we hope to show is that the apparently simple and straight-forward is really complex and convoluted. We are initially surprised because we do not begin to appreciate the number of steps involved, the number of participants whose preferences have to be taken into account, the number of separate decisions that are part of what we think of as a single one. Least of all do we appreciate the

geometric growth of interdependencies over time where each negotiation involves a number of participants with decisions to make, whose implications ramify over time. What is so hard about building a terminal and airline hangar when the money is there, the plans are signed, and the people agree that minorities are to get a share of the jobs? We will show that what seemed to be a simple program turned out to be a very complex one, involving numerous participants, a host of differing perspectives, and a long and tortuous path of decision points that had to be cleared. Given these characteristics, the chances of completing the program with the haste its designers had hoped for—and even the chances of completing it at all—were sharply reduced.[9]

This illustration suggests that we require far simpler interventions that do not depend on such complex chains of decision-making. Complex theoretical solutions, when communicated from one set of decisionmakers to another, tend to be modified and distorted in light of the needs and goals of each group. To minimize such manipulations we need to develop approaches that set some easily monitored, basic requirements, but that also allow discretion on the details of implementation. For example, it is easier to control costs through the establishment of a fixed budget, which providers must adjust to, than it is to devise complex formulas of deductibles and coinsurance and covered and uninsured services. The latter approach requires detailed monitoring and encourages both consumers and providers to distort their actions in order to gain benefits that may not be technically covered under the detailed restrictions. Under a fixed budget, providers will attempt to make reasonable allocations of the money available. Under the more complex approach, they may be induced to relabel health examinations as "acute care visits" to have the insurance pay, or they may hospitalize patients, despite their assessment that this is unnecessary, because this aspect of care is covered under the insurance contract.

In considering the failures of service bureaucracies to provide acceptable and effective services to clients, policymakers tend to see four major sources of failure: the defective recruitment and socialization of personnel, the organization of the service itself and the incentive structure affecting behavior, the business management of the organization, and the leadership.

Many believe that the problems inherent in service delivery stem from recruiting the wrong people to provide the service or from improperly training those who are chosen. For example, medical educators frequently blame poor distribution of medical care and lack of responsiveness of physicians on the methods used to recruit students for medical schools and on their medical education. If physicians are unwilling to practice in rural areas, or with the urban poor, or with minorities, educators suggest that what is needed is to recruit medical students from rural areas or from minority groups. Or they argue that students should be selected whose personality traits or values differ from those of the traditional medical student. In response to the awareness that physicians tend to choose specialties in contrast to primary care, they seek to develop new programs or specialties such as family medicine, which they hope will induce doctors to have greater interest in general medical problems. In short, those who advocate such solutions tend to view delivery problems as problems in changing people—what they believe and value, and what they know. Thus, solutions involve changes in admission practices and in educational programs, but rarely in the conditions of practice itself.

The second view—the one focusing on the incentive structure—gives far less credit to the individuals who deliver care and to how they have been trained, and far more to the way in which the organizational system in which they function affects their behavior. Solutions depend less on changing people and more on changing organizational arrangements, reward systems, and ways of coordinating the efforts of various individuals. For example, writing on service institutions, Peter Drucker argues that failures result because rewards are not effectively used to induce a high level of performance.

> Human beings will behave as they are being rewarded—whether the reward is money and promotion, a medal, the autographed picture of the boss, or a pat on the back. This is the one lesson the behavioral psychologist has taught us during the last fifty years (not that it was unknown before). A business or any institution which is paid for its results and performance in such a way that the dissatisfied or disinterested customer need not pay has to earn its income.[10]

In the chapters that follow we examine in considerable detail how the system through which physicians are paid and how the structure of practice affect responsiveness to patients. Although Drucker tends to oversimplify the problem, the reward system does have an important bearing on how participants see their work and how they relate to one another. Also, in conjunction with other aspects of the organization such as work pressures, reward systems affect the priorities established and strategies of work.

A third view—often heard in these cost-conscious times—is that the problems of service delivery are largely problems of failures in management, and a neglect of those conditions that enhance efficiency. The basic difficulty is seen as poor business practices, vague incentives promoting cost-effective behavior, and lack of accountability. Change, it is maintained, depends on introducing greater competition among providers, developing less expensive substitutes for many services, and instituting a managerial approach that rationalizes practices. This view relies heavily on the scientific management movement prevalent in industrial management and in such approaches as operations research and systems engineering.[11]

This approach tends to focus excessively on the economic aspects of care, taking little account of its symbolic and interpersonal aspects. Competition may lead to greater efficiency, but it may also encourage neglect of less tangible aspects of medical care that are more difficult to measure. It may encourage reduced cost in the pricing of one or another service, but also provide incentives for delivering many unnecessary services. I do not wish to suggest that greater efficiencies cannot be achieved in service delivery. The present system is wasteful in many ways. But achieving efficiencies depends on more than finding cheaper substitutes for one or another service. There must be evidence that such substitutes constitute adequate care and that they are acceptable to clients. In short, the management approach emphasizes neither people nor structures conducive to improved quality. It focuses simply on means to reduce or limit cost, and attempts to encourage this through competition and more efficient organization of each of the elements of medical care.

A contrasting view of management emphasizes improved leadership. Here it is maintained that the quality and effectiveness of the organization depends on those who direct it, on their abilities to gauge the capacities of their personnel and to anticipate problems of organization accurately and creatively. Since effective performance often depends on a sense of involvement among personnel, the leadership perspective emphasizes charisma—the ability to stir staff loyalties and commitment to common goals. Those who emphasize leadership are aware that more is required than an inspiring personality. It is assumed that good leaders understand how to utilize opportunities and to deal with the problems of communication and timing. Assessing organizational problems depends on the quality of organizational intelligence; loyalty from personnel and implementation of goals depend on both the effective recruitment of personnel and the use of group and other devices to encourage commitment; and correctly assessing the capacities and performance of personnel is dependent on adequate communication and monitoring.

What makes the leadership position distinctive is the faith that good leaders understand organizational needs and how to manage expectations and communication to achieve their objectives. Also, they are assumed to know people, how to gauge their capacities, and how to motivate individuals to their best efforts. Such managers are not necessarily conceptual persons, but they have had practical experience. In the usual rhetoric, they have "met a payroll."

BOUNDED RATIONALITY OR SELF-ACTUALIZATION?

There is considerable consensus that the concept of economic man, implicit in so much of economic modeling, inadequately portrays the irrational and rational factors that guide people in organizations. Economists often escape the consequences of their assumptions by using a flexible concept of utility that is adjustable after the fact; but despite this, the concept of economic man is poor guidance for understanding organizational behavior, particularly in human services organizations where emotions run deep and where altruistic expectations play no small part in the relationship between agency personnel and clients. Indeed, even in industrial organizations and business firms, where we would expect the concept of economic man to work most powerfully, there are many departures from predicted behavior resulting from peer group influences, the individual's personal goals, and the desire to control the conditions of work.[12]

In this book we are concerned with ways of organizing medicine that will bring out the best in health professionals and also achieve high quality, responsive, humane care. In addition, we wish to understand the conditions that facilitate patient responsibility and behavior consistent with maintaining a high level of health. In investigating the organizational arrangements under which these goals are achieved most effectively, we must consider our assumptions about people and their behavior, and the organizational incentives that are most likely to facilitate their capacities and fulfillment of need. To what extent should organizations define operating procedures in detail and attempt to minimize uncertainty and use of discretion, as compared with maximizing opportunities for professional and paraprofessional personnel to improvise new solutions and to carry out their responsibilities in a relatively free and spontaneous way? All organizations must have some mix of established routines and opportunities for discretion; the problem is defining the best mix for achieving the outcomes most valued. Some physicians, for example, believe that the quality of medicine can only be improved by developing clear quality control standards, communicating them to physicians, and evaluating the degree to which conformity is achieved. Other physicians—the majority, in fact—believe that they must be free to exercise their professional judgment and that it is inappropriate for an organization to prescribe detailed standards for their work. One way of examining the issue of the optimum balance between standard procedures and spontaneity is to contrast the views of two major organizational analysts, Herbert Simon and Chris Argyris.

Herbert Simon, in perhaps the most influential single conception of administrative behavior, presents the concept of bounded rationality. Taking into account human frailties and the irrational forces in decision-making, Simon argues that "the central concern of administrative theory is with the boundary between the rational and non-rational aspects of human behavior. Administrative theory is peculiarly the theory of intended and bounded rationality—of the behavior of human beings who *satisfice* because they have not the wits to maximize."[13] Simon, who brings to the field of administrative behavior a wide knowledge of organizations, psychology, and developments in the computer sciences, sees the issues relating to bounded rationality largely in terms of the limits of human beings' capacities to process information and limits of ability, attention, and knowledge. Although Simon is fully acquainted with psychodynamic thinking, he gives such factors little emphasis. Nor does he give much attention to the emergence of informal organizations, which often modifies substantially both the goals and decision-making processes in organizations.

Simon's efforts have been devoted to modifying classical concepts of rationality in light of growing knowledge and his own research on how people process information. As he notes in *Models of Man:*

> If we examine closely the "classical" concepts of rationality we see immediately what severe demands they make upon the choosing organism. The organisms must be able to attach definite payoffs (or at least a definite range of payoffs) to each possible outcome. This, of course, involves also the ability to specify the exact nature of the outcomes—there is no room in the scheme for "unanticipated consequences." The payoffs must be completely ordered—it must always be possible to specify, in a consistent way, that one outcome is better than, as good as, or worse than any other. And if the certainty or probabilistic rules are employed, either the outcomes of particular alternatives must be known with certainty, or at least it must be possible to attach definite probabilities to outcomes.

> My first empirical proposition is that there is a complete lack of evidence that, in actual human choice situations of any complexity, these computations can be, or are in fact, performed. The introspective evidence is certainly clear enough but we cannot, of course, rule out the possibility that the unconscious is a better decision-maker than the conscious. Nevertheless, in the absence of evidence that the classical concepts do describe the decision-making process, it seems reasonable to examine the possibility that the actual process is quite different from the ones the rules describe.[14]

In *Administrative Behavior,* Simon points out how the psychological environment limits human rationality by imposing certain constraints on decision-making, but he strongly argues that effective socialization and well-designed patterns of authority allow the regularization of behavior and thus limit the irrational. As he sees it, the problems of irrationality reside in fragmentary knowledge and difficulties in anticipation, the problems in placing values on consequences that can only be imperfectly anticipated, and the complexity of choice itself. Man achieves control when he can logically program decision processes. Although Simon is too acute an observer to fail to see irrational elements in organization life, his preference is clearly to focus on the rational dimensions and how they might be expanded through better understanding of problem-solving. As he notes,

> reason is the handmaiden of freedom and creativity. It is the instrument that enables me to have peak experiences unimaginable to my cat or to my dog. It is the instrument that enables me to dream and design. It is the instrument that enables me and my fellow men to create environments and societies that can satisfy our basic needs, so that all of us—and not just a few—can experience some of the deeper pleasures of sense and mind. And because we depend so heavily upon reason to create and maintain a humane world, we see the need to understand reason better—to construct a tested theory of reasoning man.[15]

A contrasting view of the conditions for effectiveness is championed by Chris Argyris, a prolific writer on organizations who has conducted many studies of management. He urges us to adopt a normative theory of self-actualization, and encourages the design of organizations that maximize trust, openness, and individuality. Argyris believes that humans have a basic motivation to be competent, to be growth-oriented, to seek novelty, and to achieve. He believes that the more people have such experiences, the more self-confidence they have, and the less likely they are to be threatened by new information or opportunities to achieve new goals. The task of the social sciences, he argues, is to create organizations where these basic human needs can become expressed more readily. Argyris has been a persistent critic of most current organizational theory in sociology and political science, maintaining that these theories overrationalize human beings and encourage hierarchical organizational structures that are conducive to mistrust and conformity.[16]

> The consequence of intendedly rational man concept, in short, is to focus on the consistent, programmable, organized, thinking activities of man; to give primacy to behavior that is related to goals; to assume purpose without asking how it has developed. Man, as a person who feels, experiences chaos; manifests spontaneity; becomes turned on without planning it or being able to explain it in terms of consistency of conscious purpose; thinks divergently; and who may strive, at times, to separate himself from his past, is not the primary concern of intendedly-rational-man organizational theorists.[17]

In his own studies of organization, Argyris has illustrated how frequently honest communication becomes blocked, and how the failure to reveal true feelings and perceptions interfere with effective decision-making. Thus, he has developed a method of working with management groups that encourages managers to express their feelings and thoughts openly and work together more cooperatively. While Argyris's work is helpful in showing how self-protective maneuvers and blocked communication often thwart cooperation and the achievement of valued goals, his normative theory of self-actualization, based on the motivational theories of Maslow and other psychodynamic theorists, remains exceedingly vague. Although Argyris repeatedly emphasizes that organizations ought to be designed to enhance self-actualization, he neglects the fact that people's motives and aspirations often come from their socialization in organizations and from the systems of reward of which they are a part, and not from immutable, built-in needs. While one can agree with Argyris that communication based on fear and suspiciousness may be highly destructive, it is not obvious that this is the natural consequence of hierarchy and authority. A hierarchical authority structure is simply a way of insuring that a job is properly done. It may serve to inspire and encourage as well as to frighten and thwart effective behavior. Like any tool, it may be used poorly and without sensitivity to people's needs and expectations. Personnel should indeed have inspiration and commitment to their tasks, but this can be achieved through effective hierarchical organization as well as through other means.

The concept of self-actualization suffers from the same looseness that characterizes much of psychodynamic thinking. People left free to follow their own instincts do not necessarily excel, and may show little ability to mobilize themselves for effective problem-solving. People can never free themselves from inducements or potential punishments. If the organization does not clearly serve as a source of values or standards of performance, people will obtain them from elsewhere; and such influences may be more or less consistent with the needs of the organization. To return to our example of physician behavior, it seems clear that if the organizations in which they work have no clear standards or guidelines, physicians will respond in terms of their prior professional training and their perceptions of what is personally rewarding. Such adaptations may be inconsistent with high quality care and the effective use of organizational resources. Similarly, if the organization is too tightly organized and too severely restricts needed discretion, much of the creativity and possible innovation in problem-solving may be lost. Discretion is particularly important when the task itself involves the management of complex personal problems. It appears, then, that the solution lies with an organizational conception that provides guidance and support to the practitioner, but also considerable opportunity for self-expression and innovation. In this regard, a model that views personal adaptation in relationship to organizational environments may be instructive.

PERSONAL ADAPTATION AND THE DESIGN
OF ORGANIZATIONAL ENVIRONMENTS

As the prior discussion indicates, organizational theory has depended on limited concepts of human personality. Much of organizational psychology depicts personality either as an outgrowth of psychobiological needs and propensities, which may be more or less thwarted by organizational restraints, or as a product of the reinforcement schedules present in the organizational environment. The former depiction, which is seen in Argyris's works, emphasizes the extent to which organizations either facilitate or frustrate the expression of human needs. The latter portrays human beings as passive actors whose behaviors are shaped almost exclusively by the reinforcement schedules the organization has devised. Both views tend to portray people in organizations as less active than they really are, and fail to take account of the reactions and the strategies people use to make organizational life more personally satisfactory. The view presented here focuses on the continuing transactions between people and their work, and the manner in which they purposely manipulate the organization to pursue their own as well as group objectives.

The chapters that follow illustrate in a variety of ways how organizational participants take organizational constraints into account in devising behavior strategies. Physicians in prepaid group practice and in solo practice situations will structure their work differently in response to the varying incentives implicit in the payment systems to which they are exposed. Patients seeking formal assistance for their problems will seek out sources of care that are compatible not only with their problems but with their social and psychological preferences. Medical researchers, faced with more stringent guidelines requiring informed consent, learn how to communicate to patients so as to maximize their willingness to provide it. Bureaucrats required to evaluate their programs by federal directives will do so in a way that insures their survival.

A useful assumption from which to proceed—and one consistent with the views of Argyris—is that individuals in organizations seek to maintain or enhance their sense of esteem and confidence. This is achieved through opportunities to exercise mastery, the presence of supportive relationships, and the extent to which the person is recognized by the distribution of material rewards, status, or other indications of acceptance by relevant groups. Thus, aspiring medical students or house officers gain confidence through actual practice, as they are supervised and encouraged by more senior physicians. As they acquire skills and experience they are increasingly rewarded not only with new opportunities but with other symbolic and material inducements. The ability of individuals to function effectively depends on the appropriateness of their skills for dealing with the major problems faced by the organization, the adequacy of the psychological techniques they use to maintain a sense of personal comfort when faced with difficult tasks, and the degree to which they feel motivated to engage in problem-solving.[18]

The exercise of skills depends on the innate ability of the person and the adequacy of that person's preparation. A major difficulty in modern organizations is the rapidity of changes in technology and the lag that develops between what is possible and what is actually done. To the extent that individuals develop appropriate adaptive skills they can face new challenges with confidence. But when preparation or the conditions for effective performance are inadequate, problem-solving becomes ritualistic, and people become threatened and defensive. When self-esteem is threatened, people may adapt in ways that are irrelevant to organizational needs or even in opposition to them.[19]

The ability of the organization to facilitate effective coping depends on certain structural characteristics—for example, mechanisms for communication and sharing of information, the adequate provision of resources to allow the job to be done, and ways of gaining access to others in the organization who can be helpful. Organizations must enable people to obtain the necessary information to get their jobs done without overloading them. Overload may come in the form of too much unnecessary information or excessive rules and procedures.[20] People who have more information than they can cope with may react by doing nothing at all.

The challenges faced by human service organizations often are of a kind that requires complex forms of cooperation. However astute or personally effective an individual might be, that individual may not do very well at particular tasks without effective sharing of information with others and efforts at coordination. For example, many different types of personnel become involved in the care of a patient with a complex illness. The quality of performance depends not only on the effectiveness of each person in doing a particular job, but also on whether individuals successfully communicate about the case and coordinate their efforts in an overall plan. It is not atypical for different medical and surgical personnel involved in a case to communicate poorly, leading to serious errors or redundant care. Difficulties in achieving cooperation may result from different personal styles, heavy work demands, or competition in viewpoint among varying personnel. Disputes over status and the relative values of varying approaches such as occur, for example, between internists and surgeons, result in mutual suspiciousness, fears of revealing oneself and making oneself vulnerable,[21] and mistrust of the intentions and actions of the other. Such competition erodes performance.

Problems of prestige and authority are important in the relationships between physicians and other health personnel, such as nurses, who are crucial in providing good patient care. Overly rigid authority lines may result in the failure of personnel to act on the basis of common sense judgment, and ritualistic conformity may substitute for intelligent behavior. The dominance of physicians over medical tasks is, in part, a conscious design to insure a clear focus of responsibility and authority. But although every team must have clearly defined leadership—and particularly those that require quick and forceful decisions—health professionals other than physicians must have greater latitude of judgment and practice and must not be conditioned to unthinking obedience. If to allow nurses to operate independently of the authority of physicians is impractical, to train nurses so that they are reluctant to exercise independent and critical judgment is equally senseless. Some of the aspects of this interesting and important issue are illustrated by a study by Hofling and his colleagues.[22]

In Hofling's experiment, carried out on 22 wards in two hospitals, nurses on duty were asked to give a patient an excessive dose of a medicine with which the nurse was unfamiliar. The medical order was transmitted by telephone (in violation of hospital policy) and was given to the nurse by a person with a name of someone on the staff, but with whom she was not personally familiar. The medication itself was not one on the ward stock list, cleared for use. Of the 22 nurses reported on in the study, 21 followed the order and were preparing to administer the medication (before being stopped by an observer) despite the fact that the dose ordered was double the maximum daily dose listed on the label.

A description of the experiment was then presented to 12 graduate nurses and 21 nursing students in a hypothetical context. The hypothetical presentation was almost identical to the actual experiment:

I should like you to imagine yourself, as vividly as possible, in this situation. You are a staff nurse, working 3:00 P.M. to 11:00 P.M. on a ward of a general hospital, and in charge of the ward during that period.

It is the official policy of this hospital that medication orders are to be written by the physician before being carried out by the nurse. This policy fairly often is not adhered to.

You are the only nurse on the ward, the head nurse and the departmental supervisor having left the hospital. None of the house doctors are on the ward, which is moderately busy.

Dr. Smith is known to be on the staff of the hospital, but you have not met him. Mr. Jones is one of the patients on your ward. At about 8:00 P.M. you receive the following telephone message: "This is Dr. Smith, from Psychiatry, calling. I was going to see Mr. Jones this morning, and I'm going to have to see him again tonight. I don't have a lot of time, and I'd like him to have had some medication by the time I get to the ward. Will you please check your medicine cabinet and see if you have some Astroten? That's ASTROTEN."

Your medicine cupboard contains a pillbox, bearing the label of the hospital pharmacy, and reading as follows:

ASTROTEN

5 mg. capsules

Usual dose: 5 mg.

Maximum daily dose: 10 mg.

You return to the telephone, and the message continues as follows:

"You have it? Fine. Now will you please give Mr. Jones a stat dose of 20 milligrams—that's four capsules—of Astroten. I'll be up within ten minutes, and I'll sign the order then, but I'd like the drug to have started taking effect."[23]

Contrary to behavior in the actual experiment, 10 of the 12 graduate nurses and all 21 nursing students indicated that they would not have followed the orders as given. While the constraints operating in a real situation are very different from the hypothetical, the magnitude of difference found in this study begs for interpretation. Hofling and his colleagues are aware of the positive functions of such obedience; unlike the Milgram experiments where subjects engage in behavior harmful to another person,[24] short-cutting the rules on medication orders is often efficient and may be of positive value to the patient. Moreover the physician-nurse relationship is a trusting one; the caller is believed to be who he says he is, and it is assumed he will do what he promises. As the authors note in commenting on the nurses' loyalty:

> The present investigation does not imply that these values should be sacrificed. Rather, it implies that it would be worth an extensive effort on the part of the nursing and medical professions to find ways in which these traditional values can be reconciled with the nurse's fuller exercise of her intellectual and ethical potentialities.[25]

As the authors see the conflict, it is one between the professionalism of the nurse, and her scientific mastery and judgment on the one hand, and her desire to be ingratiating on the other:

> the nurse retains another group of (largely conscious) motivations with respect to her relationship with the doctor. These include the wish to be liked by him, to receive his gratitude, praise and approval, and to avoid blame and recriminations. These strivings are indicated in various portions of the experimental material: in the courtesy of the telephone conversations (usually ending with a "thank you"), in the unquestioning attitudes; in the promptness of execution of the order; and in the fear of disapproval upon disclosure.[26]

Part of the difficulty is in the structure of the situation itself. Bureaucratic organizations such as hospitals often have elaborate rules that are commonly violated. For example, it is common in hospitals for nurses to act on verbal orders on the assumption that the order will be written when the physician has the time. Nurses who rigidly adhere to rules forbidding such behavior, like other bureaucrats who are formalistic in their behavior, can be extremely unresponsive to the real contingencies of hospital life. While the authority of any professional group must to some extent be bounded by that group's presumed competence and capabilities, the failure to allow discretion often leads to either a rigid unwillingness to deviate from rules or a total cynicism about rules which encourages discretion in areas in which it should be limited.

In this experimental situation, the rules are sufficiently unrealistic so that they tend not to have a deterrent effect. In discounting them, the nurse tends to be unthinking in her acceptance of the physician's authority, and insecure in her rights to question the physician and demand justification for the departure. Rules which are more limited, and which allow a range of discretion better attuned to the realities of the organization, but which also place responsibility on the nurse to exercise judgment and intelligence, are likely to induce a more independent role that is critical and more consistent with the intentions of the institution. Giving nurses responsibility with discretion, and thus making them accountable for their departures from accepted practice, provides checks and balances in the clinical situation that are likely to be conducive to improved patient care.

Nurses have undoubtedly been trained to be docile and subservient, and physicians often respond to inititative and judgment by the nurse with strong negative reinforcement. Nurses who wish to question physicians' judgments without sanctions learn to do so in an indirect way that communicates the dominant position of the physician.[27] In the future both physicians and nurses must learn new roles and responsibilities in relationship to one another.[28] The danger is that if such mutual responsibilities are not part of the socialization of doctors and nurses, and are not reinforced by the institutional setting, the situation will eventually escalate into a mindless political battle in which militancy and its consequences could have serious adverse effects on patient care.

Although competition may be an important incentive for individual effort, it often interferes with necessary cooperation. Organizational incentive systems may encourage either individual or group problem-solving and, depending on the nature of the tasks to be accomplished, it may be more advisable to develop reward structures that tie the success of any individual to the overall functioning of the unit of which that individual is a part.[29] For example, one of the difficulties in implementing the use of health practitioners other than physicians in the private practice of medicine is the fear of the medical profession that such practitioners will compete with them and erode their economic position. However, when medical units such as prepaid practices are reimbursed on a capitation basis for each patient enrolled, and when the economic rewards of each practitioner are tied to the economic functioning of the group as a whole, there is likely to be more receptivity to the use of practitioners other than physicians that allow the medical group to meet patient demand at reduced cost. The full potential of such possibilities is eroded by restrictive licensing of varying types of practitioners, but interest is growing in a form of institutional licensure that will allow licensed medical programs to meet patient needs in the most efficient and effective way. To the extent that the welfare of each member is tied to the effective performance of the group as a whole, the chances for effective manpower substitution are enhanced. The development of such reward systems can lead to problems with "free riders"—individuals who enjoy their share because of the efforts of others, but who do not do their part[30]—but this can be limited by careful group evaluation of each member's performance.

To the extent that they deal with problems that are difficult or have uncertain solutions, or when they are exposed to impossible or conflicting expectations, personnel experience considerable insecurity and anxiety. For example, physicians are expected to provide good technical care and also to deal sensitively with patients' psychosocial problems. But their time is limited, and they often feel inadequate in dealing with psychosocial problems. Successful coping is likely to depend on the capacities of the individual to control such anxieties in a manner that does not detract from task performance. Physicians often adapt to the uncertain demands involved in dealing with difficult psychosocial issues by ignoring them or denigrating their importance. Such adaptations may reduce the physicians' anxieties, but they interfere with good care. To deal with the stresses of such work without withdrawing into routinized solutions or denying that the problems exist, physicians must be able to call on support systems that are responsive to the stresses of organizational work. When they are able to recognize and face the stresses and problems they experience, individuals are more able to deal with uncertainty, and with their emotions, and to persist in effective work.

But regardless of those who adhere to the self-actualization perspective, it is not enough to provide a context to express emotions. The problems that create anxieties in the first place must be explicitly analyzed, and more effective ways of solving them must be developed. The solutions may be in the form of changed organizational procedures and routines or new behavioral strategies taught to the personnel involved. Good organizational management must be able to recognize the conditions of work that arouse adverse emotions or ineffective behavior and develop explicit mechanisms to deal with the problems or to provide support to personnel as they attempt to cope more adequately. One of the most wasteful features of many modern organizations is the failure to assist personnel in overcoming difficulties of work. The approach has relied more on monitoring and threatening than on facilitating greater mastery in problem-solving. We tend to think of improving performance as a problem of regulation rather than one of self-improvement. As I argue in the chapter on evaluation, threatened personnel learn how to thwart evaluation and regulation; it may be more fruitful to structure such evaluation efforts in a way that allows each person involved to strive for self-improvement without defensiveness. Too many organizations have individuals who are no longer functioning effectively, who suffer from self-derogation and low self-esteem, who engage in numerous maneuvers to protect themselves from feared retribution, and who obtain whatever gratifications of work they can from ancillary activities largely irrelevant to the goals of the organization. A strict regulatory approach only brings out the defensiveness and anxieties of such people.

The fuel of organizations is the incentive structure that fires human motivation and that directs people's energies to tasks. In our society we depend mostly on material rewards and prestige, and less on appeals to people's inherent goodness, loyalty, or commitment to the greater good. The difficulty with material incentives is that people learn to do what is measured, often neglecting less tangible and visible needs. Organizations can be far more effective if they can achieve a high degree of commitment and loyalty and arouse enthusiasm. This is more likely to be achieved when people feel that they are important to the efforts of the organization, that their contributions are valued, and that they participate in an important way. They must also feel that the management of the organization cares about their welfare. For committed individuals, an organization is a source of emotional as well as material rewards.

WHAT MANNER OF MAN?

In sum, neither bounded rationality nor self-actualization adequately defines the needs of individuals within organizations. Human beings often derive their goals and aspirations from organizational ideologies, and the effective performance of members not only aids the organization but also serves to enhance their own esteem. Thus, it may be less important that members have autonomy than a sense of commitment to valued goals, the means to solve problems effectively, and supportive relationships that encourage workers' efforts, that recognize their anxieties, and that nurture their sense that they are valued persons.

The source of organizational values depends on the larger historical and social context and the ideologies that prevail. Perhaps the most difficult question of all is how to promote the creation of new settings based on a humane, social ethic and one involving a greater sense of sharing and sacrifice. Numerous indications suggest that our society, and even our helping institutions, are becoming more bureaucratic and less humane. Helping organizations are part of a larger organizational field and cannot readily sustain more humane settings without significant support from society at large. Attempts to create new organizational settings, and ones that direct attention to the intimate concerns of people, continually confront the existing economic and political values and the reward structures that are prevalent in the society. Thus, even small, innovative attempts to develop a new kind of medical program, hospital, or medical school frequently encounter hostile environments.

The creation of new settings involves an extraordinary amount of planning and understanding of the constraints imposed by the outside world.[31] It is not a job for romantics and utopians, but one requiring the application of our very best organizational and political skills and our keenest understanding of organizational processes. The creation of new settings must come to terms with the fact that human beings are adaptive creatures who do not simply react to the incentive structures developed, but who also try to mold those structures in their own images and with their own intentions. Thus, organizational design must be directed not only to how tasks will be accomplished, but also to the climate of organizational life. In Part II of this book we examine the climate of medical practice and how varying forms of medical organization affect the adaptations of doctors and patients alike.

NOTES

1. H. Simon (1957), *Administrative Behavior,* 2d ed. (New York: Free Press).

2. B. Ehrenreich and J. Ehrenreich (1971), *The American Health Empire: Power, Profits and Politics* (New York: Random House).

3. C. W. Mills (1956), *The Power Elite* (New York: Oxford University Press).

4. Robert A. Dahl (1961), *Who Governs: Democracy and Power in an American City* (New Haven: Yale University Press).

5. R. Alford (1972). "The Political Economy of Health Care: Dynamics Without Change," *Politics and Society,* **2**:127–164.

6. Ibid., p. 164.

7. T. Bice et al. (1972), "Socio-Economic Status and the Use of Physician Services: A Reconsideration," *Medical Care,* **10**:261–271.

8. A. Rivlin (1972), "Why Can't We Get Things Done?" *Brookings Bulletin,* **9**:5–9. For quotation, see p. 6.

9. J. Pressman and A. Wildavsky (1973), *Implementation* (Berkeley: University of California Press), pp. 93–94.

10. P. Drucker (1974), *Management: Tasks, Responsibilities, Practices* (New York: Harper), p. 146.

11. For critical review of these movements, see I. Hoos (1972), *Systems Analysis in Public Policy: A Critique* (Berkeley: University of California Press); and N. P. Mouzels (1968), *Organization and Bureaucracy: An Analysis of Modern Theories* (Chicago: Aldine), especially Chapter 4.

12. For example, see M. Dalton (1959), *Men Who Manage* (New York: Wiley); and G. Homans (1950), *The Human Group* (New York: Harcourt Brace).

13. H. Simon (1957), op. cit., p. xxiv.

14. H. Simon (1957), *Models of Man* (New York: Wiley), pp. 245–246.

15. H. Simon (1973), "Organization Man: Rational or Self-Actualizing?" *Public Administration Review,* **33**:352.

16. C. Argyris (1972), *The Applicability of Organizational Sociology* (Cambridge: Cambridge University Press).

17. C. Argyris (1973), "Some Limits of Rational Man Organizational Theory," *Public Administration Review,* **33**:261.

18. D. Mechanic (1974), "Social Structure and Personal Adaptation: Some Neglected Dimensions," in G. V. Coelho et al., eds., *Coping and Adaptation* (New York: Basic Books).

19. See, for example, R. Merton (1952), "Bureaucratic Structure and Personality," in R. Merton et al., eds., *Reader in Bureaucracy* (New York: Free Press).

20. See D. Mechanic (1973), "The Sociology of Organizations," in S. Feldman, ed., *The Administration of Mental Health Services* (Springfield, Ill.: Thomas).

21. C. Argyris (1967), *Some Causes of Organizational Ineffectiveness Within the Department of State* (Washington, D.C.: Center for International Systems Research, Department of State).

22. C. K. Hofling et al. (1966), "An Experimental Study in Nurse-Physician Relationships," *Journal of Nervous and Mental Disease,* **143:**172–180.

23. Ibid., p. 173.

24. S. Milgram (1974), *Obedience to Authority: An Experimental View* (New York: Harper & Row).

25. Ibid., p. 178.

26. C. K. Hofling et al. (1966), op. cit., p. 178.

27. W. A. Rushing (1964), *The Psychiatric Professions: Power Conflict and Adaptation in a Psychiatric Hospital Staff* (Chapel Hill: University of North Carolina Press); W. A. Rushing (1963), "Social Influence and the Social Psychological Function of Deference," *Social Forces,* **41:**142–148.

28. Institute of Medicine (1972), *Educating for the Health Team* (Washington, D.C.: National Academy of Sciences).

29. M. C. Deutsch (1949), "An Experimental Study of the Effects of Cooperation and Competition Upon Group Processes," *Human Relations,* **2:**199–232; M. C. Deutsch (1973), *The Resolution of Conflict: Constructive and Destructive Processes* (New Haven: Yale University Press).

30. M. Olson, Jr. (1968), *The Logic of Collective Action: Public Good and the Theory of Groups* (New York: Schocken Books).

31. S. Sarason (1972), *The Creation of Settings and the Future Societies* (San Francisco: Jossey-Bass).

II
PATIENT BEHAVIOR
AND THE DESIGN OF
MEDICAL CARE
ORGANIZATION

Chapter 5

The Health Maintenance
Organization:
Background
Considerations

In the previous chapter we examined various diagnoses of the failure of
human service organizations and different conceptions about how they can
be designed more effectively. The delivery of health care services has been
frequently criticized on most of the bases discussed in that chapter. It has been
maintained that the organization of health care is inefficient and wasteful; that
it is unresponsive to the needs of clients and often provides services in an inhumane fashion; that health care lacks imaginative management and leadership;
that medicine attracts the wrong kinds of people and fails to allocate them
properly to the roles they are expected to perform. The health maintenance organization is one of the most frequently advocated antidotes to these difficulties.

The HMO type of organization is said to offer access to high-quality medical
care and to have reasonable costs at the same time. The concept, originally
conceived with the large, prepaid group practices in mind, has now been
expanded to include the medical foundation programs. These programs have
grown as a response to medical societies' fears of government intrusion in the
organization and governance of medical practice. Since medical foundations are
less well known than prepaid group practices, it is useful to review their major
characteristics.

Services are offered on a prepaid basis by a corporation established through a local or state medical society.[1] However, enrollees may obtain their medical services from any eligible participant. Doctors agree to provide services under the terms established by the medical society, and the corporation is responsible for utilization and quality review and cost containment. With the passage of Professional Standards Review Organization legislation, mandating review of care in federally financed programs, foundations can also provide the mechanism through which medical societies retain administrative and operative control over such review. In the foundation program consumers pay for services on a prepaid basis. Physicians are remunerated for services rendered. The corporation may establish a fee schedule.

Of the many claims made for the values of the HMO by government officials and other advocates, some can be taken seriously and others can be discounted as rhetoric. Some realists maintain that the major consideration is cost-containment, and that advocacy for the HMO mechanism arises simply from the realization that large prepaid group practices have lower rates of hospitalization and surgery than competing forms of practice. In a period of rising costs, any means to meet demands for access and also contain costs are attractive. Others argue more generally in favor of prepaid group organization, citing their organizational advantages over more conventional forms of practice.[2,3] In any case, advocates' claims must be evaluated seriously, since these claims are being used to sell HMOs to the public.

The medical foundations are relatively new, and we know little about their performance in contrast to prepaid group practices. But even in the prepaid group practice field, most of what we know comes from a few large prototypes such as Kaiser-Permanente. Information on other variants of the concept is limited. Very few groups exclusively provide prepaid services, and most have only limited prepaid activity. The American Medical Association, on the basis of its survey of American medical groups in 1969, reported that only 22 per cent of medical groups with prepaid practice activity have greater than 50 per cent of prepaid work, and 45 per cent of groups with some prepaid activity have less than 5 per cent of such activity.[4] Moreover, 57 per cent of the groups providing prepaid services had 5 or fewer physicians, and 80 per cent had 15 or fewer physicians. The larger groups were more likely to have significant amounts of prepaid activity. Thus, the data on the large prototypes may tell us little about the substantial number of smaller groups providing some prepaid care. A study by Hetherington and his colleagues in Los Angeles[5] found impressive differences in performance between a large and small prepaid practice.

Similarly, the large prototypes may be atypical on a variety of organizational features such as the ownership and relationship to hospital facilities, the scope of specialty services under their control, internal governance and incentive systems, conditions of work and monitoring of practice, economic organization, leadership and administrative supervision, special services and programs available, and on other dimensions as well. The data on the prototypes probably provide a more favorable picture of the national scene than reality warrants. Of course, the large prototypes also probably exaggerate certain problems of care that are less likely to be observed in smaller and less bureaucratic programs.

A prepaid group practice may be an available option within a foundation program, but the incentives that are believed to encourage more efficient organization in prepaid group practice are probably less effective in respect to other providers of care within the foundation.[6] The attractiveness of the medical foundation for many doctors is that they can continue to practice in their usual way, even though some cost and quality controls are involved. Given the motivation to continue current patterns of practice, the foundation is less likely to bring about economies of scale, innovative uses of manpower, or the special programs possible in more organized settings.

THE CLAIMS FOR HEALTH MAINTENANCE ORGANIZATIONS

One way of abstracting the claims for HMOs is to consider the reasons given by the Department of Health, Education, and Welfare for making it part of the Government's health strategy. These reasons are not unique to HEW, but generally are taken from the writings of HMO proponents. In the words of the HEW White Paper, *Toward a Comprehensive Health Strategy for the 1970's,*

> HMO's simultaneously attack many of the problems comprising the health care crisis. They emphasize prevention and early care; they provide incentives for holding down costs and for increasing the productivity of resources; they offer opportunities for improving the quality of care; they provide a means for improving the geographic distribution of care; and by mobilizing private capital and managerial talent, they reduce the need for federal funds and direct controls.

Perhaps most questionable of all is the contention that HMO organization "maintains health." The HEW document states that:

> Because HMO revenues are fixed, their incentives are to keep patients well, for they benefit from patient well-days, not sickness. Their entire cost structure is geared to preventing illness and, failing that, to promoting prompt recovery through the least costly services consistent with maintaining quality. In contrast with prevailing cost-plus insurance plans, the HMO's financial incentives encourage the least utilization of high cost forms of care, and also tend to limit unnecessary procedures.[7]

Claims are also made for potential continuing education and innovative teaching programs, the use of new technologies and management tools, the effective delegation of tasks to supporting personnel, and professional review and quality control in the colleague group. As noted earlier, the idea for the HMO was originally derived from the large, prepaid group practices. The extent to which the alleged advantages are intended to apply to medical foundations as well is unclear, since the foundation form appears to have been grafted onto the HMO idea.

Since data for testing these claims are already available in several excellent reviews,[8] I want to examine the larger issues posed by these claims. Data on costs and utilization of services are relatively good; on most other matters our information is scanty. Later in this section of the book, data from some of our own studies are presented to illustrate some of the neglected areas for research on HMOs.

DO HMOs PROMOTE HEALTH?

In theory, prepaid groups reimbursed on a capitation system (a fixed payment per person for a specified period) have an economic incentive to keep people well. The theory assumes that the medical group is motivated to avoid serious, costly episodes of illness and thus gives special effort to early treatment and prevention of disease in their patients. At a more modest level, it is also argued that the elimination of most economic barriers to access to care characteristic of prepaid group practice encourages patients to seek medical care early and more readily to use preventive services, thus avoiding more serious illnesses that require more extensive and expensive service. Finally, it is frequently maintained that the comprehensive scope of benefits provided at one site of care tends to promote continuity of information and service that enhances the quality of care.

Advocates for the health maintenance position have presented very little data to support the claim; indeed, the entire argument rests upon some limited studies carried out at the Health Insurance Plan of New York some years ago. Thus, it is useful to consider what processes must occur in theory to make the claim plausible. First, we must assume that early intervention and adequate treatment will in fact prevent serious later morbidity in a significant number of cases. Although there are clearly instances where this assumption is valid, it does not follow that prepaid group practice differs significantly from other medical contexts in the extent to which such instances are identified and dealt with promptly. No doubt, economic barriers keep people who need medical care from getting it and they may suffer as a result; but the extent of negative consequences of delayed care, which would have been preventable through earlier care, is not apparent. But even if the effects of earlier care are large, we cannot assume that prepaid group practices do not replace economic barriers with other types of barriers to access, a problem on which I will elaborate later. In fact, prepaid group practice may delay access to care in some ways more than typical fee-for-service medicine.

Since the different outcomes of prepaid group practice allegedly operate through incentives affecting the physician, we must examine how these organizational incentives are perceived and responded to by individual physicians in the group. Most of what we know about physician behavior, and the emphasis doctors place on clinical judgment, would alert us to the probability that an incentive structure as vague as the health maintenance one is likely to be uncertain in its effect, and that the behavior of physicians is more likely to be affected by their own needs and training and the practice pressures to which they are subjected. Similarly, the assumption that comprehensive coverage increases continuity of care is based on the belief that when a plan provides a wide range of services, the services are more likely to be coordinated through time. More comprehensive plans may involve a wider range of personnel, however, and although there may be continuity within the plan, breakdowns in communication may be more likely to develop and to interrupt the pattern of care.

HOW PREPAID GROUP PRACTICES
ACHIEVE ECONOMIES

Although the evidence, in general, supports the contention that prepaid group practices achieve economies through lower rates of admission to hospitals, lower rates of surgical intervention (especially in more discretionary areas), and in some cases shorter lengths of hospital stay, the dynamics through which these economies are achieved are not fully understood. To some extent, the magnitude of savings is exaggerated by the sociodemographic composition of prepaid group practice populations, which would lead one to anticipate lower medical need for surgical intervention and hospital care. Also, many estimates take into account only the costs to the prepaid plan, and neglect the additional cost of services obtained outside the program which are not covered by the contract. Even so, evidence shows that significant economies are achieved in the prepaid context. Some studies suggest that the savings are particularly large in the area of discretionary care—tonsillectomy, hysterectomy, and the treatment of respiratory disease, for example—but these findings are not always consistent.

Perhaps the most salient fact about the large prepaid group practices is that hospital use is constrained by the relatively small number of beds that have been available to physicians within the plans. Kaiser-Permanente, for example, maintains a far lower bed to population ratio than is characteristic of competing practice structures in the same geographic areas. Much of the hospital cost containment observed in HIP could be explained by the tight bed supply available to HIP physicians during much of the plan's history, although it is not clear that this is still the case.[9] The single best predictor of the magnitude of hospital use is the degree to which beds are available. Not only are physicians more likely to use a hospital bed in a marginal case when they are in ample supply, but physicians are often pressured to use hospital facilities when occupancy rates are low. To the extent that the economic advantage of prepaid group practice merely reflects the looseness or tightness of hospital bed supply, it can probably be achieved through a variety of alternative structural arrangements.

Medical foundation programs will provide an opportunity to examine whether such economies can be maintained outside a group structure using peer review and economic incentives for the physician. One possibility accounting for some hospital economies in prepaid group practice is the economic incentive available to medical groups to keep their hospital costs low. Medical foundations that do not control access to hospital beds, as Kaiser-Permanente does, must rely on these control mechanisms and on communications to physicians that it is in their economic interest to use hospital facilities more sparingly. Such incentive structures, of course, pose certain dangers as well as potential advantages. As we noted in an earlier chapter, in the marginal case the physician's interest is to some extent balanced against the patient's interest, and evaluation of incentives must consider not only samples of cases that lead to hospitalization but also instances where hospitalization may be required but does not occur. Economic pressures lead to an emphasis on identifying unnecessary hospitalization and surgery; the other side of the coin involves those patients whose best interests may be neglected by the failure to provide assistance that could be made available. A prudent policy would require that we evaluate medical work within the entire context of practice.

Although HMO theory suggests that ambulatory services are substituted for hospital services as a means of achieving economies, and that they are provided early so as to prevent illness, we do not know for sure that this is the way prepaid practices actually function. To the extent that managers are tempted to achieve even greater economies, restrictions on access can be imposed on hospital care and on ambulatory care at the same time. This possibility has escaped even such sophisticated analysts as Roemer and Shonick, who note that if one considers the "influence of substantial ambulatory diagnostic and treatment facilities found in a group practice setting, as well as a restriction on available beds, one may expect a *relatively* higher level of ambulatory, compared with hospital utilization under the PGP type of HMO."[10] In support of this argument they cite a study by Roemer and his colleagues that found that the ratio of doctor visits to hospital use was almost double (6.3 to 3.6) in the group practice studied in comparison to other practice settings. What they fail to comment on, and this may be by far the more important and telling fact, is that in the Blue plans studied there were 3984 doctor visits per 1000 persons per year; the comparable figure in group practice was 3324. Whatever the ratios, patients in ambulatory group practices had lower rates of utilization.

Although the idea that more comprehensive insurance is likely to lead to substitution of one type of service for another is intuitively compelling, in most instances it has not held up when examined empirically. For example, it was widely believed that the structure of Blue Cross–Blue Shield plans that paid for services within hospitals, but did not cover outpatient care, created an incentive for unnecessary hospitalization. The theory argued that if these programs were extended to outpatient care, ambulatory services would then be substituted for unnecessary hospital services. As recently as July 1974, Alice Rivlin, former assistant secretary of HEW, wrote in the *New York Times*:

> the system is biased toward high-cost care, discourages preventive medicine and does nothing to promote efficiency. Since many patients are covered for hospitalization but not for other forms of care, doctors have a tendency to order hospitalization in order to reduce the patient's bill even when treatment at home, in the doctor's office or in an outpatient clinic would be cheaper and just as effective.[11]

The difficulty with the argument is that it does not conform with actual experience. Almost every study that compares the effects of plans offering only hospital coverage with those providing similar hospital benefits and additional ambulatory coverage shows that when ambulatory services are extended, outpatient utilization increases and hospital utilization increases slightly as well.[12]

It is not difficult to understand why the intuitive theory fails in practice. The effect of extending ambulatory benefits acts most directly on the consumer who responds to the elimination of economic barriers to care by increased utilization of physicians' services. The actual insurance benefits of the patient have relatively little influence on the physician's strategies of evaluating and managing patients; indeed, Lewis and Keairnes[13] found that most physicians were not aware of their patients' insurance benefits. To the extent that patients are more likely to seek ambulatory medical services, and to the extent that other controls are not affecting the physician's behavior, one would anticipate that some of the additional ambulatory utilization would lead to hospitalization. In short, the extension of the insurance benefit package, without specifically designed controls on the physician's behavior, is likely to result in higher rather than lower costs. Even if all physicians were well informed about the insurance coverage of their patients, it is not clear that substitution of ambulatory for hospital services would take place without additional incentives for the physician or strict utilization review.

In comparing prepaid with other practice structures, we unfortunately depend heavily on reported statistics of such items as doctor visits. This is, of course, a quantitative index that tells us almost nothing about the substance of the visit. One might contend, for example, that the prepaid patient obtains more substantive care in a given visit, and thus the low rates of ambulatory utilization in many prepaid practices are deceptive. Unfortunately, little data are available to evaluate such a claim, although anecdotal data would lead us to doubt its validity. Prepaid physicians work under greater time pressures in seeing patients than fee-for-service physicians, and give less time to each patient. Moreover, Freidson,[14] in studying physicians in a large prepaid practice, has noted that doctors faced with heavy patient demand may send the patient for a diagnostic test or X ray and ask the patient to reschedule a later visit as a means of controlling their time expenditures relative to the number of patients they have to see. Hetherington and his associates,[15] in their comparative study of insurance plans, note that doctors in a large prepaid practice ordered a larger number of diagnostic tests. They suggest that this is done in part as a management device in response to practice pressure. The extent to which this occurs more frequently in prepaid practice than in other practice organizations would support the hypothesis that there is relatively less substance per visit in prepaid practice.

It is difficult to anticipate how nongroup physicians would respond to similar pressures since they are faced with competing incentives. Repeated visits in a fee-for-service structure may be consistent with physicians' economic interests. They are paid for each visit, and so might be motivated to break visits into smaller substantive units. But fee-for-service physicians also work with the realization that patients tend to be suspicious of the doctors' motivation when they suggest repeated visits, and thus they may make a special effort to provide more substantive care per visit. The data presented in later chapters indicate that physicians in nongroup practice respond to practice pressures by increasing their hours seeing patients, while prepaid physicians process their patients more quickly; this suggests that fee-for-service physicians, if they wish, are probably in a stronger position to maintain the substantive integrity of a patient visit. Research is clearly necessary on this point.

A distressing fact about many prepaid group practices is that they replace economic barriers with other significant, noneconomic barriers that interfere with patients obtaining desired service. This varies a great deal with the context and depends on the financial structure of the plan. The Columbia Plan,[16] for example, servicing a sophisticated, demanding upper-middle-class community, has a high level of ambulatory utilization; but the contract at Columbia is both more comprehensive and expensive than most. The larger plans that market more economical contracts than Columbia or the Harvard Plan achieve economies through a variety of means that limit the levels of ambulatory care and hospital care available.

HOW PREPAID GROUP PRACTICES
LIMIT PATIENT AMBULATORY DEMAND

HMOs can be thought of as large chain stores, like Sears, Penney's or Wards, that market medical services rather than consumer goods. As their customers know, there are advantages and disadvantages to shopping at chain stores. Customers feel some confidence that such stores sell products at prices that are generally competitive. Moreover, many different products can be purchased at the same location, and the general reliability of the stores saves customers the effort needed to obtain product information that will protect them from being cheated by a dishonest dealer. Nevertheless, it is often difficult to find store personnel to ring up a sale, sales persons tend to be ignorant about the products they market, and consumers who want to buy something may waste some time and experience some frustration. But even though certain amenities associated with more exclusive stores are absent, many customers feel that the products they buy are a "good deal for the money." Customers who value their time highly or who expect responsive, knowledgeable sales help are not particularly attracted to chain stores.

For economic and other practical reasons, all systems of medical care, even those that offer comprehensive benefits and promise full access, must to some extent control the demands clients make on them. No system of care can allow completely uncontrolled access and remain economically viable for long. Therefore, some means of rationing the distribution of services must be introduced. In the fee-for-service system, the economic barriers to care serve this purpose, but prepaid plans must develop functional alternatives.

Other than the fee, there are basically three alternative means to limit services: by controlling the resources that are made available to the system of care; by imposing various controls on providers, or providing incentives for them, so that they serve as effective gatekeepers in the allocation of services; and by requiring patients to pay other than economic costs to obtain services. Such costs may involve time, distance, or the need to confront bureaucratic barriers. While some of these controls help ration services in a fashion consistent with medical conceptions of need, others impose new irrationalities and impediments to implementing medical concepts of quality. Thus, we should consider the advantages and disadvantages of each of these means of rationing services.

The most usual means for rationing services in prepaid group practice is to limit the provision of facilities and personnel. Such rationing may also occur more by happenstance than by design; for example, prepaid practices may encounter difficulties in recruiting primary care practitioners, and thus offer less primary care than planned. Given a fixed allocation of resources, prepaid group practices then develop queues for various services when demand is large. Most prepaid group practices develop around a limited number of medical groups who provide a lower ratio of physicians, specialists, and hospital beds relative to the populations they serve than is the case in the community as a whole. We have already noted that this control over resources may be the main factor explaining the economies achieved by the large prepaid practices. In addition, since services are provided at limited sites of care, the average subscriber will live further from the site of care than does the average patient using fee-for-service physicians. Data from Kaiser-Permanente in Portland show that utilization declines with distance from the site of care.[17]

Rationing by control over the provision of resources is the major means used by socialized systems of medical care. The National Health Service of England, for example, controls costs by central budgeting decisions that affect each of its constituent units. When demand is too great, queues develop, particularly in the case of discretionary services. Unlike rationing through a fee that places a special burden on those with most limited incomes, rationing by limiting resources potentially allows for allocation decisions to be made on medical rather than on social and economic criteria. In the case of hospital and surgical care, for example, which depend on physician decision-making, rationing by controlling resources allows a queuing process that may be organized around such concepts as severity of problem, patient need, or efficacy of the desired care. Obviously, if rationing is too severe, needy patients will be denied service.

To say that a particular rationing device offers the potential for rationing on a medical basis does not imply that this in fact occurs. Medical care organizations and providers, like any others, are susceptible to political pressures, to the force of special interests, and to the demands of more vocal and exacting consumers. A rational queuing process may well break down under the pressure of such forces. The British experience suggests that rationing works in particular units such as hospitals or in general practitioners' panels. But larger decisions involving the allocation of funds to different functions, building and locating new facilities, and redistribution of resources among geographic areas appear to be far more susceptible to political influences. Although there is anecdotal evidence that some persons have discovered strategies for jumping ahead in the queue, this appears to be a minor problem. But the English have a strong sense of fair play, and queuing might not work as well in other countries. In any case, it should be possible to audit the pattern of care under a system that rations resources to determine to what extent persons who require certain services from a medical standpoint are denied them because of either economic measures or irrationalities in setting priorities. Although making such determinations is far from an exact science, it should be possible to develop standards that allow examination of whether the queue is operating in a rational manner or whether it is being subjected to various nonmedical pressures by more aggressive patients or by variabilities in physician orientations.

Rationing resources that affect access to the system of medical care presents special problems. Unlike rationing in such areas as hospitalization, surgery, or the use of expensive diagnostic and treatment modalities, which are under the control of physicians, the decision to seek access to the medical system is under the control of the patient and the various social, cultural, and psychological forces that affect the help-seeking process. Rationing access to physicians by having relatively limited first-contact care facilities allows various irrational forces, rather than medical need, to predominate in determining who has access to care. As with economic barriers, rationing of first-contact services will have uneven effects and is likely to keep needy people from obtaining services vital to their health.

Thus I believe strongly that prepaid group practices have a major responsibility to provide a relatively liberal resource base in ambulatory medical care that is consistent with HMO theory on the one hand and with the contractual promises they make on the other. There is growing indication that some large prepaids have been less than generous on this dimension; much more attention ought to be given to the effective use of less expensive practitioners in insuring greater and more rapid access to care among program enrollees.

The second means of rationing is exercised through providers, either by having them serve as gatekeepers to more expensive services or by providing incentives or controls that attempt to limit the extent to which providers use more expensive services. The gatekeeper function is relatively simple, and is commonly used in nationalized systems to control access to specialized care. In the United States, patients can choose any specialist, or even a specialized hospital facility, and seek services directly. But in England, for example, National Health Service patients are expected to see a nonhospital-based general practitioner when they require care. Referrals to hospital, to specialists, or to other diagnostic or rehabilitative facilities occur through the general practitioner. Thus the general practitioner is viewed as a gatekeeper who insures that patients who do not require complex services do not flood more specialized and expensive facilities. Provision of access to the general practitioner is relatively inexpensive, and patients know there is someone they can reach if they have any special difficulty. The reality departs somewhat from the theory. Many specialists and hospital departments, for example, criticize general practitioners for not screening patients strictly enough and for allowing patients access to more specialized services too readily. This criticism must, however, be examined in perspective, since the specialty services do not have an epidemiological view of the larger population of illnesses and problems from which the general practitioner selects patients for referral. Compared with more open systems in which patients can go directly to specialty services and hospitals, the English system works fairly well in coping with most problems within the general practice setting.

The success of the gatekeeper function depends on the degree to which it is reinforced by other incentives. It has been argued, for example, that since

British GPs are paid on a capitation basis, they have little incentive to work up patients themselves rather than referring them to a specialty service. A somewhat different economic incentive structure may retard this tendency, but the danger is that if the structure is too rewarding for nonreferral, GPs may keep patients they should more appropriately refer. There are other forces operating against the tendency for capitation physicians to refer too readily. Given their training, professional orientations, and interests in a diverse practice, such doctors probably find it stimulating to handle a more complex case, and thus it is not obvious that capitation payment will induce overreferral. The fact that there is some acrimony between GPs and more specialized services may, in part, reflect their different views of the world and of patients, and the varying populations they serve.

The prepaid group practice structure attempts to control overreferral to more specialized services through economic incentives. In Kaiser-Permanente, for example, the medical group has an economic incentive to limit referral to the hospital service, and if they use such facilities too generously the group may lose remuneration potentially available to them. As Scott Fleming notes:

> The amount of incentive compensation—which generally varies within fairly narrow limits—depends upon, and thereby constitutes an incentive for, the effective operation of the total program. It recognizes that the performance of individual physicians not only influences the efficiency of group operations as such but also influences the economy and effectiveness of the total program—hospitals, health plan and supporting services as well as medical groups.[18]

There are no adequate data that allow us to assess how effective this incentive is, since other factors operate at the same time to limit hospital use. Should such incentives be highly effective, they pose potential problems of underreferral, and an assessment of the extent to which this occurs requires careful auditing and evaluation studies. I tend to doubt that incentives this vague can have much effect on physician behavior.

The competitive fee-for-service system has implicit incentives discouraging referral. Physicians, often conscious of the possibility of losing both fees and patients, may continue to care for patients whose problems are beyond their capacities. Many general practitioners continue to perform major surgery when better trained surgeons are available and frequently underutilized. And even though we cannot maintain that they are less skilled at surgery than are better trained physicians, we do know that general practitioners are more likely to undertake questionable or unnecessary surgery.[19] Similarly, physicians devise various means to protect themselves from losing patients to specialists to whom they refer. To assure that patients will return, they may be referred to specialists at major centers outside one's practice area. In many communities nongroup physicians will not make referrals to group specialists on the assumption that reciprocity is lacking, since group specialists tend to make referrals within their own group. Of course, this is all anecdote; it is difficult to know how pervasive such tendencies are but the fact that they exist illustrates the principle.

Unfortunately, there has been little sociological study of referral networks among physicians;[20] in my experience, this is an issue on which physicians offer considerable resistance to investigation. The economics of referral have been sufficiently problematic for physicians to encourage development of some form of sharing fees. Although fee-splitting is now regarded as unethical, it continues in subtle forms, and reflects strains characteristic of the referral process and the system of reciprocity that develops within different medical communities. It is not unusual for surgeons in receiving a referral to invite the general practitioner to assist in the operation so that the GP also receives a fee. As William Nolen notes in his book, *A Surgeon's World:*

> Usually fee-splitting isn't done in quite so flagrant a style. A slightly more sophisticated approach is that in which the surgeon asks the internist to help him supervise the postoperative management of the case, even though the surgeon could easily handle it for himself. The internist drops in to see the patient for each of the seven or eight postoperative days and puts in a fifteen-dollar charge for each visit. The surgeon then reduces his customary fee by the amount the internist charges. . . . The American College of Surgeons had made rule after rule in a zealous attempt to stamp out fee-splitting. Every time they close one loophole, another opens up. Some rules are simply ignored. There's a rule, for example, that the referring doctor shall not assist the surgeon at an operation. I pay no attention to that one. . . . I always ask the referring doctor to help me; and, of course, he charges for his services.[21]

A common problem shared by administrators of prepaid health plans is how to ration services dispensed by physicians such as prescription drugs and devices, or diagnostic procedures used in the evaluation of the patient. In the fee-for-service situation, unless the patient has insurance for such services, the cost to the patient may serve as some deterrent to unnecessary use. In prepaid systems, however, patients may expect prescriptions or certain procedures performed, and physicians may accede to such demands despite their judgment that they are unnecessary. In the National Health Service of England, for example, there is great concern about the costs of prescription drugs and various means are used to attempt to control costs. The NHS has a prescription charge that is viewed as a deterrent against the patient incurring unnecessary prescription costs or using the physician to obtain nonprescription drugs at no cost. Also, the NHS audits the costs of prescriptions written by general practitioners, visiting doctors who either have very high costs or who overuse certain classes of drugs. Although this is a relatively minor administrative procedure, the presence of the mechanism may affect the physician's behavior and may have an educational function as well. What is most clear about the auditing program, which essentially identifies doctors who deviate from the statistical averages of prescription behavior and has a government physician discuss the issue with them, is that it results in considerable resentment and ill-will between many GPs and the Department of Health and Social Security.

Large, prepaid group practices in the United States make administrative attempts to control the use of diagnostic procedures and referrals, but we know very little about them. The only study of such controls is Eliot Freidson's study of a large medical group.[22] and it is clear from his description that physicians do not accept the authority of the administration in controlling what they view as their clinical behavior. The administration of the group Freidson studied received relatively little support from physicians when they attempted to control what they felt was excessive use. Doctors see such control as interference with their professional judgment and tend to reject its legitimacy. Of course, prepaid practices, perhaps partly for these reasons, have had difficulties in recruiting physicians; but if this type of practice becomes more popular among physicians, and if administrators can be more forceful, control mechanisms might have greater influence. In any case, Professional Standards Review Organizations will be attempting to use such administrative devices to control utilization and quality. It remains to be seen to what extent this can be managed successfully.[23]

The third general means of rationing—the various noneconomic obstacles that are placed in the way of patients using contracted services—are generally those patients find most infuriating. Such noneconomic means have the effect of keeping people who may need assessment or services, or those who are less aggressive and less demanding, from obtaining access, and thus are probably most irrational from a medical standpoint. Think of a patient who has some problems and who attempts to make an appointment to see a physician. The person may reach the general switchboard and be told to hold on until one of the receptionists is available. After some waiting the call may be transferred with further delay. Usually, it is impossible to talk with one's physician on the phone; messages may not be delivered or answered. The patient who attempts to make an appointment to see a particular physician may be told that the first available place is from five to seven weeks ahead. Patients are usually given the alternative to come to urgent care, but will not see their own physician there. In urgent care, the patient will be seen by a doctor who is probably not familiar with the case history, leading possibly to diagnostic work the patient's own physician, familiar with the case, would not do. And there may be further delays in getting a specialty referral, or a specific diagnostic procedure performed, and so on. This runaround may not be typical of or unique to prepaid group practice. The only point I wish to make is that bureaucratic barriers are exaggerated in large, prepaid group practices and contribute to patient perceptions that they are not fully responsive or caring.

Individual responses to such noneconomic barriers vary. The higher status, more affluent patient, who is more educated and more capable of dealing with bureaucracy, knows better how to "play the system," to make demands, to insist on services, to accept "no nonsense." The more passive consumer, or less sophisticated ones, are more "put off" by the bureaucratic response, become more easily discouraged, and accept the situation more readily. The finding by Hetherington and his associates[24] that the large prepaid group they studied gave relatively more physician services to the affluent client is a matter of grave concern to any planner who views the HMO as a major element in the strategy for developing a more equitable and effective pattern of service. The bureaucratic barriers characteristic of large group practices stand in the way of the fulfillment of medical need. The commonsense theory that those who are really sick will somehow gain access has no evidence to support it, and serves as a rationalization to tolerate unacceptable practices.

In the chapters that follow, I elaborate on some of the problems discussed here, as well as some others, in reporting on two sets of studies examining physician performance and patient reactions in prepaid practice as compared with other organizational settings. Chapter 6 describes the concerns motivating these investigations as well as some of our findings, and Chapter 7 describes in detail a study of patients using different medical plans in Milwaukee, Wisconsin.

NOTES

1. R. Egdahl (1973), "Foundations for Medical Care," *New England Journal of Medicine,* **288**:491–498.

2. See, for example, P. Ellwood et al. (1971), "Health Maintenance Strategy," *Medical Care,* **9**:291–298.

3. M. I. Roemer and W. Shonick (1973), "HMO Performance: The Recent Evidence," *Milbank Memorial Fund Quarterly,* **51**:271–317.

4. R. J. Walsh (1972), *Socio-Economic Issues of Health* (Chicago: Center for Health Services Research and Development, American Medical Association), p. 73.

5. R. Hetherington, C. Hopkins, and M. Roemer (1975), *Health Insurance Plans: Promise and Performance* (New York: Wiley-Interscience).

6. An interesting possible exception is the Health Maintenance Program designed by Wisconsin Physicians Service, Blue Shield. Within this program patients obtain a prepayment plan but select any eligible primary care physician. The primary care physician is reimbursed on a combination capitation-fee-for-service system with incentives for avoiding "unnecessary costs." The system is relatively unique in that patients may not seek additional medical services within the plan except through their primary care physician, and thus the physician is a "gatekeeper" to more expensive services. While this expectation is communi-

cated to patients, it is not necessarily enforced. Investigation is necessary to determine how effective this plan is in cost containment.

7. U.S. Department of Health, Education, and Welfare (1971), *Toward a Comprehensive Health Policy for the 1970's: A White Paper* (Washington, D.C.: Government Printing Office), pp. 31, 32.

8. Three studies by A. Donabedian are examples: (1965), *A Review of Some Experiences with Prepaid Group Practice,* Bureau of Public Health Economics Research Series No. 12 (Ann Arbor: School of Public Health, University of Michigan); (1969), "An Evaluation of Prepaid Group Practice," *Inquiry,* **7**:3–27; and (1973), *Aspects of Medical Care Administration* (Cambridge: Harvard University Press). Two studies by H. E. Klarman are: (1963), "Effect of Prepaid Group Practice on Hospital Use," *Public Health Reports,* **78**:955–965; and (1971), "Analysis of the HMO Proposal—Its Assumptions, Implications, and Prospects," in Proceedings of the 13th Annual Symposium on Hospital Affairs, *Health Maintenance Organizations: A Reconfiguration of the Health Services System* (Chicago: Graduate Program in Hospital Administration and Center for Health Administration Studies), pp. 24–38. Finally, see M. Greenlick (1972), "The Impact of Prepaid Group Practice on American Medical Care: A Critical Evaluation," *Annals of the American Academy of Political and Social Science,* **399**:100–113; and notes 3 and 5 above.

9. H. E. Klarman (1971), op. cit.

10. M. I. Roemer and W. Shonick (1973), op. cit., p. 290.

11. A. Rivlin (1974), "Agreed: Here Comes National Health Insurance," *New York Times Magazine,* July 21.

12. C. Lewis and H. W. Keairnes (1970), "Controlling Costs of Medical Care by Expanding Insurance Coverage: Study of a Paradox," *New England Journal of Medicine,* **282**:1405–1412.

13. Ibid.

14. E. Freidson (1976), *Doctoring Together* (New York: Elsevier).

15. R. Hetherington et al. (1975), op. cit.

16. M. L. Peterson (1971), "The First Year in Columbia: Assessments of Low Hospitalization Rate and High Office Use," *Johns Hopkins Medical Journal,* **128**:15–23.

17. J. Weiss and M. Greenlick (1970), "Determinants of Medical Care Utilization: The Effect of Social Class and Distance on Contacts with the Medical Care System," *Medical Care,* **9**:296–315.

18. S. Fleming (1971), "Anatomy of the Kaiser-Permanente Program," in A. Somers, ed., *The Kaiser-Permanente Medical Care Program: A Symposium* (New York: Commonwealth).

19. School of Public Health and Administrative Medicine, Columbia University (1961), *The Quantity, Quality and Costs of Medical and Hospital Care Secured by a Sample of Teamster Families in the New York Area.*

20. For an exception, see S. M. Shortell (1972), *A Model of Physician Referral Behavior: A Test of Exchange Theory in Medical Practice,* Research Series No. 31 (Chicago: Center for Health Administration Studies, University of Chicago).

21. William A. Nolen (1970), *A Surgeon's World* (New York: Random House), pp. 211–212.

22. E. Freidson (1976), op. cit.

23. Institute of Medicine (1974), *Advancing the Quality of Health Care* (Washington, D.C.: National Academy of Sciences).

24. R. Hetherington et al. (1975), op. cit.

Chapter 6

The Design of Medical Care Organization and Responsiveness to Patients

In Chapter 5 the suggested advantages of Health Maintenance Organizations were examined, as were varying forms of rationing services in different practice settings. To give us a better understanding of how economic incentive systems and the features of medical organization affect how physicians practice and, more specifically, how they deal with patients, this chapter reports on our studies of physicians in several types of practices.

PATIENTS' NEEDS AND BEHAVIOR

To be effective, the design of medical services clearly must take very carefully into account the behavior of patients who seek services and the nature of their needs. Organizations designed to provide highly personal services to clients must pay attention not only to technical issues, but also to the conditions that lead patients to seek services, to why some people with a particular illness seek care while others do not, why seeking care occurs at particular points in time, and how the needs of patients and their motivation for medical care interact with the organization of services. I regard these issues of sufficient importance to devote Part III of this book to studies of such problems. The brief discussion here is intended to provide a necessary context for our discussion and understanding of physician behavior and difficulties in achieving physician responsiveness to certain needs of patients.

Even a cursory examination of the potential population with illness suggests that there are many untreated patients with similar problems for every patient who seeks medical care. Using relatively conservative estimates of the occurrence of physical symptoms in the population—that is, symptom reports based on an action criterion such as taking bed rest or medication—it is apparent that a large proportion of the population, approximately three-quarters, have symptoms in any given month comparable to those that physicians see every day.[1] Approximately only one in three of these patients will seek a consultation with a physician. These estimates are based largely on acute and chronic physical illness and do not consider the high prevalence of psychiatric problems in the population. Estimates of psychiatric problems are difficult to provide since they vary so substantially from one study to another, depending on the criterion used.[2] Obviously, if the criterion is too loose, the category becomes too inclusive. Various studies suggest that an estimate that from 5 to 10 per cent of the population have serious psychiatric problems requiring care—depression, alcoholism, and the like—would be conservative.[3] Some epidemiological studies have reported that up to 60 per cent of the population suffers from psychological impairments.

Differences in response to symptoms depend on how problems develop and their severity, on social and cultural background and experience, and on the immediate contingencies of patients' life situations.[4] But before elaborating on each of these points, we should consider what people mean by health and how health relates to medical conceptions.

Although persons in Western nations have a fairly sophisticated view of health and illness, it is quite different from the professional viewpoint of physicians. Medicine makes abstract distinctions among diseases that affect how the physician evaluates and treats patients. Patients, however, react to illness experientially and in a way that usually does not distinguish between feeling states and specific symptoms. Perceived health is an overall experience and not a specific assessment of the absence of one or another disease entity. Thus, when the correlates of persons' perceptions of their physical health are examined, psychological distress is one determinant of how they see themselves.

People generally seek care when they experience symptoms that disrupt their ability to function and interfere in some fashion with their life. Investigators have consistently observed that illness is most noticeable when it is disruptive to usual functions, activities, and routines.[5] However, the seriousness of symptoms from a medical perspective may or may not be related to their salience or disruptiveness.

Patients are also more likely to define symptoms as worthy of care when bodily indications are unfamiliar and frightening and when they lack an interpretation that allows "normalization" of the symptom. Some symptoms are far more easily accounted for than others; chest pains might be attributed to indigestion, muscle ache to physical activity, or headaches to tension and stress.

How people react to symptoms is also related to their prior learning and experience and to the cultural and social definitions of the groups within which they live. Some groups encourage the expression of distress; others expect stoicism and denial. Some cultural groups have a detailed psychological vocabulary to conceptualize and describe personal problems; others communicate disapproval of any such suggestion.[6] These norms not only differ among social and ethnic groups but also may vary for men and women, and children and adults. Such norms—and experience in reference to them—come to have an important effect on how persons define their difficulties in functioning and how they adapt to life problems.

Going to a doctor is only one of many possible responses for persons suffering pain and distress or disruption in life activities. In some of our studies we have attempted to measure in a rather crude way the varying propensity of persons to go to a doctor when they face illness. In some subgroups persons learn to seek out physicians readily when they have a problem, to have faith in doctors, and to have little skepticism about the value of medical care. In other contexts, learning experiences lead to delay in seeking medical care, denial of symptoms, and little trust in doctors. These propensities are not fixed or unchanging, but frequently interact with the organization and typical response of the health care system and other factors in the individual's environment.

Various studies indicate that life difficulties and psychological distress are frequently present among persons seeking medical care.[7] Such stressful life situations have been said to contribute to the occurrence of illness, and this indeed may be the case.[8] But as Balint and his coworkers maintain,[9] life difficulties and psychological distress frequently trigger the use of physician services, although a physical symptom might be presented as a justification for coming to see the doctor. Thus the high rate of psychological distress among patients seen may result either because such distress contributes to symptoms and illness, or because it contributes to illness behavior and help seeking, or both. Our research suggests that psychological distress appears to have a larger influence among patients with high readiness to use physician services. Among patients with less readiness and greater skepticism of medical care, psychological distress may result in other forms of coping.

There are limits within which discretion in help seeking operates. When symptoms are sufficiently acute and severe, the impact of definitional processes is limited. But when symptoms are milder and do not seriously disrupt daily life, such social processes may be crucial. Since much of ambulatory care is for nonincapacitating symptoms, social definitions and response have an important impact on the content and process of primary care.

In part, patients who seek medical care as a result of life difficulties and high readiness to depend on physicians may present their problems in a variety of ways, and underlying problems are frequently identified only with difficulty. At one extreme are the patients who have a highly developed psychosocial vocabulary and who present their problems to the doctor in psychosomatic and psychosocial frames of reference. They may complain of family conflict, depression, difficulties on the job, or whatever. Studies indicate that such patients tend to be better educated city dwellers from backgrounds that encourage a psychological vocabulary—from Jewish populations, for example. A second type of patient chronically complains of diffuse physical symptoms that are characteristic of both psychological and physical disorder: loss of appetite, difficulty sleeping, fatigue, aches and pains, and so on. Such patients are more likely to be of rural origins, to have less education, and to come from cultural backgrounds that discourage the open expression of emotions and complaints. Various data suggest that these patients subject themselves to considerable diagnostic work and to a high prevalence of surgical procedures. Other types of presentations fall between these two extremes. A common complaint by patients is "nerves," a category between a physical and psychological presentation. Patients describing their problem as one of "nerves" frequently resist any interpretation that directly implicates factors in their immediate life situations, but seem to recognize their problems as somewhat different than more conventional physical disorders. Many patients presenting self-limited acute complaints of mild or moderate severity may have come to the doctor as much because of life difficulties as of the symptom presented. The fact that physicians cannot really know contributes enormously to the difficulty of their task. Let us consider how this all appears from the physician's perspective.

PHYSICIANS' RESPONSES TO PATIENTS' COMPLAINTS

The capacity of the doctor to cope effectively with typical primary medical care problems depends not only on his or her personality, attitudinal orientations, and prior preparation, but also on the practice pressures and incentives the doctor faces and the manner in which care is organized. To get through the day's work, physicians must manage not only their patients but also their own time. In addition, they hope to be reasonably responsive to their patients. How they do this will depend on both the organization of the practice and on incentives implicit in how the doctor is paid.

The discussion that follows is exploratory since there is little research on

how practice structure affects the physician's behavior. Our studies of physicians in varying settings are unique but also have certain limitations. Most
seriously, they are cross-sectional and nonexperimental, and depend exclusively
on physicians' report. Thus, when one observes an association between a mode
of practice and other behavior, it is impossible to separate to what extent the
outcome is attributable to organizational effects from the extent to which
persons with specific behavioral orientations select particular modes of practice.
Also, without independent observations, self-reports of physicians concerning
their own work must be viewed with some skepticism. Wherever possible, I
have sought data from other studies that either strengthen or contradict my
conclusions, but I emphasize that the types of investigations I discuss cannot
prove my contentions.

When I first became interested in general medical practice in England and
Wales in the early 1960s I was impressed by the frequency with which practitioners complained of the triviality and inappropriateness of medical consultations. As I inquired into the issue it became clear that the conventional explanations for such complaints appeared to be inconsistent with existing information. Although perceptions of triviality were attributed to the fact that the National Health Service was free—and thus the argument that the absence of economic barriers leads to exploitation of the doctor—the available data on practitioner utilization could not sustain this contention. Average medical utilization
was not substantially higher in England than in the United States, nor was it
likely that differences in utilization or patients' behavior from one practitioner
to another could account for their widely varying reports of triviality. Also,
doctors with larger panels complained more vigorously of trivial patients, even
though existing data suggested that their patients had lower average per capita
utilization of medical services than patients of doctors with smaller panels. I
came to the same conclusion as Ann Cartwright,[10] who was working on similar
issues at the time, that the attributions of triviality told us more about doctors
and their practices than about the objective characteristics of patients or the nature of their problems.

The reports of official bodies—such as the Gillie Committee[11] or the Royal
Commission on Medical Education[12]—explain the dissatisfaction of physicians
and their frustrations by such factors as a lack of a hospital affiliation, the
absence of group practice or adequate ancillary help, or the unsatisfactory
educational preparation of the general practitioner. When we studied a national sample of general practitioners in 1965-66 we could find little evidence
in support of any of these arguments except that doctors with training in psychiatry and behavioral science seemed somewhat more content.[13] We cannot determine whether this results from such training or from the types of people who
select to have such training. Our sample of 800 general practitioners did not
provide many who were working in modern practice structures, with the ad-

vantages usually attributed to group or health center practice or to the effective use of paraprofessional manpower. Thus, the diagnosis of these official committees could conceivably be correct. But within the prevalent variations then existing—and still existing—I am frankly skeptical.

A large number of variables was examined in the study of English general practitioners. Most variables describing doctors' backgrounds or modes of practice had little effect on how they viewed their patients or on their own satisfactions and dissatisfactions. Only one factor appeared to matter very much—patient demand. The more patients the doctor saw, the more likely the doctor was to describe them as trivial and inappropriate. The influence of patient demand was pronounced even when controlling many other variables simultaneously.

Such an association is, of course, open to a variety of interpretations. We were able to exclude some of these since we had collected a great deal of data on various aspects of the doctors' practices. One could not account for the differences on the basis of geographic area or the doctors' descriptions of the social class characteristics of their patients. Nor is it likely that the different perceptions of triviality reflect real differences in the distribution of morbidity or help seeking in varying doctor's panels, although this issue deserves more study. Therefore, I came to the following interpretation of these findings.

English general practitioners, paid on a weighted capitation basis, develop some concept of how much time they ought to devote to their practices. Although they may adjust to varying patient demands in their practice, they do this within their views of what constitutes an equitable workweek. They then establish fixed office hours within which they accommodate the patients who wish to see them. Doctors who have larger practices, and who schedule more limited office hours relative to patient demand, must practice an assembly-line medicine that depends on symptomatic treatment. As patient demand grows, doctors must practice in a more hurried way to get through the daily queue. One way of coping is to increase office hours substantially; but a capitation system of payment provides no incentive for this response. Obviously, some doctors do so because of their own compulsiveness or sense of obligation, but our concern here is with the average tendencies, not the exceptions.

The general practitioner sees many patients with psychosocial problems and who are suffering from significant psychological distress, as has been well documented by the studies of general practice carried out by Michael Shepherd and his group.[14] These patients may present common physical complaints to justify their consultations, but their visits may be motivated by underlying distress. Such patients are difficult to care for under the best of circumstances, but in busy offices doctors have little time to talk with them and explore in any detail the nature of their concerns.

In treating such patients symptomatically, doctors are aware of their failures to explore the problem and thus feel frustrated. The attribution of triviality is probably a reflection of this feeling. Indeed, we find that doctors who report that a large proportion of their patients are trivial also report that they frequently do not have time to do an adequate examination and to do what is necessary for the patient. They also report more frequently than other doctors that they more commonly issue prescriptions without seeing the patient and give patients certificates although unconvinced that the patient is too sick for work.[15] In short, I am suggesting that British general practitioners define patients as trivial because the nature of their practice induces them to treat patient complaints as if they are trivial.

Anticipating that fee-for-service arrangements would create different incentives for the doctor's behavior, we carried out a similar investigation of a national sample of 1500 general practitioners, internists, pediatricians, and obstetricians in the United States.[16] Although perceptions of triviality are not uncommon in the United States, such reports are much less frequent than in British practice. In general, doctors in the United States see many fewer patients, and are expected to give the patient more time than in typical British practice. We anticipated that in fee-for-service practice, doctors would be subject to a larger extent to what Freidson has called "client control"—that is, they would feel pressured by patient expectations to spend a reasonable amount of time with them and to provide certain amenities. Because of the fee-for-service incentive, we anticipated that doctors would be more likely to respond to such patient expectations by increasing their office hours. Indeed, this is what we and others find. Doctors in fee-for-service practice, who face large patient demand, work very long hours.[17, 18] Unlike the British practitioner, the doctor is rewarded for every additional patient seen.

We further anticipated that physicians in large, prepaid group practices in the United States would be exposed to incentives very much like those characteristic of English general practice. Although our sample of doctors in prepaid groups was a small percentage of our national sample, our data suggested that they responded very much like the English general practitioners, and that they were much more likely to attribute triviality or inappropriateness to the patients seen.

This provocative finding led us to select still another national sample of physicians who practice in prepaid groups. This second sample included only general practitioners and pediatricians. The analysis of these data suggests a complex and differentiated response that has been described elsewhere.[19] For our purposes here I only note that consistent with our previous survey of U.S. physicians, general practitioners and pediatricians in prepaid group practice are more than three times as likely as nongroup, fee-for-service practitioners to indicate that 50 percent or more of their patients are trivial or inappropriate (see Table 6.1). While only 9 per cent of nongroup general practitioners report

Table 6.1   Reports Concerning Trivial Consultations in Varying Practice Settings

	Reporting 50% or More Patients Are Trivial %	Reporting 10% or Less Patients Are Trivial %
British general practitioners (N = 772)	24	12
All nongroup U.S. primary care physicians (N = 1148)[a]	7	36
All group U.S. primary care physicians (N = 310)[a]	10	36
Nongroup U.S. general practitioners (N = 604)	9	33
Group U.S. general practitioners (N = 113)	13	27
Nongroup U.S. pediatricians (N = 136)	9	31
Group U.S. pediatricians (N = 43)	9	33
Prepaid U.S. general practitioners (N = 108)[b]	32	7
Prepaid U.S. pediatricians (N = 154)[b]	29	14

[a] Includes general practitioners, pediatricians, internists, and obstetricians.

[b] Includes physicians in practices involving 50 per cent or more prepaid practice activity.

this many patients as trivial, 32 per cent of general practitioners in prepaid practice give such a report. The comparable figures for pediatricians are 9 per cent and 29 per cent. More general practitioners and pediatricians in prepaid practice in the United States report 50 per cent or more of their patients as trivial than the 24 per cent of British general practitioners who give such reports.

Of course, prepaid patients may exploit medical care in the absence of economic barriers, and perceptions of triviality may reflect such abuse. We have carefully examined existing data involving studies of prepaid practice and utilization data reported by the large prepaids such as HIP and Kaiser-Portland. In some cases, average utilization in prepaid practice is higher than in other forms of practice; in some cases, there are no clear differences; and in some cases there is evidence of lower rates of utilization than in the population at large.[20] This should not be surprising. As we noted in the previous chapter, there are many noneconomic barriers that control rates of utilization: the resources made available, distance to the outpatient facility, difficulty in making an appointment, waiting time, and the responsiveness of care once one arrives.

On the basis of our two earlier surveys we suspected that physicians in prepaid contexts viewed themselves as working on a contractual basis. They receive a fixed salary for a defined period of work and, unlike fee-for-service physicians, had no incentives to increase substantially the amount of time they spend seeing patients. Thus we suspected that when prepaid practices face large patient demands, they schedule extra patients within the physician's defined hours of work rather than have the physicians work longer hours. This would result in a practice less responsive to the patient. Studies of consumers of prepaid practice also report that they are more likely than fee-for-service patients to feel that practitioners are less responsive to their needs and seem less interested in them,[21, 22] and this is consistent with the overall argument.

When we more closely examined the specific components of the physician's satisfactions and dissatisfactions in our U.S. samples we found support for this interpretation. Fee-for-service physicians have longer workweeks than prepaid physicians and complain the most of their long hours of work and lack of leisure time. Prepaid group practitioners are more satisfied with their overall workweek, but they tend to be more dissatisfied with the amount of time for each patient.

We have also found that attributions of triviality are associated with concern about people bringing less serious disorders to doctors and more readily seeking help for problems in their family lives, and with less overall satisfaction. Attributions of triviality are consistently higher among physicians who report that they are dissatisfied with the amount of time they have for each patient and among those who report seeing more patients on a busy day. We suspect that attributions of triviality reflect the reactions of a technically inclined physician burdened by a heavy patient load and with few incentives to be responsive to the psychological and social concerns that are associated with many patient consultations.

THE ELABORATION OF A TENTATIVE MODEL OF PHYSICIAN BEHAVIOR

As our research progressed, we wanted to organize our thinking about the factors affecting the physician's strategies for managing patients and practice. Thus we developed the model described in Figure 6.1. The appropriate application of this model requires some discussion.

To understand the skills and orientations necessary for physicians, one must have an idea of the challenges that will be characteristic of their future work.[23] It is worth reiterating the obvious fact that medical education results in different pathways that call for varying intellectual capacities, technical skills, and personal orientations and characteristics. Moreover, we have no clear way of

108

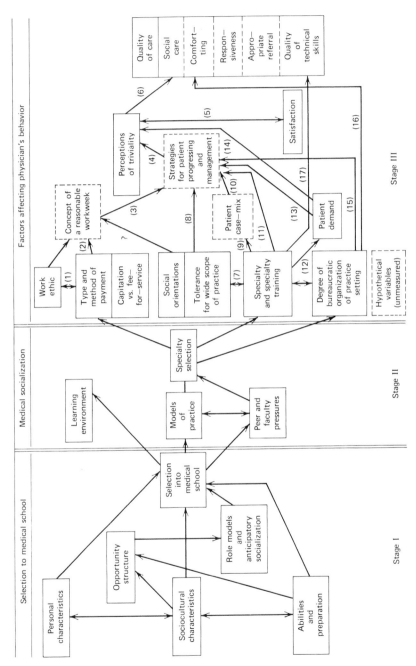

Figure 6.1

predicting the results of physician sorting into various occupational tasks, or the way in which changes in knowledge, biomedical capacities, or in social and cultural conditions will modify the pattern of medical care in the future. Therefore, models of training necessarily develop within a context of uncertainty about future medical practice. To some extent this uncertainty can be limited by defining more clearly to what types of practice discussions of physicians' attributes, training, and the practice contexts that increase the probability of high quality, responsive medical care refer. The model presented here refers only to physicians engaged in office-based primary care, and not to more highly specialized practitioners.

One of the difficulties in discussing models of medical education and practice is the diversity of medicine. Medicine embodies certain common skills, but also others that vary greatly from one context to another. Medical education has adapted to the growth of knowledge and the elaboration of technology by increasing specialization and subspecialization around various technical areas, bodily systems, or population groups. Until very recently, it has been implicitly assumed that any doctor in the course of medical education and postgraduate training has acquired the skills necessary to perform as an adequate primary care physician. Therefore, the generalist is often seen as a second-class doctor, not as a specialist who faces unique problems and requires special skills and conditions of work.

The work of primary care physicians differs considerably from the model of practice students observe in caring for seriously ill patients in teaching hospitals. Primary care physicians must have sufficient grasp of problems in general medicine, pediatrics, obstetrics-gynecology, and psychiatry to identify and handle many common problems in these areas. But many of the problems they deal with are not easily encompassed within disease classifications characteristic of hospital patients.[24] If one attempts to define the work of primary care physicians in terms of the types of patients that select themselves for care from a community at risk, and their morbidity as compared with the illnesses of persons who do not seek care, it becomes evident that the social dimensions of the doctor's role are extremely significant.

Figure 6.1 is divided into three stages. Only rough and incomplete representations of the processes involved in the first two stages are presented since they are not directly pertinent to our concerns here. Stages 1 and 2 are included only to indicate that the behavior of the physician is influenced by the sociocultural, personality, and intellectual sorting processes that bring selected students to medical school and to various types of medical activity.[25] The characteristics of students then interact with the learning environments, models of practice, and faculty and peer pressures that medical students confront.[26] Both the selection and socialization factors obviously have an important influence on how physicians respond in the practice setting, but since the data we have cannot illuminate these issues, they remain as part of the background of the model.

Physicians, of course, vary in their personal needs, inclinations, and aspirations. They may drift until they find a suitable work context,[27] trying one or another form of practice, seeking situations particularly compatible with their interests and experience, and structuring their work settings in terms of their special needs. Any reasonable model of practice must certainly assume some turnover as physicians sort themselves into organizational arrangements compatible with their needs, orientations, and competing opportunities.

Since the literature includes very little data on the characteristics of physicians seeking particular work settings, it is difficult to know to what degree the effects of practice structure are confounded with the types of people selected to particular types of practices. In recent years, group practice has been a more popular alternative form of practice, and more doctors are going into it than leaving it. Data on multispecialty groups show relatively low turnover and consistent growth.[28] Although only a minority of doctors is in group practice, there is no evidence of any major differences in overall satisfaction between doctors in such settings and those in other forms of practice.[29]

The advantages of organized group practice for the physician have been frequently described, but difficulties sometimes develop concerning the distribution of remuneration, institutionalized patterns of shared responsibility, and relationships among physicians within the group. Both Ross[30] and Prybil,[31] in studying terminators from multispecialty group practice, found problems of remuneration foremost among the factors motivating a shift to other forms of practice. Problems included the amount of remuneration and distribution among the specialties with varying income generating potential; some doctors left because economic opportunities were better elsewhere. However, most doctors do not terminate, and those who leave for economic reasons may have special interest in their incomes or have especially poor remuneration. In any case, these findings suggest that doctors are likely to base their ideas of adequate income on their knowledge of opportunities elsewhere.

An important cause of dissatisfaction in large groups is the requirement that doctors fit their behavior into an organized system. As medical groups become larger and more bureaucratic, physicians must yield to some extent to organizational necessity and administrative authority. Inevitably, some physicians may balk at these requirements. Particularly in prepaid practices, patients have a contractual arrangement with the group. Unlike fee-for-service doctors, group physicians cannot deal with the demanding and troublesome patient by imposing a fee barrier or by suggesting the patient go elsewhere. Since the group is responsible for the patient's care, physicians who encourage the difficult patient to leave impose a burden on their colleagues. Thus, as Freidson[32] notes, the bureaucratic physician must develop new strategies for dealing with such patients.

Freidson identifies three types of demanding patients: those with complaints for which the physician can find no cause or about which little can be done, those who attempt to use "pull" to reinforce their demands for service, and the bureaucratic patients who demand services from the physician as a contractual right. Freidson argues that the bureaucratic patient is the most difficult type for physicians to handle in prepaid practice.

> They posed demands which the physicians were unaccustomed to dealing with, for the demands stemmed from the contractual framework of practice in the medical group and were generic to the role of the bureaucratic client rather than the customer or layman. Perhaps this is why they seemed so outrageous and insulting, for such demands treated the physicians as if they were officials rather than "free professionals."[33]

Even though they may have had few "demanding patients," Freidson found that many of his physician respondents explained their departure from the prepaid group in terms of their intolerance for such patients.

ADDITIONAL FACTORS AFFECTING DOCTORS' EFFORTS AND RESPONSIVENESS

I have already described what I believe to be the major ways in which the payment system and patient demand affect the physician's response to patients, particularly to those who are demanding or difficult to manage effectively. Responsiveness also depends on other factors related to the doctors' attitudes and training and the incentives of practice. Physicians clearly vary a great deal in their attitudes about how much effort should be devoted to their practices. We saw that those who are reinforced by fee-for-service payments work longer hours. Attitudes toward medical work are changing, however; there is a growing impression among medical school faculty members that more students and house officers have different work orientations from those of earlier classes. As physicians become more reluctant to assume continuing responsibility for patients, organizational innovations will be required to ensure that the patient in need can receive responsive care at any time.

Our studies also show that doctors in prepaid practice, compared with nonsalaried doctors, are less likely to agree that physicians should work long hours and be prepared to sacrifice their own interests for patients' welfare. In addition, prepaid doctors are less tolerant of the patient with alcoholism, obesity, and other psychosocial problems—that is, they tend to have a lower social orientation to care. Low social orientation, combined with having too many patients and little incentive for increased effort, contributes to unresponsive care.

Other factors about which little is known may help reinforce a lack of physician responsiveness to patients' concerns. One such factor is the patient mix in various types of practice; another is the range of work of the primary care doctor. How much variety in primary care cases is necessary for physicians to maintain their interest? It is possible, even likely, that when their practices become too loaded with certain types of patients, and with too many patients for whom no clear-cut action leading to successful intervention can be taken, doctors are more likely to become frustrated and alienated from their work. Is there a minimal number of more complex cases necessary to maintain a physician's confidence and self-image? Our study of internists, pediatricians, and primary care physicians in prepaid practice shows that their practices are organized to carry out only a limited range of primary care functions. Such physicians, for example, are less likely to report that they tape sprains, excise simple cysts, suture lacerations, do proctoscopic or sigmoidoscopic exams, do uncomplicated obstetrics, or set simple fractures.[34, 35] Also, general practitioners in prepaid practice, as compared with nonprepaid GPs, do many fewer diagnostic procedures. It would be useful to know how the patient mix and range of functions in primary care affect the doctor's perceptions and behavior. It would also be useful to understand better how the bureaucratic organization of ancillary personnel affects the physician's work pattern. Some prepaid doctors complain that their ability to serve their patients better is limited by the scheduled work hours of ancillary personnel and facilities.

IMPROVING THE FIT BETWEEN PATIENTS' NEEDS AND EXPECTATIONS AND MEDICAL SETTINGS

In identifying some of the problems of responsiveness in prepaid practice I have emphasized the negative features. Potentially, however, more organized settings allow for effective use of paraprofessionals, efficient use of new technologies, and greater physician interaction. Each type of practice organization has distinctive advantages and disadvantages. Prepaid practices pose many problems; fee-for-service practices present even more serious problems due to the incentive to carry out marginal or unnecessary care.[36] Since the criteria of quality care are uncertain, we are hard pressed to be clear on what the optimal incentives are.[37] At the very least, however, we should seek to minimize the most obvious distortions that result from the fee-for-service incentive, and those that result from capitation. This can only be achieved by experimenting with various incentive arrangements and evaluating their relative impacts.

In considering alternatives we must understand that all health services research is to some extent limited by the fact that it deals with particular groups of patients and doctors at specific times and places. In the United States, doctors and consumers are accustomed to fee-for-service settings. Future physicians and patients, brought up with different expectations and having different experiences, may find bureaucratic settings for providing and receiving care highly acceptable. Crossnational research suggests that many practice structures are satisfactory to doctors and patients, who tend to support the system they know. We should remember this as we consider the long-term effects of modifying organizational arrangements.

Some of the problems typical of prepaid practice should be seen in the light of the low number of physician hours relative to patient demand. As we have seen, salaried physicians have little motivation to increase their work hours. Furthermore, prepaid practices may achieve savings beyond those associated with lower hospitalization and surgical rates by limiting the resources available for ambulatory medical care relative to demand. This pattern of practice, when it exists, requires the physician to process patients more rapidly, results in long waiting times between requests for service and seeing one's physician, and leads to unnecessary dependence on delivery of urgent care services, that is, medical consultations where patients are unlikely to see their own physician. The growing dependence on urgent care facilities in prepaid practices—with regular appointment waiting times of six and seven weeks—promotes neither continuity of care nor patient perceptions of responsiveness. The urgent care alternative sidesteps primary care relationships, and thus is neither the most effective way to reassure patients nor the most efficient way to use the information about the patient already available to the primary care physician. It is possible to estimate acute care needs of populations and to schedule physician time to maximize the opportunities of patients with acute needs to see their own physician. This accomplished, the urgent care route can be used only as a last resort, rather than as a usual coping device.

Prepaid group practices can also improve their services a great deal by more effective use of paraprofessionals. Such personnel have been particularly underutilized in the care of psychosocial and psychiatric disorders, where patients require both time and a willingness to listen to them. The vast majority of psychiatric difficulties are treated not by psychiatrists or other mental health specialists but by primary care physicians. No matter how effective psychiatric services are, and they are far from optimal, much responsibility will continue to rest with the primary care doctor. Many patients with mild and moderate problems of a psychosocial kind could be served effectively on a continuing basis by nurse practitioners supported by the primary care doctor.[38]

There is increasing evidence that providing psychiatric assistance to chronically complaining patients is related to an overall reduction in medical and hospital utilization.[39] However, since these studies tend to be nonexperimental it is difficult to project whether the same outcomes can be achieved among chronic complainers who presently resist psychiatric care or a psychiatric interpretation of their problem.[40] Such patients are probably best managed by the primary care physician. Physicians, of course, have an obligation to satisfy themselves that patient complaints have no basis in detectable organic disease, but if they are not to exaggerate such physical detection processes, they must also be attentive to patients' psychological states and provide an opportunity for relevant psychological and social information to become salient. Many complaining patients are significantly depressed and anxious, but do not feel free to discuss these feelings unless the physician provides an appropriate opening.

There is growing evidence that indicates that dealing with many psychosocial problems requires more than the social support and encouragement that help reduce feelings of anxiety and distress.[41] In many circumstances patients require specific instructions that assist them in dealing with their life circumstances. Such instructions, to be effective, must be relevant to patients' problems, consistent with their experiences, and psychologically and culturally credible. The growing utility of behavior modification approaches offers some promise for the practitioner dealing with problems of child care, obesity, phobias, and the like. In many areas of behavior it is not clear what directions for behavior change are credible, but it is valuable for the practitioner to keep in mind not only the needs of the patient to maintain greater psychological comfort but also the necessary instructions and skills required for the patient to cope with his or her life situation.

I emphasize the dimension of credibility since every practitioner knows that there is a substantial difference between recognizing a patient's level of psychological distress and obtaining the acceptance of the patient that this is part of the problem. Many persons resist psychological interpretations of their distress because of ingrained cultural inhibitions or existing social norms in their important primary groups. Physicians who force a definition on a patient that the patient is unprepared to accept achieve little, and may undermine themselves as trusted sources of help. To achieve results, physicians must work patiently and subtly within the patient's frame of reference.

If giving such help is indeed part of the responsibility of primary care physicians, it is not difficult to understand why a technically efficient and operationally hurried practice may not be conducive to its fulfillment. The realities of care require certain trade-offs between optimally responsive care and the need to meet demands for access to the physician, but we would do well to recognize what is sacrificed and attempt to develop appropriate models of care that are better fitted to the forces that create concern in the population and that bring patients into medical care.

The problem in meeting patient expectations is inherent in the different conceptions of physician and patient and in the conflict between giving patients more comprehensive care in contrast to seeing more patients. Physicians who take a broad view of their responsibilities and devote time to exploring life situations and providing support and advice must limit their patient load. Patients have diverse needs and orientations, and no simple, uniform assumptions will allow physicians to proceed effectively. To respond to the patient as an individual, the physician must know that patient and be sensitive to his or her changing needs, and this requires time and continuity. Physicians, of course, complain that they lack the time and, in any case, they are not sure that such investments yield much in the way of tangible benefits. Thus physicians focus on identifying and treating recognizable disease states that are relatively clear-cut, subject to routinization, and consistent with the models of behavior the physician has learned to feel comfortable with.

The more specialized approach to the patient has other consequences as well. Focusing on the search for disease is largely a technical activity, one that depends little on the patient's cooperation and involvement. The patient becomes an object whose wishes do not require much attention; the doctor proceeds independently, making decisions on the tests to order, the procedures to use, and the expenses involved. Even with such major decisions as hospitalization, length of stay, and the use of discretionary procedures, the involvement of the patient is usually limited to providing nominal or legal consent. Most medical activity leaves the patient with the impression of being worked on and is hardly conducive to maximizing the patient's choices.

The existing pressures toward the specialization and institutionalization of medical work—and the emphasis on efficiency and productivity—make it difficult to reorder priorities in a way that insures patients care that is responsive to them as persons rather than as objects, that maximizes opportunities for expression and choice, and that provides occasions for participation and instruction in relationships with professionals. But if one measures the success of medical care by its effective implementation rather than by the number of consultations and number of procedures performed, then what now appears inefficient and wasteful may turn out not to be as costly as alleged. Current medical practice is characterized by frequent disruptions in communication, by differing expectations of patients and physicians, and by frequent failure to conform with medical advice.[42] Care that is responsive to patient perceptions and expectations, that provides the patient an opportunity to be heard, and that instructs patients in a fashion consistent with knowledge of life situations and problems may result in greater cooperation and implementation of medical care. Chapter 11, describing a study by Bonnie Svarstad, indicates some of the complexities in this area.

One should not underestimate how little we know about managing human problems in the context of medical care. Serious research in this relatively neglected area is of high priority. From the perspective of human values, however, medicine has a social role that far transcends the technical procedures that doctors know how to perform. To deny these needs and motivations is to debase the practice of medicine and its traditions. But neither should we minimize the practical issues. The implementation of comprehensive medicine depends on a more adequate distribution of medical personnel, better models for organizing health care tasks between physicians and among health workers generally, and the development of new educational settings in which the larger problems of medical practice are given attention as a major priority in the work of faculty and the training of students. This is not possible without fundamental changes in medical education and medical practice and in the reward structures that influence behavior.

NOTES

1. K. L. White, T. F. Williams, and B. G. Greenberg (1961), "The Ecology of Medical Care," *New England Journal of Medicine,* **265**:885–892.

2. B. S. Dohrenwend and B. P. Dohrenwend (1969), *Social Status and Psychological Disorder* (New York: Wiley-Interscience).

3. E. Gardner (1970), "Emotional Disorders in Medical Practice," *Annals of Internal Medicine,* **73**:651–652.

4. D. Mechanic (1972a), *Public Expectations and Health Care* (New York: Wiley-Interscience), pp. 203–222.

5. D. Mechanic (1968), *Medical Sociology* (New York: Free Press), pp. 145–146.

6. D. Mechanic (1972b), "Social Psychologic Factors Affecting the Presentation of Bodily Complaints," *New England Journal of Medicine,* **286**:1132–1139.

7. M. Shepherd (1966), *Psychiatric Illness in General Practice* (London: Oxford University Press).

8. L. E. Hinkle, Jr. (1974), "The Effect of Exposure to Culture Change, Social Change, and Changes in Interpersonal Relationships Upon Health," in B. S. Dohrenwend and B. P. Dohrenwend, eds., *Stressful Life Events: Their Nature and Effects* (New York: Wiley-Interscience).

9. M. Balint (1957), *The Doctor, His Patient and the Illness* (New York: International Universities Press).

10. A. Cartwright (1967), *Patients and Their Doctors: A Study of General Practice* (London: Routledge).

11. Great Britain Ministry of Health (1963), *The Field of Work of the Family Doctor* (London: Her Majesty's Stationery Office).

12. Great Britain Royal Commission on Medical Education (1968), *1965–68 Report* (London: Her Majesty's Stationery Office, Cmnd. 3569).

13. D. Mechanic (1970), "Correlates of Frustration Among British General Practitioners," *Journal of Health and Social Behavior,* **11**:87–104.

14. M. Shepherd (1966), op. cit.

15. D. Mechanic (1970), op. cit.

16. D. Mechanic (1972c), "General Medical Practice: Some Comparisons Between the Work of

Primary Care Physicians in the United States and England and Wales," *Medical Care,* **10**:402–420.

17. Ibid.

18. For a discussion of the complexity of the production of physician services, see R. M. Bailey (1970), "Philosophy, Faith, Fact and Fiction in the Production of Medical Services," *Inquiry,* **7**:37–53.

19. D. Mechanic (1975), "The Organization of Medical Practice and Practice Orientations Among Physicians in Prepaid and Nonprepaid Primary Care Settings," *Medical Care,* **13**:189–204.

20. Health Insurance Plan of New York (1970), *H.I.P. Statistical Report: 1968* (New York: Division of Research and Statistics); E. Saward et al. (1968), "Documentation of Twenty Years of Operation and Growth of a Prepaid Group Practice Plan," *Medical Care,* **6**:239–244; Columbia School of Public Health and Administrative Medicine (1962), *Family Medical Care Under Three Types of Health Insurance* (New York: Foundation on Employee Health, Medical Care and Welfare, Inc.); Committee for the Special Research Project in the Health Insurance Plan of New York (1957), *Health and Medical Care in New York City* (Cambridge: Harvard University Press); B. J. Darsky et al. (1958), *Comprehensive Medical Services Under Voluntary Health Insurance* (Cambridge: Harvard University Press); O. W. Anderson and P. B. Sheatsley (1959), *Comprehensive Medical Insurance: A Study of Costs, Use and Attitudes Under Two Plans* (New York: Health Information Foundation Research Series), no. 9.

21. E. Freidson (1961), *Patients' Views of Medical Practice* (New York: Russell Sage Foundation).

22. A. Donabedian (1965), "A Review of Some Experiences with Prepaid Group Practice," *Bureau of Public Health Economics Research Series,* no. 12 (Ann Arbor: School of Public Health, University of Michigan).

23. D. Mechanic (1972a), op. cit.

24. K. White (1970), "Evaluation of Medical Education and Health Care," in W. Lathem and A. Newberry, eds., *Community Medicine: Teaching, Research and Health Care* (New York: Appleton-Century-Crofts); R. Huntley (1963), "Epidemiology of Family Practice," *Journal of the American Medical Association,* **185**:175–178; J. Fry (1966), *Profiles of Disease: A Study in the Natural History of Common Diseases* (Edinburgh: E. and S. Livingstone, Ltd.).

25. H. Gough (1971), "The Recruitment and Selection of Medical Students," in R. Coombs and C. Vincent, eds., *Psychosocial Aspects of Medical Training* (Springfield, Ill.: Thomas); H. Lief (1971), "Personality Characteristics of Medical Students," ibid.

26. S. Bloom (1963), "The Process of Becoming a Physician," *Annals of the American Academy of Political and Social Science,* **346**:77–87; H. Becker et al. (1961), *Boys in White: Student Culture in Medical School* (Chicago: University of Chicago Press); R. Merton et al., eds. (1957), *The Student Physician* (Cambridge: Harvard University Press).

27. S. Miller (1970), *Prescription for Leadership: Training for the Medical Elite* (Chicago: Aldine).

28. M. McNamara and C. Todd (1970), "A Survey of Group Practice in the United States," *American Journal of Public Health,* **60**:1303–1313.

29. D. Mechanic (1971), "Physician Satisfaction in Varying Settings," presented at the National Center for Health Services Research and Development Manpower Conference, Chicago.

30. A. Ross, Jr. (1969), "A Report on Physician Terminators in Group Practice," *Medical Group Management,* **16:**15–21.

31. L. Prybil (1970), "Physicians in Large, Multi-Specialty Groups: An Investigation of Selected Characteristics, Career Patterns, and Opinions," University of Iowa Graduate Program in Hospital and Health Administration.

32. E. Freidson (1973), "Prepaid Group Practice and the New 'Demanding Patient'," *Milbank Memorial Fund Quarterly,* **51:**473–488.

33. Ibid., pp. 482–483.

34. D. Mechanic (1972c), op. cit.

35. D. Mechanic (1975), op. cit.

36. M. Roemer (1962), "On Paying the Doctor and the Implications of Different Methods," *Journal of Health and Social Behavior,* **3:**4–14; U.S. Department of Health, Education, and Welfare (1971), *Toward a Comprehensive Health Policy for the 1970's: A White Paper* (Washington, D.C.: Government Printing Office).

37. A. Donabedian (1973), *Aspects of Medical Care Administration: Specifying Requirements for Health Care* (Cambridge: Harvard University Press).

38. C. E. Lewis and B. A. Resnik (1967), "Nurse Clinics and Progressive Ambulatory Patient Care," *New England Journal of Medicine,* **277:**1236–1241.

39. W. Follette and N. A. Cummings (1967), "Psychiatric Services and Medical Utilization in a Prepaid Health Plan Setting," *Medical Care,* **5:**25–35; I. D. Goldberg et al. (1970), "Effect of a Short-term Outpatient Psychiatric Therapy Benefit on the Utilization of Medical Services in a Prepaid Group Practice Medical Program," *Medical Care,* **8:**419–428.

40. W. Follette and N. Cummings (1968), "Psychiatric Services and Medical Utilization in a Prepaid Health Care Setting, Part II," *Medical Care,* **6:**31–41.

41. H. Leventhal (1970), "Findings and Theory in the Study of Fear Communications," *Advances in Experimental Social Psychology,* **5:**119–186; L. D. Egbert et al. (1964), "Reduction of Postoperative Pain by Encouragement and Instruction of Patients: A Study of Doctor-Patient Rapport," *New England Journal of Medicine,* **270:**825–827.

42. P. Ley and M. S. Spelman (1967), *Communicating with the Patient* (London: Trinity Press).

Chapter 7

Consumer Response in
Varying Practice Settings

David Mechanic and Richard Tessler

In the preceding chapter attention was focused primarily on how various practice organizations affect the work of physicians and their responsiveness to the needs of patients. In this chapter we examine how patients respond to medical care organized in varying ways and under different auspices. We report on a study of a newly established prepaid group practice, and compare the reactions and satisfactions of members of this group with comparable consumers using other sources of care. Increasingly, federal legislation and administrative policy require the evaluation of medical care programs receiving government subsidy. Most evaluation in medical care has dealt with the quality of care provided by physicians as judged by physician reviewers. To be adequate, however, assessment must also encompass how patients respond to programs, the extent to which they find their care acceptable and responsive, and the impact of different delivery modes on the health of the population.

We also wish to illustrate how to evaluate consumer reactions. Government officials, health professionals, and purchasers of medical insurance should be able to ascertain how well particular health programs are doing from the consumer's perspective, and the strong and weak points of programs. Such information allows for more intelligent choices and locates areas that can be improved. Since a major difficulty in comparing health plans is the possibility that consumers with special needs and characteristics are attracted to particular programs, we also examine the extent to which there is significant selection into prepaid insurance programs among persons who feel their health is vulnerable or who are particularly health conscious. In short, we want to achieve a better understanding of how consumers choose among health programs, how they perceive and use medical care services, and how these behavioral orientations interact with the organization of the health delivery system.

At the invitation of a committee of the Medical Society of Milwaukee, and with the cooperation of Blue Cross and a prepaid medical group, we examined the response of consumers to a prepaid group practice insurance program (Compcare) as compared with alternative health insurance policies marketed by Blue Cross and Surgical Care–Blue Shield. The prepaid health program is sold by Blue Cross to employee groups in a dual choice situation. The insurance alternatives may be either more traditional Blue Cross–Blue Shield coverage, or comparable insurance made available by a private insurance company.

The scope of benefits and employee cost of these alternatives vary from one situation to another. Because of this variability, and the manner in which the prepaid program is marketed, it was not feasible to compare a random sample of employees in Milwaukee enrolled in Compcare with a random sample of employees enrolled in other programs. In such a study the non-Compcare comparison groups would have varying benefit structures and a different balance of employer-employee contributions. Moreover, persons in such a study would have had varying exposure to the Compcare experience, thus complicating the analysis. Therefore, we decided to study particular employer groups providing their employees with an option between Compcare and another Blue Cross-Blue Shield alternative.

The first study, which we call the *choice* study, was a telephone survey of City of Milwaukee employees who had recently chosen between Compcare and an alternative Blue Cross–Blue Shield policy. The aim of this study was to examine the reasons respondents give for their choices and to assess selective influences in choice based on sociodemographic factors, residence, prior health history, and attitudes toward health and health care. Further studies of two major employers in Milwaukee, which we call the *satisfaction* studies, were based on a household interview that assessed use of health care services, perceived access and satisfaction, and a variety of health attitudes, behavior, and experiences of persons enrolled in Compcare and other programs. In all three studies, our data are derived from the reports and perceptions of those interviewed, and we have no independent means to assess the accuracy of these reports in most areas of concern. Thus, these are studies of people's feelings and reactions, not necessarily of the objective reality.

THE COMPCARE HEALTH PROGRAM

This prepaid group practice program serves approximately 18,000 persons, and was developed by Blue Cross–Surgical Care Blue Shield. Care is provided by a multispecialty practice. Approximately half of the patients in the group are enrolled in the program; the other half obtain services on a fee-for-service basis. Enrollees in the Compcare program receive a fairly comprehensive benefit package on a prepayment basis including outpatient visits, specialty services, consultation services outside the group at the request of a group physician, diagnostic and laboratory procedures, physical examinations and immunizations, and eye examinations by an ophthalmologist (but not lenses or frames). Among the services excluded from coverage are drugs, dental care, most cosmetic care, and sterilization services. Inpatient services are comparable to Blue Cross policies generally except that hospital services, excluding emergencies, must be provided by the hospital with which the group is associated.

ALTERNATIVE BLUE CROSS–BLUE SHIELD PLANS

The alternatives involved in this study provided reasonably liberal outpatient benefits. In Firm 1, the alternative to Compcare provided emergency medical care, accident care within 48 hours, $200 diagnostic services per year, outpatient surgical procedures, and X-ray and radiation therapy. As of May 1973, Major Medical was added for all firm employees, which included a $100 deductible and 20 per cent coinsurance thereafter up to a $10,000 maximum per person. The alternative in Firm 2 included emergency medical care, accident care with no time limit, outpatient surgical procedures, unlimited diagnostic services, and X-ray and radiation therapy. Firm 2 had similar Major Medical coverage to the one described above except that there was a $50,000 maximum per person. The alternative available for City of Milwaukee employees included emergency medical care, accident care within 72 hours, outpatient surgical procedures, X-ray and radiation therapy, and $200 diagnostic services per year. Major Medical involved a $50 deductible and 20 per cent coinsurance thereafter with a $20,000 maximum per person.

DESCRIPTION OF THE GROUPS STUDIED

Firm 1

Compcare was first offered to employees as of July 1, 1972, providing one year of experience with the Prepaid Medical Group among Compcare subscribers. The firm pays the entire premium for Compcare, and the employees studied are primarily semiskilled and skilled hourly employees. We included in our study all subscribers who joined Compcare in July 1972 and who were still eligible to receive care at the prepaid group at the time of the interview. As a comparison group, we selected a random sample of employees who were eligible for

Compcare but who chose the Blue Cross–Blue Shield program as of July 1, 1972.

Firm 2

Compcare was first offered to Firm 2 salaried personnel effective June 1971. Thus, except for the small number who shifted in 1972, the Compcare sample includes two years of experience with the Prepaid Medical Group. During the 1972 reenrollment period, only 5 of 200 employees did not reenroll in Compcare, and during the following year only 2 more employees left this program when given an opportunity to change. Thus the original group is largely intact. Like Firm 1, this firm pays the entire premium. Unlike Firm 1, however, this sample is a salaried, white-collar group of higher socioeconomic status. Our study includes all Compcare subscribers who were eligible to receive services as of June 1972 and whose eligibility continued to the time of interview. A random sample of comparable employees eligible for Compcare but who retained the Blue Cross–Blue Shield alternative was also studied.

City Employees of Milwaukee

The City of Milwaukee first offered Compcare to its employees in June 1973, to be effective July 1, 1973. Because of ongoing contract negotiations, the police were not offered this option. In contrast to the other employee groups, City of Milwaukee employees who selected Compcare were required to pay $11.77 per month for a family and $4.03 per month for a single plan. The city, however, paid the entire Blue Cross–Blue Shield premium. Of approximately 7000 city employees, 183 (2.6 per cent) selected Compcare, and this entire group was included in our study. A random sample of Blue Cross–Blue Shield subscribers was also selected as a comparison group. Interviewing began soon after the choice situation, usually before those in Compcare had any experience with the prepaid group. This study was carried out through a telephone interview and included both blue- and white-collar workers. Because additional payments are required of those selecting Compcare, the study should bring into sharp focus individual and family characteristics that affect the selection of prepaid group practice.

DATA COLLECTION

The interviews were carried out in the summer of 1973 by the Wisconsin Survey Research Laboratory, which maintains a field office in Milwaukee. To make the order in which persons in the subsamples were interviewed as random as possible, interviews were staggered. A concerted attempt was made to achieve a high response rate and, overall, more than 90 per cent of eligible respondents in the three studies were successfully interviewed. In the telephone study, a household interview was attempted when cooperation could not be elicited by phone. The response rate in each of these samples is higher than those generally obtained in comparable studies, and minimal error can be attributed to nonresponse.

FACTORS AFFECTING THE SELECTION OF PLANS IN THE DUAL CHOICE SITUATION

Previous studies of enrollment in prepaid versus other plans indicate the importance of such features as breadth of insurance coverage, emphasis on preventive medicine, and the availability of comprehensive medical care at a single location. Among the reasons people give for not selecting prepaid practice options are preexisting ties with a private physician, concern about possible impersonality of care, and physical distance from the prepaid facility.[1-3]

It is particularly important to understand the extent and nature of selective biases in choices among alternative plans. From a practical standpoint, the relative costs and benefits of one alternative versus another depend on the health needs and characteristics of persons in various plans, and how they regard and use medical services. Knowledge of such selectivity is also important in evaluating research findings comparing alternative health care programs. For pragmatic reasons almost all of what we know about the performance of alternative plans comes from cross-sectional studies of persons who have selected a particular health care program. When we observe differences in the performance of plans, or the behavior of patients within them, it is difficult to know to what extent the results reflect real differences in performance, and to what extent they reflect the special characteristics of patients choosing one or another health care program. Information on the selection process, although it does not compensate for the lack of randomized controlled trials, informs our interpretation of results from cross-sectional studies.[4,5] For example, in studies of mortality among patients in the Health Insurance Plan, as compared with alternative populations, we are hard pressed to know to what extent the results are a product of the special organizational characteristics of the HIP program, and to what extent they can be traced to characteristics of consumers of this program.[6,7]

One important type of selectivity that we examine concerns individuals and families who anticipate or require, because of preexisting conditions, higher than average needs for medical care. This is commonly known as the risk-vulnerability hypothesis.[8-11] The notion is that people who estimate the risk of illness as great, and who feel vulnerable to high costs for medical care, are predisposed to enroll in prepaid plans because of the protection provided against out-of-pocket costs. Although various studies have addressed the issue, most of them concentrate on sociodemographic characteristics as substitute measures for need, and do not directly examine data on health status or health consciousness. In talking with researchers who have investigated this issue, we have also come to suspect that the research literature probably is biased in the direction of overestimating the health selection effects into prepaid group practice. Investigators probably expect to find differences between prepaid and nonprepaid group practice; when such differences are not found, the data are probably seldom written up or submitted for publication.

There is evidence in the literature that prepaid group enrollees are more likely to be older, married, and to have young children than people choosing alternative options.[12–16] Yedidia[17] reports that the age composition of prepaid group practice enrollees is not distinctive, however, and on this basis questions the proposition that high risk families are attracted to prepaid plans. More direct evidence concerning the relative vulnerability of enrollees in prepaid group practice comes from studies that include measures of health status and illness. Anderson and Sheatsley[18] report no differences in the perceived health status of members of families enrolling in prepaid group practice and an alternative insurance plan. They also found that individuals selecting the prepaid option were no more likely than those in the comparison group to have experienced an expensive illness prior to enrollment. Hetherington and colleagues[19] found higher proportions of families with chronic and acute illnesses in prepaid than in alternative plans, but whether such differences existed at the time of the choice is not clear. Bice,[20] studying a lower income area in Baltimore, found that families who had previously lacked an alternative other than episodic outpatient care were more likely to enroll in a prepaid group practice if they had higher as compared with lower previous utilization.

Of course, prepaid group practice, and the populations given an opportunity to enroll in them, may vary on many important dimensions; therefore, the findings vary from one study to another. An overall assessment must be based on the research literature as a whole, and cannot depend on any single study or study population.

Another selective bias to be examined concerns the possibility that people who enroll in prepaid plans bring with them distinctive attitudes and orientations toward illness and medical care. Anderson and Sheatsley[21] were unable to find any consistent differences between health attitudes of individuals participating in prepaid and fee-for-service insurance plans. However, they did not probe systematically for the possibility that enrollees in prepaid group practice are more oriented toward health maintenance and preventive health utilization. Other studies have reported evidence of high rates of preventive health utilization in prepaid plans,[22–24] but it is not clear to what extent such differences reflect the organization of the plans or the prior attitudes of their enrollees.

In addition to examining the above issues, we also consider the possible effect of neuroticism[25] on choice behavior. We wish to examine indirectly the allegation that prepaid group practice tends to attract a large number of "worried wells," people who are prone to present problems that physicians regard as trivial,[26] a contention that may be very much exaggerated.[27] The "worried well" hypothesis, however, may be supported in part by the finding of Hetherington and colleagues[28] that "hypersensitivity" to physical symptoms was higher among subscribers in a large group practice than in other insurance plans, but careful inspection of the data throws this in doubt. Hetherington and his associates had physicians rate various symptoms in terms of the extent to which they required medical care. Symptoms were then classified as high and low need. The measure of hypersensitivity took into account symptoms for which patients indicated they would seek medical care despite low need ratings by the physicians. Low need symptoms included insomnia, "nerves," general fatigue, and the like. Who is to say whether seeking care for such symptoms should be regarded as "trivial," or as the behavior of the "worried well"?

The sociodemographic characteristics of prepaid group practice and Blue Cross respondents are presented in Table 7.1. A significantly larger proportion of respondents who enrolled in Blue Cross–Blue Shield were married and selected family plans. Prepaid group practice respondents were significantly better educated than those retaining Blue Cross–Blue Shield health insurance. There were no significant differences in the two groups in age, sex, employment status, religion, family income, or number and ages of children. Comparable patterns were replicated in the satisfaction studies. Although the educational difference echoed that in the choice study, it was not statistically significant.[29]

EXPLICIT REASONS FOR CHOICE

To assess respondents' reasons for their choices, we asked in an open-ended way why they made the decisions they did. We then suggested various reasons for making the choice and asked respondents to indicate how important each reason was for their family. Finally, we asked respondents to select the single reason among those suggested that was of greatest importance to their family.

In the open-ended question,[30] Blue Cross–Blue Shield respondents indicated most frequently that they were satisfied with Blue Cross coverage (32 per cent), that they had inadequate information about the choice (22 per cent), that they were satisfied with their present doctor (21 per cent), that they did not wish to assume the additional cost to enroll in the prepaid plan (15 per cent), and that the prepaid practice clinic was inconveniently located for them (14 per cent). Other reasons given were inertia (15 per cent), preference for a wider choice of doctors or hospitals (9 per cent), and concern about a clinic atmosphere at the

Table 7.1 Sociodemographic Characteristics of Prepaid Group Practice and Blue Cross Enrollees

Sociodemographic Factors	Blue Cross (N = 165) (%)	Prepaid Group Practice (N = 168) (%)	p^a
Respondent—married	77	57	$<.001$
Family health plan	80	62	$<.001$
Number of children			
0	46	55	
1–2	32	23	NS
3 or more	22	22	
Number of children under 12			
0	71	76	NS
1 or more	29	24	
Age of respondent			
30 or less	24	29	
31–45	34	30	NS
46–55	27	30	
56 or more	15	11	
Sex of respondent—female	73	73	NS
Respondent employed	72	80	NS
Education of respondent			
Some high school or less	19	14^b	
Completed high school	52	41	$<.01$
Some college or more	28	46	
Religion of respondent			
Protestant	37	25	
Catholic	51	56	NS
Other	12	19	
Respondent—black	11	6	NS
Family Income			
Under $8000	7	13	
$8000–$10,999	39	34	NS
$11,000–$14,000	27	29	
Over $14,000	27	24	

^{a} Statistical significance is computed using the χ^2 distribution. The criterion used is the .05 level.
^{b} Percentages may not add to 100 per cent because of rounding errors.

prepaid practice (5 per cent). Those selecting prepaid group practice most frequently referred to the more comprehensive coverage this program provided (30 per cent) and to the fact that at the time of choice they lacked a continuing or adequate relationship with a physician (23 per cent). Other reasons given included the fact that the plan covered office visits (15 per cent), that it was a "good deal" for the money (14 per cent), that physical exams were paid for (13 per cent), that they knew about particular doctors at the prepaid practice clinic (13 per cent), that a family member had a condition requiring a great deal of medical attention or the possibility of this occurring (9 per cent), that the prepaid plan offered complete care at one location (7 per cent), and that it provided preventive medicine (8 per cent).

Table 7.2 shows the reactions of respondents to eight possible reasons for their choice. Except for the item dealing with size of family, responses differed among respondents choosing each of the two options. Those retaining the Blue Cross–Blue Shield policy were more likely to rate as important the location of the prepaid practice clinic and the fact that the family physician would be restricted to the prepaid group practice. The Blue Cross group saw these as disadvantages; to those selecting the prepaid plan, they were advantages. For example, 87 per cent of the Blue Cross sample saw the prepaid practice's location as a disadvantage, 81 per cent saw its association with a particular hospital a disadvantage, and 90 per cent saw the restriction of their family physician to the prepaid practice group as a disadvantage. In contrast, 76 per cent in the prepaid plan said the location of the clinic was an advantage, 97 per cent said its association with a local hospital was an advantage, and 93 per cent indicated that it was an advantage that their family physicians would be part of the prepaid group practice. A majority of respondents choosing both options agree that having one's medical care in one place was an advantage—100 per cent of prepaid practice respondents, and 69 per cent of the Blue Cross respondents.

Table 7.2 also shows the proportions in the subgroups who indicate each reason as the most important one. The pattern of response differs significantly for the two subgroups. For Blue Cross respondents, the most important reasons for their choice were the restriction of their family physician to the prepaid group practice and the location of the clinic. Prepaid group practice respondents rated the fact that all of the family's care would be provided in one place, knowing medical care costs in advance, and the availability of medical care on nights and weekends as most important. Although more prepaid practice respondents rate as very important the chance that a member of their family might need a lot of medical care, an identical proportion in the two groups—14 per cent—rate it as most important.

Table 7.2   Proportion of Respondents in the Choice Study Rating Fixed Alternative Items as Very Important in Choice

	Blue Cross–Blue Shield (N = 165)		Prepaid Group Practice (N = 168)		
	% Rating Item Very Important	% Saying It Is Most Important Reason	% Rating Item Very Important	% Saying It Is Most Important Reason	p^a
Location of prepaid practice clinic	37	25	28	8	NS[b]
Prepaid practice clinic's association with specific hospital	16	2	22	3	< .05
In Compcare, all the family's medical care would be provided in one place	24	7	58	24	< .001
In Compcare, your family physician would be a member of the prepaid group	48	34	27	12	< .001
Availability of medical care at night and on weekends at prepaid clinic	22	9	56	18	< .001
Knowing in advance what your medical care costs would be for the year	18	2	45	19	< .001
Importance of the size of your family in choosing health plan	19	7	24	3	NS
Chance that a member of your family might need a lot of medical care	29	14	40	14	< .05

[a] Statistical significance computed by the χ^2 statistic and the criterion used is the .05 level. In this table the probability figures shown refer to the ratings of importance of each item and not to the ratings of the single most important item.
[b] Probability is <.06.

SELECTIVITY DUE TO HEALTH STATUS

To determine whether there were any differences in health status between families enrolling in prepaid group practice and families retaining their Blue Cross–Blue Shield policies, respondents were questioned about their medical histories and current health problems, and about those of other family members. As one indicator of selectivity due to health status, respondents were presented with a list of 34 chronic health problems and, for each problem, were asked if anyone in their family had ever had that problem. Table 7.3 presents the mean number of chronic problems reported for Blue Cross and Prepaid Practice respondents, their spouses, and children. The results show that prepaid group practice respondents reported significantly more chronic conditions than Blue Cross–Blue Shield respondents. As Table 7.4 shows, 14 per cent of prepaid practice respondents reported five or more chronic illnesses, in contrast to 7 per cent in the Blue Cross group.[31]

Although Blue Cross and prepaid practice respondents do not differ much in the percentage who report chronic illnesses, any addition of enrollees with a high level of chronic illness can result in considerable use of service. Analysis of the relationship between chronicity and utilization was undertaken with data drawn from the satisfaction study. The results are presented in Table 7.5. The results reveal significant relationships between respondents' reports of their own chronicity and various indicators of medical care utilization. Respondents with five or more chronic illnesses were overrepresented among those making four or more office visits in the past year, those spending six or more days in the hospital, those with the highest total cost of hospitalization, and those undergoing surgery.

Although there were no overall differences among spouses and children of prepaid and Blue Cross respondents in number of chronic problems reported (see Table 7.3), differences did tend to emerge in a direction consistent with the risk-vulnerability hypothesis for low income families for whom we would expect degree of chronicity to have its greatest impact on perceived vulnerability to medical care expenditures. Tables 7.6 and 7.7 show the distribution of reports of chronic illnesses among spouses and children of Blue Cross and prepaid practice enrollees whose family income was less than $11,000. Forty per cent of the prepaid practice spouses were reported to have two or more chronic illnesses as compared to 23 per cent of the Blue Cross spouses. Thirty-two per cent of the prepaid respondents, in contrast to 21 per cent of the Blue Cross respondents, reported two or more chronic illnesses among their children.[32]

Indicators of health status other than chronicity were all unrelated to choice of health plan (see Table 7.3). When asked to assess health status on a scale ranging from excellent to poor, prepaid and Blue Cross respondents did not differ in their ratings of their own health, their spouse's health, or the health status of each of their children. The number of days family members spent in bed because of illness within the last three months was not significantly different for prepaid

Table 7.3   Health Status of Families Selecting Blue Cross and Prepaid Practice Options

Health Status Indicator	Blue Cross $\bar{X}$	Prepaid Practice $\bar{X}$	p^a
1. Chronic problems			
a. respondents (N = 333)	1.67	2.12	<.05
b. spouses (N = 221)	1.24	1.33	NS
c. children (N = 164)[b]	.71	.84	NS
2. Perceived health			
a. respondents (N = 333)	1.61	1.61	NS
b. spouses (N = 221)	1.64	1.56	NS
c. children (N = 164)	1.35	1.36	NS
3. Bed disability days			
a. respondents (N = 333)	.42	.44	NS
b. spouses (N = 221)	.36	.13	NS
c. children (N = 164)	.34	.43	NS
4. Major illnesses			
a. respondents (N = 333)	1.08	1.09	NS
b. spouses (N = 221)	1.07	1.02	NS
c. children (N = 164)	.01	.05	NS
5. Hospital days			
a. respondents (N = 333)	1.26	1.26	NS
b. spouses (N = 221)	1.17	1.00	NS
c. children (N = 164)	.25	.72	NS
6. Perception of family's medical problems (N = 333)	1.52	1.51	NS
7. Perception of family's utilization patterns (N = 333)	1.51	1.54	NS

[a] Statistical significance is based on unstandardized regression coefficients, employing the F distribution. The criterion used is the .05 level.

[b] The total number of chronic illnesses among all children in the family, coded 0, 1, 2 or more, is represented here. All other figures for children included in this table are based on the average score for children in each family.

Table 7.4   Number of Chronic Illnesses Reported by Respondents in Blue Cross and Prepaid Practice Plans[a]

Reported Chronic Illness	Blue Cross ($N = 165$) (%)	Prepaid Practice ($N = 168$) (%)
No chronic illnesses	28	23
One	26	21
Two	23	25
Three	11	13
Four	5	5
Five	4	6
Six or more	3	8

[a] $\chi^2 = 6.53$; $df = 6$; $p > .05$.

Table 7.5   Relations Between Chronicity and Use of Services Among Respondents in the Satisfaction Study ($N = 989$)

	Numbers of Chronic Illnesses					
	0	1	2	3–4	5 or more	
	($N = 272$) (%)	($N = 276$) (%)	($N = 180$) (%)	($N = 182$) (%)	($N = 79$) (%)	p^a
Office visits						
0	39	32	21	24	10	
1–3	48	48	52	41	33	< .001
4 or more	13	20	28[b]	35	57	
Days in hospital						
0	89	90	90	84	75	
1–5	8	5	5	9	8	< .01
6 or more	3	6	5	7	17	
Cost of hospitalization						
0	89	90	90	84	75	
less than $1019	10	6	8	11	14	< .01
$1019 or more	1	4	2	5	10	
Surgery						
yes	4	4	3	9	16	< .001
no	96	96	97	91	84	

[a] Statistical significance is based on the chi square distribution.
[b] Percentages may not add up to 100 per cent because of rounding.

Table 7.6   Number of Chronic Conditions Reported for Spouses by
Insurance Plan Among Families with Incomes of Less Than $11,000[a]

Number of Chronic Illnesses	Blue Cross $(N = 44)$ $(\%)$	Prepaid Practice $(N = 25)$ $(\%)$
0	41	32
1	36	28
2 or more	23	40

[a] $\chi^2 = 2.31$; $df = 2$; $p > .05$.

practice and Blue Cross respondents. No consistent differences emerged when
respondents were questioned about the total number of days spent in a hospital
in the preceding year, or about major illnesses in the past three months (indicated by reports of illnesses for which a physician was seen five or more times).
Nor were there significant differences in respondents' ratings of the seriousness
of their family's medical problems as compared with other families, or the extent
to which their families were prone to utilize medical services. Each of these
analyses was repeated for those in the low income groups, but no relationship
worthy of note emerged.

Thus far the health status results have been presented separately for individual
health status measures, employing respondents, spouses, and children as units of
analysis. Another approach was undertaken in which individual measures of
health status were aggregated into a summary index with the family employed as
the unit of analysis. For respondents who had a spouse and at least one child

Table 7.7   Number of Chronic Conditions Reported for Children by
Insurance Plan Among Families with Incomes of Less Than $11,000[a]

Number of Chronic Illnesses	Blue Cross $(N = 28)$ $(\%)$	Prepaid Practice $(N = 25)$ $(\%)$
0	64	44
1	14	24
2 or more	21	32

[a] $\chi^2 = 1.13$; $df = 2$; $p > .05$.

covered by the insurance plan, an index of overall family risk was constructed. Five pieces of information concerning the health status of family members prior to the interview were employed: number of chronic illnesses, perceived health status, bed disability days, major illnesses, and days spent in a hospital. Each item was available for respondents, spouses, and children. The empirical distributions on each were examined, and extremes on the end of each distribution were designated as high risk categories. One point was then assigned to a family whenever any member's score fell into a high risk category. The total possible range on the risk index was 0 to 15.

Table 7.8 shows that overall family risk was not significantly related to choice of health care plan, though the difference in the highest risk category is in the direction predicted by the risk-vulnerability hypothesis. Twenty per cent of the families enrolling in prepaid practice, in contrast to 16 per cent of the families retaining Blue Cross–Blue Shield health insurance, received scores of 7 or more on the risk index. These differences are small and could represent chance variations.

A comparable analysis was carried out on the satisfaction study sample to determine whether the same trend would emerge.[33] But since a measure of major illness was not included in the satisfaction study, the risk index was based on four rather than five types of information about respondents, spouses, and their children, and thus had a range of 0 to 12. The same cutoff points for assigning risk points were used. Table 7.9 shows that a similar trend emerged in the cross-validation sample, though once again it is weak and not statistically significant. Eleven per cent of the families participating in the prepaid practice, in contrast to 7 per cent of the families participating in Blue Cross, received the highest scores on the risk index.

Table 7.8   Scores on 15-Point Family Risk Index Based on the Choice Survey[a]

Score on Risk Index	Blue Cross ($N = 85$) (%)	Prepaid Practice ($N = 65$) (%)
0–3	4	3
4	28	31
5	29	23
6	22	23
7 or more	16	20

[a] $\chi^2 = .46$; $df = 4$; $p > .05$.

Table 7.9   Scores on 12-Point Family Risk Index Based on the
Satisfaction Survey[a]

Score on Risk Index	Blue Cross (N = 309) (%)	Prepaid Practice (N = 301) (%)
0–1	1	1
2	27	24
3	28	29
4	22	23
5	13	13
6 or more	7	11

[a] χ^2 = 2.48; df = 5; p > .05.

SELECTIVITY DUE TO HEALTH ATTITUDES AND BEHAVIOR

In evaluating the possible relationship between orientations toward preventive health practices and the choice of prepaid group practice, we questioned respondents about their propensities to use medical services under varying circumstances for both themselves and their children, their perceptions of the importance of regular checkups, when they last had a routine checkup, and whether they owned a medical reference book. We also asked more general questions concerning perceived control over illness, faith in doctors, and skepticism about medical care. The results (presented in Table 7.10) show no significant differences. As with the health status data, each of the analyses was repeated with the lower income families. None of the resulting coefficients were statistically significant.

We did find, however, one exception to the general proposition that there is no selectivity due to preventive health attitudes and practices. Unlike the choice study, the satisfaction study included items designed to determine whether children covered by alternative insurance plans had received specific immunizations. Evidence for selectivity in immunization patterns is clearest for children 5 years old and over who had been participating in the prepaid program for one year only. These respondents were asked when, if ever, each of their children had been immunized against measles, polio, rubella, and mumps. The results, presented in Table 7.11, show that 32 per cent of the children in the prepaid program, in contrast to 23 per cent of those covered by Blue Cross health insurance, were reported to have received all four of the immunizations more than

Table 7.10 Reports on Use and Attitudes Toward Preventive and Other Services

Measures of Use and Attitudes Toward Preventive and Other Services	Blue Cross (N = 165) $\bar{X}$	Prepaid Practice (N = 168) $\bar{X}$	p^a
1. Propensity to use medical services for oneself	12.77	13.09	NS
2. Propensity to use medical services for young children[b]	13.46	12.86	NS
3. Importance of physical checkups	3.08	3.11	NS
4. Months since last checkup	48.98	38.89	NS
5. Importance of physical checkups for young children	2.64	2.58	NS
6. Perceived control over illness	8.93	9.01	NS
7. Faith in doctors	3.11	3.01	NS
8. Skepticism about medical care	8.50	8.75	NS
9. Possession of a medical reference book	1.59	1.54	NS

[a] Statistical significance is based on unstandardized regression coefficients, employing the F distribution. The criterion used is the .05 level.
[b] Items 2 and 5 were only asked of respondents with children under 12 (N = 93).

Table 7.11 Reports of Number of Immunizations Received One Year or More Prior to Interview by Children 5 Years of Age and Over[a]

Number of Immunizations Received	Blue Cross (N = 373) (%)	Prepaid Practice (N = 445) (%)
None	6	4
1	22	18
2	20	19
3	29	26
All 4	23	32

[a] $\chi^2 = 11.47$; $df = 4$; $p < .025$.

a year prior to the interview. Children currently covered by the prepaid plan were more likely to be fully immunized prior to prepaid practice enrollment than children of families choosing to retain Blue Cross health insurance.

A final question was whether people with psychoneurotic symptoms would enroll in disproportionate numbers in a prepaid group practice plan. The results indicate that prepaid group practice respondents were no more neurotic ($\bar{X} = 7.86$) than Blue Cross–Blue Shield respondents ($\bar{X} = 7.88$). Nor were there significant differences in neuroticism in the satisfaction study, comparing prepaid practice and Blue Cross respondents.

In sum, the risk-vulnerability hypothesis received little support in this study. Sociodemographic indicators of risk vulnerability (age, number of children, etc.) did not predict enrollment. Indeed, the relationship that emerged between marital status and enrollment is contrary to some of the implications of the risk-vulnerability hypothesis. Similarly, most of the data on health status do not support the risk-vulnerability formulation. There was little sign of selectivity due to perceived health status, bed disability, major illnesses, or hospitalization either when these variables were examined separately or when they were examined as part of an index of overall family risk.

Some support for the risk-vulnerability formulation came from analyses of the distribution of chronic illnesses in the two groups. Prepaid practice respondents reported more chronic illnesses than Blue Cross respondents, and although the overrepresentation of respondents with chronic illnesses in the prepaid program was not large, our data suggest that persons with many chronic illnesses tend to be heavy users of medical services. From a practical point of view, therefore, any overrepresentation of persons with chronic illnesses is a significant matter. There was also a tendency for spouses and children of lower income families enrolling in prepaid group practice to have more chronic illnesses than spouses and children of lower income families who chose to retain the Blue Cross plan.

The evidence for selectivity due to preventive health attitudes and behavior was somewhat mixed. In the choice study there was no evidence of selectivity in choice due to health attitudes and propensities. The enrollment decision was unrelated to several questions designed to tap health consciousness and readiness to use medical services. If a conclusion is to be drawn on the basis of this study alone, it would be that prepaid group practice and Blue Cross enrollees are basically the same in their propensities to use preventive services and in their attitudes toward care. On the other hand, retrospective data drawn from the satisfaction study concerning immunization of children participating in alternative insurance plans indicated that children of prepaid practice respondents were more fully immunized at the point of enrollment than children of respondents who chose to retain Blue Cross–Blue Shield.

There was no evidence of selectivity due to neuroticism. Thus the results provide no support for the proposition that prepaid practices tend to attract disproportionate numbers of "worried wells."

It is important to emphasize that this is basically a case study. Any conclusions about degree of selectivity into prepaid plans must be made on the basis of cumulative experience in varying social settings. The people studied were drawn from an employed population and the Blue Cross–Blue Shield alternative was liberal in its outpatient coverage. Selective influences on choice may prove to be greater in other populations where the saving in costs resulting from enrollment in prepaid group practice plans is more obvious and clear-cut for individuals and families at risk.

CONSUMER SATISFACTION WITH PREPAID GROUP PRACTICE: A COMPARATIVE ANALYSIS

As was noted at the beginning of Part II, the primary goals of prepaid group practice are to guard against unnecessary hospitalization and surgery through financial disincentives to providers, to foster efficiencies through the pooling of resources and the more effective use of allied health manpower, and to encourage early and preventive medical care utilization through comprehensive benefits made available to consumers on a prepaid basis. A necessary condition for the realization of these goals is consumer acceptance and support, for if prepaid practice is to remain viable it must attract consumers in the marketplace and satisfy its clients. Moreover, since there may be major gaps between the theory of prepaid group practice and its actual operations, it is necessary to appraise critically the performance of different prepaid practice settings. Because entities described as prepaid group practices differ on a variety of important dimensions, it is difficult to generalize from one setting to another.[34] However, information on the performance of a variety of prepaid practices operating in different contexts can help us understand both the advantages and potential difficulties of this form of organization.

Reviewers of previous studies of consumer satisfaction have concluded that the vast majority of prepaid group practice participants are satisfied with their care.[35-38] Weinerman, for example, in his review of relevant research observes that "samples of patients in the Montefiore Medical Group, the Permanente Group in Oakland, and the Labor Health Institute of St. Louis each contain only 7 per cent who expressed strong dissatisfaction, with varying proportions of the other 93 per cent reflecting partial or complete satisfaction."[39]

There is, however, some difficulty in evaluating these high levels of reported satisfaction. Most people in consumer surveys report that they are satisfied with their care, regardless of the medical care setting, but tend to be much more critical of physicians and medical care in general. These high levels of personal satisfaction to some extent reflect a natural reluctance to believe that one's source of care is less than adequate; indeed, if people felt this way they would be likely to change physicians. A second complication arises from the fact that the inadequacies of medical care do not reach people's awareness until they have a need for care and find the expected care lacking. But at any given time only a minority of patients find themselves in a situation that seriously tests the health care system, and longer time periods studied cross-sectionally do not capture the fact that dissatisfied patients may have changed their source of medical care, or that their dissatisfaction is not salient when they are questioned.

One limitation of research on prepaid practice has been the fact that few studies have employed comparison groups, making it difficult to evaluate the significance of varying levels of reported satisfaction and dissatisfaction. By comparing patients receiving care in different settings, particular problems associated with one or another type of practice are more easily recognized and understood.

The existing evidence on relative satisfaction with prepaid group practice is inconsistent. Roemer et al.[40] reported less dissatisfaction in a prepaid group practice plan relative to the level of dissatisfaction expressed by consumers in plans involving fee-for-service practice. Anderson and Sheatsley,[41] in contrast, report significantly more dissatisfaction among prepaid group practice consumers than consumers of more traditional health insurance. Gartside et al.,[42] in a study comparing Medicaid recipients enrolled in a prepaid group practice plan with such recipients receiving care in other settings, report no significant differences in satisfaction. Such inconsistencies should not be unexpected because the entities under consideration from one study to another may vary in important ways and the unique circumstances of each situation are likely to affect performance.

In examining satisfaction with different practice plans, we consider the relative importance of structural features as compared with other factors that affect satisfaction and dissatisfaction among consumers. Differences in satisfaction are often a product of varying expectations, experiences, and personal attributes as well as a feature of the actual services provided. Among the factors considered in addition to health plan are sociodemographic variables, health status, life distress, and attitudes toward various facets of medical care.

A related issue is whether differences in reported satisfaction between consumers of prepaid group practice and consumers of fee-for-service health insurance are in fact attributable not to structural characteristics that distinguish the two types of practice but rather to characteristics that distinguish individuals who choose one type or the other.[43] Unless possible selective biases are taken into account, individual difference effects may be mistaken for structural effects.

A relatively specific operational definition of satisfaction is employed in this discussion. Our satisfaction measures reflect a common concern with consumers' subjective reactions to the medical care they receive. For example, consumers were asked to indicate their satisfaction with the amount of privacy in the doctor's office, the amount of time the doctor spends with them, the doctor's concern about their health, and so forth. Thus our focus is on the acceptability of medical care once it is obtained. In defining satisfaction in this way, we reserve for independent analysis the question of access to medical care—the ease with which the physician can be reached and a consultation initiated, taking into account difficulty in arranging appointments, convenience in traveling to the site of medical care, and waiting time on arrival. Consumers' thoughts and feelings about these aspects of medical care utilization are referred to collectively as access-centered satisfaction.

Although the literature describes access-related complaints among prepaid group practice participants[44] and includes indictments of prepaid group practice plans based in part on their presumed inaccessibility,[45] little comparative data exists. Again, the seriousness of the problem of inaccessibility of care within prepaid group practice plans must be assessed in relation to the magnitude of the problem elsewhere. A final objective of the present study, therefore, was to collect data that would permit precise comparisons to be drawn between prepaid group practice participants and those in alternative plans on the question of access-centered satisfaction.

SOME DIFFERENCES IN SATISFACTION

Satisfaction with medical care received was indicated by 11 items dealing with specific aspects of medical care. These items are presented in shortened form in Table 7.12. The satisfaction items were asked only of people who had received some medical services under their plan in the past year, and thus had had some recent experience on which to base their responses. As indicated in Table 7.12, there was no significant difference between Blue Cross and prepaid practice participants with respect to use of any medical services in the past year.[46] Thus minimal error can be expected due to variation on that point.

Table 7.12 indicates that the majority of all respondents are very satisfied with their care and that this level of expressed satisfaction holds up over a broad range of items. Although prepaid practice participants were on the whole satisfied with their medical care, Blue Cross participants indicated significantly higher levels of satisfaction on most items.

We also asked respondents with children under 12 about their satisfaction with the care their children had received under the plan in the past year.[47] The items designed to measure satisfaction with child care are presented in shortened form in Table 7.13. They are comparable in content to the satisfaction items presented in Table 7.12, but rephrased to be appropriate for child care.

Examination of Table 7.13 indicates a pattern of results similar to those presented in Table 7.12.[48] There was no significant difference in contact with medical services between children of Blue Cross and prepaid practice enrollees.

Table 7.12   Reports on Satisfaction with Medical Care Among Prepaid Practice and Nonprepaid Practice Subscribers

Measures of Satisfaction	Blue Cross $(N = 354)$ $(\%)$	Prepaid Practice $(N = 356)$ $(\%)$	p^a
Proportion of respondents receiving services in past year	73	70	NS
Per cent very satisfied among respondents receiving services in past year			
With amount of privacy in doctor's office	92	86	NS^b
With the amount of time the doctor spends with you	82	74	< .05
With the doctor's concern about your health	85	70	< .001
With the doctor's warmth and personal interest in you	83	67	< .001
With the amount of information given to you about your health	81	64	< .001
With the doctor's training and technical competence	93	78	< .001
With the doctor's friendliness	89	79	< .001
With friendliness of nurses, receptionists, etc.	84	81	NS
With quality of medical care received	88	77	< .001
With adequacy of office facilities and equipment	93	84	< .001
With the doctor's willingness to listen when you tell him about your health	86	78	< .05

^{a} Statistical significance computed by the χ^2 statistic using the .05 criterion for statistical significance.
^{b} < .07.

Table 7.13   Reports on Satisfaction with Medical Care for Children Under 12 Among Prepaid Practice and Nonprepaid Practice Subscribers

Measures of Satisfaction	Blue Cross (N = 197) (%)	Prepaid Practice (N = 189) (%)	p^a
Proportion of respondents with children under 12 who received services in past year	85	87	NS
Per cent very satisfied among respondents with children receiving services in past year			
With the amount of privacy in doctor's office	94	88	NS
With the amount of time the doctor spends with your children	84	74	NS[b]
With the doctor's concern about your children's health	89	75	<.001
With the doctor's warmth and personal interest in your children	88	73	<.001
With the amount of information given you about your children's health	84	73	<.001
With the doctor's training and technical competence	94	82	<.05
With the doctor's friendliness	90	77	<.001
With the friendliness of nurses, receptionists, etc.	87	84	NS
With the quality of medical care that your children have received	92	80	<.05
With adequacy of office facilities and equipment	92	87	NS
With the doctor's willingness to listen when you tell him about your children's health	87	77	<.05

[a] Statistical significance computed by the χ^2 statistic using the .05 criterion for statistical significance.
[b] <.06.

The large majority of prepaid participants were very satisfied with all aspects of child medical care about which we inquired. Although the absolute level of satisfaction with child care expressed by prepaid practice participants appears high, relatively less satisfaction was expressed by prepaid enrollees than by Blue Cross enrollees across a number of items.[49]

CONSTRUCTION OF THE SATISFACTION INDICES

Thus far data have been presented for the respondent's satisfaction with her own medical care and with the care her children have received in terms of a number of separate indicators of satisfaction. A more parsimonious way to present these results is to construct summary indices. This presupposes, however, the presence of a single underlying dimension of satisfaction common to each of the items.

To assess the unidimensionality of the satisfaction items, factor analyses of the measures of satisfaction presented in Tables 7.12 and 7.13 were carried out. Utilizing a principal components procedure with a varimax rotation, single factors emerged for both sets of items. Since these results suggested single dimensions underlying responses to the measure of satisfaction with own care and to the measures of satisfaction with child care, we proceeded to construct two summary indices and to treat them as dependent variables in subsequent analyses.

Thus, for each respondent, responses to individual measures of satisfaction—with 3 indicating very satisfied, 2 indicating somewhat satisfied, and 1 indicating not satisfied at all—were added and a single summary score was assigned. For the index of satisfaction with own medical care, the possible range was 11 to 33. The mean score obtained was 30.48, and the standard deviation was 4.05. For the index of satisfaction with child care, the possible range was the same. The obtained mean was 30.76, and the standard deviation was 4.21.

When summary indices are employed, the satisfaction differences noted between Blue Cross and prepaid practice participants in prior analyses emerge once again. Health plan membership accounts for 4.22 per cent of the variance in the index of satisfaction with own care, and for 4.62 per cent of the variance in the index of satisfaction with child care. For the respondent's satisfaction with her own medical care, greater satisfaction was expressed by Blue Cross participants ($\overline{X} = 31.32$) than by prepaid participants ($\overline{X} = 29.65$). Similarly, for satisfaction with children's medical care, greater satisfaction was indicated by participants in fee-for-service plans ($\overline{X} = 31.64$) than by participants in the prepaid group practice plan ($\overline{X} = 29.83$). It is also clear that when the results are expressed in terms of mean differences in summary indices significant differences do emerge, but they occur on the upper end of the distribution of possible satisfaction scores (recall that the highest possible score is 33). Most people report that they are very satisfied with their health care, regardless of which plan they are enrolled in.

INDIVIDUAL DIFFERENCES AND SATISFACTION

Here we present data bearing on the question of the extent to which satisfaction, in addition to being affected by participation in different health care plans, is also conditioned by individual differences. To generate the results, the two satisfaction indices were regressed independently on groups of independent variables. For example, we regressed each of the satisfaction indices on all measured sociodemographic variables simultaneously. The independent variables were entered into the regression equation as free variables, and a .05 level of probability for exclusion was designated. Omitted from the resulting equations therefore were variables that did not achieve the .05 level of significance. The same procedure was followed for other groups of measured independent variables—attitudes, life distress, and health status indicators.

Table 7.14 presents data relevant to the respondent's satisfaction with her own medical care. The following sociodemographic variables were entered into the regression equation: number of family members covered by the insurance plan, respondent's age, sex, respondent's educational attainment, spouse's

Table 7.14   Individual Difference Variables and the Index of Satisfaction with Medical Care (N = 712)

Individual Difference Variables	Partial Correlation Coefficient[a]	Coefficient of Determination (R^2) for Entire Group
1. Sociodemographic		
marital status	− .09	
housewife	.12	.016
2. Attitudes		
skepticism toward		
medical care	− .21	
faith in doctors	.15	
readiness to seek care	.10	.088
3. Distress		
spirits in general	.13	
major life change	− .08	.022
4. Health status		
subjective health		
assessment	− .12	.014
5. All individual difference		
variables		.121

[a] All partial correlation coefficients are significant, $p < .05$.

educational attainment, head of household's occupational prestige, family income, religion, ethnicity, race, marital status, and respondent's employment status. Section 1 in Table 7.14 shows that the only sociodemographic variables that were not excluded from the regression equation were marital status and a dummy variable for housewife. Married respondents expressed lower levels of satisfaction than respondents who were not currently married; housewives expressed greater satisfaction than respondents who were employed outside the home. As indicated in column 3, these two sociodemographic variables accounted for less than 2 per cent of the variance in satisfaction.[50]

The attitudinal variables examined in relation to satisfaction with own care were internal-external control, social desirability bias, neuroticism, skepticism toward medical care, faith in doctors, and readiness to seek health care. Inspection of the results in section 2 shows that all but the last three variables were excluded from the regression equation, and that as a group these three variables accounted for approximately 9 per cent of the variance in satisfaction—explaining more of the variance in satisfaction than any of the other individual difference groupings considered. Satisfaction was lower among those with greater skepticism toward medical care, less faith in doctors, and lower readiness to seek medical care. The index of skepticism toward medical care consisted of six items employed in previous research.[51] A typical skepticism item is: "Do you often doubt some of the things doctors say they can do?" Faith in doctors was indicated by an item that asked respondents to choose between the following alternatives: (a) "I have great faith in doctors," (b) "In general, I think doctors do a good job," (c) "In general, I think most doctors are overrated," and (d) "I distrust doctors." Readiness to seek help was measured by responses on the likelihood of seeking medical care in eight hypothetical situations involving pain and symptomatology.[52]

Several indicators of life distress were introduced into the regression equation for satisfaction with own care. Introduced into the equation were a subjective assessment of personal distress, an index of uncomfortable feelings and emotions, an index of life worries, indicators of positive and negative life events, a subjective assessment of mood, and an indicator of major life changes. As shown by the partial correlations presented in section 3, all but the last two indicators of life distress were excluded from the regression equation. Both of these showed negative relationships with satisfaction. People who report that in general their spirits are low are less likely to express satisfaction with medical care than those reporting higher spirits. Similarly, people who experienced a major life change (either positive or negative) in the past year report less satisfaction with medical care than people who did not experience such a change. These two indicators accounted for approximately 2 per cent of the variance in satisfaction.[53]

Satisfaction with medical care received was examined in relation to three indicators of physical health—chronic problems, bed disability, and subjective health status. The only health indicator that was not excluded from the regression equation was subjective health status, and it accounted for a little more than 1 per cent of the variance in satisfaction. Respondents were asked: "How about your personal health? Would you say that overall it is excellent, good, fair, or poor?" The results show that the more unfavorable an individual's assessment of her personal health, the less likely she was to express satisfaction with her medical care.

Associations between each of the individual difference predictors of satisfaction with own care are presented in Table 7.15. Inspection of the correlation coefficients shows some covariation among items, including some covariation among items representative of different types of individual difference groupings. To take account of these relationships, a final regression equation was constructed in which all of the individual difference predictors were introduced simultaneously as free variables into a single regression equation. The results of this analysis show that with the single exception of major life changes, each of the individual differences remained in the equation.

Turning to the index of satisfaction with child care, the same sociodemographic, attitudinal, life distress, and health indicators employed in the foregoing analyses were introduced systematically into a set of regression equations for satisfaction with care received by children under 12. As reported in section 1 of Table 7.16, the only sociodemographic variable not excluded from the first regression equation was age of respondent, with older respondents expressing more favorable reactions to child care than younger respondents. Age of respondent accounted for about 2 per cent of the variance in satisfaction with child care.

Three attitudinal variables remained in the second regression equation presented in Table 7.16. The respondent's skepticism toward medical care in general was inversely related to satisfaction with child care. Readiness to seek care for children, based on a format similar to that employed with reference to the respondent but tailored for children's symptoms, was positively related to satisfaction with child care. And finally, an eight-item indicator of social desirability bias was positively related to satisfaction with child care. This index consisted of a subset of eight items drawn from the Crowne-Marlowe need for social approval scale.[54] The scale is designed to measure individual propensities to stretch the truth in order to make oneself look good. As a group, the three attitudinal variables that remained in the regression equation accounted for approximately 6 per cent of the variance in the index of satisfaction with child care.

When satisfaction with child care was regressed against indicators of respondent health status, each of the indicators was excluded from the equation; hence health status does not appear as a category in Table 7.16.

The only indicator of life distress that was not excluded from the next equation (see section 3 in Table 7.16) was an index of worries, and it accounted for about

Table 7.15 Zero-Order Correlations Among Individual Difference Predictors of Satisfaction with Own Care (N =712)

	Marital Status	Housewife	Skepticism	Faith in Doctors	Readiness To Seek Care	Spirits	Major Life Changes	Subjective Health Status
Marital status								
Housewife	.334***							
Skepticism	.050	−.002						
Faith in doctors	−.023	.020	−.177***					
Readiness to seek care	.002	.004	−.094*	.074*				
Spirits	−.060	−.024	−.074*	.031	.007			
Major life changes	.101**	.082*	.123***	−.053	−.085*	.065		
Subjective health status	−.022	.012	.046	−.056	.129***	−.281***	−.020	
Satisfaction with own care	−.053	.090*	−.242***	.186***	.121***	.123***	−.075*	−.117**

* p < .05.
** p < .01.
*** p < .001.

Table 7.16 Individual Difference Variables and the Index of
Satisfaction with Child Care ($N = 385$)

Individual Difference Variables	Partial Correlation Coefficient[a]	Coefficient of Determination (R^2) for Entire Group
1. Sociodemographic age of respondent	.15	.024
2. Attitudes skepticism toward medical care	−.15	
readiness to seek care for children	.14	
social desirability bias	.10	.057
3. Distress index of respondent's worries	−.11	.011
4. All individual difference variables		.080

[a] All partial correlation coefficients are significant, $p < .05$.

Table 7.17 Zero-Order Correlations Among Individual Difference
Predictors of Satisfaction with Child Care ($N = 385$)

	Age	Skepticism	Readiness To Seek Care	Social Desirability Bias	Worries
Age					
Skepticism	−.179***				
Readiness to seek care	−.103*	.092			
Social desirability bias	.139**	−.179***	.080		
Worries	.064	.065	−.027	−.249***	
Satisfaction with child care	.153**	−.161***	.127*	.142**	−.105*

* $p < .05$.
** $p < .01$.
*** $p < .001$.

1 per cent of the variance. Respondents were asked to indicate how much worry various problems such as financial problems and lack of enough social contact with others had caused them during the past year. The more worries the respondent indicated, the less satisfied she was with her children's medical care.

Zero-order correlations for all individual difference predictors of satisfaction with child care are presented in Table 7.17. Once again, some covariation between different types of individual difference variables is evident. To consider the joint impact of all individual differences for satisfaction with child care, all of the individual difference variables appearing in Table 7.17 were introduced simultaneously into a single regression equation. Excluded from this equation because it did not achieve the .05 level of significance was the index of social desirability bias. All of the other individual difference predictors of satisfaction with child care remained in the regression equation.

EFFECTS OF HEALTH CARE PLAN ON SATISFACTION INDICES, CONTROLLING FOR INDIVIDUAL DIFFERENCE CORRELATES

The fact that the satisfaction indices have a variety of significant correlates raises the question of whether the effect of health care plan on satisfaction will disappear or be substantially reduced if one or more of these groups of correlates is controlled. To investigate this possibility, means for satisfaction were adjusted

Table 7.18   Effect of Plan on Index of Satisfaction with Medical Care Controlling for Groups of Variables (N = 712)

Control Variables	Adjusted Means[a]		Unstandardized Regression Coefficient[b]
	Blue Cross	Prepaid Practice	
1. None	31.32[c]	29.65	−1.66
2. Sociodemographic	31.31	29.66	−1.65
3. Attitudes	31.24	29.73	−1.51
4. Distress	31.31	29.66	−1.65
5. Health status	31.30	29.67	−1.63
6. All controls	31.21	29.76	−1.44

[a] Means adjusted through regression analysis using control variables indicated in the far left-hand column.

[b] All regression coefficients for plan listed in the far right-hand column are statistically significant, $p < .001$.

[c] Actually unadjusted means, since no controls.

Table 7.19 Effect of Plan on Index of Satisfaction with Child Care
Controlling for Groups of Variables (N = 386)

Control Variables	Adjusted Means[a]		Unstandardized Regression Coefficient[b]
	Blue Cross	Prepaid Practice	
1. None	31.64[c]	29.83	−1.81
2. Sociodemographic	31.64	29.83	−1.82
3. Attitudes	31.59	29.88	−1.71
4. Distress	31.61	29.86	−1.74
5. All controls	31.57	29.90	−1.67

[a] Means adjusted through regression analysis using control variables indicated in the far left-hand column.
[b] All regression coefficients for plan listed in the far right-hand column are statistically significant, $p < .001$.
[c] Actually unadjusted means, since no controls.

through regression analysis to take account of possible differences between Blue Cross and prepaid practice respondents on the variables in question. Inspection of Table 7.18 and Table 7.19 shows that adjustment of the means for satisfaction had only minimal effect on the mean satisfaction scores, even (as in the last row of each table) when all significant correlates of satisfaction were controlled simultaneously. Irrespective of what controls are employed, the unstandardized regression coefficient associated with health care plan remains highly significant.[55] It appears that the individual difference correlates of satisfaction are random with respect to participation in Blue Cross or prepaid group plans and therefore that the relationships observed between health plan and the two satisfaction indices are not significantly affected when these variables are taken into account.

ACCESS-CENTERED SATISFACTION

Table 7.20 compares the responses of Blue Cross and prepaid practice respondents who have received some medical care in the past year (N = 712) to various questions concerning access. The first two questions deal with distance and traveling time to the doctor's office. Blue Cross respondents reported traveling time to be approximately 16 minutes; for prepaid respondents, it was about 27 minutes. Consistent with these different estimates, responses to the second question included in Table 7.20—"In general, how convenient is it for you to get

Table 7.20   Reports of Access to Medical Care Among Prepaid and
Nonprepaid Subscribers (N = 712)

	Means			
Measures of Access	Blue Cross (N = 354)	Prepaid Practice (N = 356)	Unstandardized Regression Coefficient	p
1. Reported time to get to doctor in minutes	15.57	26.86	11.28	.001
2. Reports it is inconvenient to get to a doctor	1.22	1.68	.46	.001
3. Reported number of days wait to get an appointment (except in emergencies)	8.31	10.30	1.99	.025
4. Reports difficulty in getting appointments	1.19	1.36	.17	.001
5. Reported waiting time at doctor's office in minutes	37.81	26.86	−10.95	.001
6. Reports that waiting time at doctor's office is too long	1.46	1.31	−.15	.01

to a doctor; is it convenient, somewhat inconvenient, or very inconvenient?"—indicate that it was more convenient for Blue Cross respondents than
prepaid practice respondents to get to a doctor.

The next two items presented in Table 7.20 deal with the scheduling of appointments. In response to question 3 in the table ("Except in emergencies,
about how many days do you usually have to wait for an appointment?") Blue
Cross respondents reported an average of about 8 days. For prepaid practice
respondents, the average was about 10 days. Respondents were also asked:
"Would you say it is easy, somewhat difficult, or very difficult for you to get an
appointment to see a doctor?" The means in row 4 show that Blue Cross
respondents reported less difficulty than prepaid respondents in obtaining an appointment.

Items 5 and 6 in Table 7.20 deal with waiting on arrival at the doctor's office and suggest a different pattern of results from those presented above. When asked "About how long do you usually have to wait there before you see the doctor?" Blue Cross respondents reported waits of approximately 38 minutes; prepaid practice respondents reported waiting time as less than 27 minutes. We also asked for subjective reactions to waiting times ("After getting there, do you feel that the time you usually have to wait to see the doctors is not too long, somewhat too long, or much too long?"). Blue Cross respondents indicated significantly more dissatisfaction over waiting time at the doctor's office than prepaid practice respondents.

PERCEIVED ACCESS AND SATISFACTION WITH MEDICAL CARE

Thus far we have considered perceived accessibility and satisfaction with care as separate dependent variables without taking account of possible relations between them. Not surprisingly, these two types of consumer beliefs and attitudes are interrelated.

The relations between the various measures of access and the two satisfaction indices are presented in Table 7.21. With only three exceptions, perceived access and satisfaction are significantly related. In general, perceived barriers to access tend to be associated with consumer dissatisfaction with medical care received. When all six measures of access are considered simultaneously in a regression equation, they account for 15.06 per cent of the variance in the index of satisfaction with own care and for 13.27 per cent of the variance in the index of satisfaction with child care.

The effects of membership in different health care plans on the two satisfaction indices remain statistically significant when the Blue Cross and prepaid practice samples are adjusted to take account of differences in perceived accessibility, though in the case of the index of satisfaction with own care the magnitude of the previously reported effect is substantially reduced. With the six measures of access controlled, health plan membership accounts for 1.70 per cent of the variance in the index of satisfaction with own care and for 2.95 per cent of the variance in the child care index.

The two satisfaction indices were also examined in relation to each of their individual difference correlates while controlling for the six measures of access. Each individual difference variable listed in Tables 7.14 and 7.16 was entered into regression equations for satisfaction with own and child care that already included the six measures of access. All but two of the individual difference correlates of satisfaction with own care, and all but two of the individual difference correlates of satisfaction with child care, remained statistically significant when the six access measures were controlled. The individual difference variables that

Table 7.21   Zero-Order Correlations Between Measures of Access and the Two Satisfaction Indices

Measures of Access	Index of Satisfaction with Own Care ($N = 712$) (r)	Index of Satisfaction with Child Care ($N = 385$) (r)
1. Reported time to get to doctor in minutes	$-.130$**	$-.130$*
2. Reports it is inconvenient to get to a doctor	$-.234$**	$-.276$**
3. Reported number of days wait to get an appointment	$-.073$	$-.072$
4. Reports difficulty in getting appointments	$-.303$**	$-.175$**
5. Reported waiting time at doctor's office in minutes	$-.034$	$-.186$**
6. Reports that waiting time at doctor's office is too long	$-.212$**	$-.226$**

* $p < .01$.
** $p < .001$.

were reduced to insignificance when the samples were adjusted for differences in perceived accessibility were marital status and major life changes for the index of satisfaction with own care, and respondent worries and readiness to seek medical care for children for the index of satisfaction with child care.

Since annual reenrollment periods coincided with the data collection period, we were able to examine the extent to which differences in satisfaction observed to exist between prepaid practice and Blue Cross participants would also translate into overt behavior. The results of the reenrollment period decisions showed that approximately 6 per cent of the prepaid practice enrollees chose to switch over to the Blue Cross insurance option. Less than 1 per cent of the Blue Cross participants changed their insurance coverage to the prepaid group practice plan. Thus the vast majority of prepaid practice respondents decided to remain with the plan rather than to change their insurance coverage. In comparison with Blue Cross participants, however, relatively fewer prepaid practice participants were willing to reenroll. These results are consistent with differences observed in consumer satisfaction. The fact that so few actually changed health plans must be attributed in part to inertia. When we asked in our survey about intentions concerning reenrollment, approximately twice the proportion of respondents who actually shifted in prepaid practice and Blue Cross indicated an intention to change plans.

What significance should be attached to the differences observed in reported satisfaction and in reenrollment behavior between prepaid and Blue Cross participants? One interpretation of the satisfaction and reenrollment results is that they arise from the fact that this study was based on a relatively new prepaid group practice. Participants had only between one and two years of experience with the plan, and for many of them prepaid group practice was probably relatively new and unfamiliar. The Blue Cross participants, on the other hand, were in the main continuing old and tried doctor-patient relationships. Thus the comparison of prepaid and Blue Cross participants may have been confounded by differences in length of exposure to the two plans and to participating physicians. Levels of satisfaction among prepaid participants may increase over time, and the differences in satisfaction between plans may ultimately disappear as prepaid participants establish continuing relationships with staff physicians. Consistent with this, one study has shown that satisfaction among prepaid group practice participants does increase over time.[56]

A contrary analysis is suggested by the writings of Eliot Freidson.[57, 58] Freed of client controls, physicians in prepaid group practice are said to be less responsive to their clients than physicians in conventional private practice. This is consistent with findings discussed in the previous chapter that physicians on capitation plans facing heavy patient work loads are more likely to characterize their patients as "trivial." In the study reported here some of the largest satisfaction differences observed involved questions dealing with physician responsiveness. In particular, prepaid practice participants were less satisfied with their doctor's apparent concern about their health (as well as their children's health), with the doctor's warmth and personal interest, and with the amount of information he or she tended to give.

Freidson also suggests that consumer dissatisfaction with prepaid group practice plans is a consequence of the attempt to rationalize the delivery of medical care through bureaucratic organization, with its rules and regulations (and associated mix-ups and confusions) and administrative personnel intervening between doctor and patient. Responses to two items not included in the satisfaction indices are consistent with Freidson's analysis of the negative impact of bureaucratization on consumer satisfaction. Prepaid participants were more likely than those enrolled in Blue Cross plans to indicate that the setting in which they receive their medical care has a clinic atmosphere that makes them feel like charity cases, and that their medical care setting is not well organized. When variation in these perceptions is controlled, the relations observed between health care plan membership and the two satisfaction indices are substantially reduced, though they remain statistically significant.

Although the specific findings are not reported here, the prepaid practice studied, like many others, has been successful in maintaining lower hospital admission rates, lower hospital costs, and significantly reduced out-of-pocket expenditures among enrolled members as compared with the competing Blue Cross–Surgical Care plans. These and other findings reinforce the point that each form of practice organization offers distinctive advantages and potential problems. The challenge we face is how to develop practice contexts and physician incentives that maximize the advantages of prepaid practice organization but that are also responsive to consumer perceptions and expectations.

Finally, this study examined the relationship between type of health care plan and access to medical care. Distances from the site of medical care were clearly different; prepaid practice respondents reported greater travel time and inconvenience than Blue Cross participants. Of course, in the metropolitan area in which the study took place prepaid group practice participants have only a single site for medical care, and people enrolled in Blue Cross plans are unrestricted in their choice of physicians and services. If prepaid group practice grows, and satellite clinics are established, we can expect some reduction in the differences observed between Blue Cross and prepaid practice participants with respect to travel time and inconvenience.

In addition, prepaid practice respondents were more likely than Blue Cross participants to report difficulty in obtaining an appointment, as well as a longer interval before getting the appointment. On the other hand, Blue Cross enrollees were significantly more likely than prepaid practice enrollees to complain about the waiting time at the doctor's office, and reported significantly higher average waiting times than did prepaid practice participants.

These results suggest a kind of trade off between the scheduling of appointments and waiting time on arrival. The prepaid plan may have adhered to a rigid appointment schedule, while fee-for-service physicians may have been more willing to try to squeeze people in even at the price of long waiting periods in the doctor's office. The two delivery systems appear to be dealing with a common problem (too many consumers relative to the supply of health care personnel) in different ways, with prepaid practice eliciting more consumer complaints about the scheduling of appointments and fee-for-service physicians eliciting more consumer complaints about waiting time on arrival.

This study has dealt with a particular practice context, and generalization to other contexts should be made with greatest care. Prepaid group practices differ from one another, but by studying a variety of such practices we will develop a better understanding of the assets and liabilities of this approach in the organization and financing of medical practice.

In this chapter we have focused on the gross relationship between type of health care plan (prepaid group practice versus fee-for-service) and consumer choice and response. One limitation, which is suggested by the previous chapter, is that we have not differentiated between the effects of prepaid practice as an organizational device and the effects flowing from the financial aspects of prepayment and salaried practice. A health care plan combines organizational and financial features. Health foundations, for example, provide patients with a prepayment plan, but tend to keep traditional patterns of organization and physician payment intact. Similarly, some group practices have many of the organizational features of prepaid practice, but operate on a fee-for-service basis. As refinements in evaluation efforts grow, we should examine more specifically the independent effects of group organization of physicians, the manner in which the physician is reimbursed, and the manner in which patients pay for their care.

NOTES

1. O. W. Anderson and P. B. Sheatsley (1959), *Comprehensive Medical Insurance: A Study of Costs, Use, and Attitudes Under Two Plans* (Chicago: Health Insurance Foundation), Research Series no. 9.

2. C. A. Metzner and R. L. Bashshur (1967), "Factors Associated with Choice of Health Care Plans," *Journal of Health and Social Behavior,* **8:**291–299.

3. B. Wolfman (1961), "Medical Expenses and Choice of Plan: A Case Study," *Monthly Labor Review,* **84:**1186–1190.

4. D. Mechanic (1972), *Public Expectations and Health Care* (New York: Wiley-Interscience), pp. 102–111.

5. D. Mechanic (1974), "The Comparative Study of Health Care Delivery Systems," *Research and Analytic Report Series,* 12–74, Center for Medical Sociology and Health Services Research, University of Wisconsin, Madison, Wisconsin.

6. S. Shapiro, S. L. Weiner, and P. M. Densen (1958), "Comparison of Prematurity and Perinatal Mortality in a General Population and in the Population of a Prepaid Group Practice Medical Care Plan," *American Journal of Public Health,* **48:**170–187.

7. S. Shapiro et al. (1967), "Patterns of Medical Use by the Indigent Aged under Two Systems of Medical Care," *American Journal of Public Health,* **57:**784–790.

8. R. L. Bashshur and C. A. Metzner (1967), "Patterns of Social Differentiation Between Community Health Association and Blue Cross-Blue Shield," *Inquiry,* **4:**23–44.

9. R. L. Bashshur and C. A. Metzner (1970), "Vulnerability to Risk and Awareness of Dual Choice of Health Insurance Plan," *Health Services Research,* **5:**106–113.

10. C. A. Metzner, R. L. Bashshur, and G. Shannon (1972), "Differential Public Acceptance of Group Medical Practice," *Medical Care,* **10:**279–287.

11. T. W. Bice et al. (1974), "Risk, Vulnerability and Enrollment in a Prepaid Group Practice and Disenrollment from a Prepaid Group Practice," unpublished manuscript, Center for Metropolitan Planning and Research, The Johns Hopkins University.

12. C. A. Metzner and R. L. Bashshur (1967), op. cit.

13. B. Wolfman (1961), op. cit.

14. A. T. Moustafa, C. E. Hopkins, and B. Klein (1971), "Determinants of Choice and Change of Health Insurance Plan," *Medical Care,* **9**:32–41.

15. T. W. Bice (1973), "Enrollment in a Prepaid Group Practice," unpublished manuscript, Department of Medical Care and Hospitals, The Johns Hopkins University.

16. R. Hetherington, C. E. Hopkins, and M. I. Roemer (1975), *Health Insurance Plans: Promise and Performance* (New York: Wiley-Interscience).

17. A. Yedidia (1959), "Dual Choice Programs," *American Journal of Public Health,* **49**:1475–1480.

18. O. W. Anderson and P. B. Sheatsley (1959), op. cit.

19. R. Hetherington, C. E. Hopkins, and M. I. Roemer (1975), op. cit.

20. T. W. Bice et al. (1974), op. cit.

21. O. W. Anderson and P. B. Sheatsley (1959), op. cit.

22. A. Donabedian (1969), "An Evaluation of Prepaid Group Practice," *Inquiry,* **6**:3–27.

23. M. I. Roemer and W. Shonick (1973), "HMO Performance: The Recent Evidence," *Milbank Memorial Fund Quarterly: Health and Society,* **51**:271–317.

24. R. Hetherington, C. E. Hopkins, and M. I. Roemer (1975), op. cit.

25. S. B. G. Eysenck and H. J. Eysenck (1964), "An Improved Short Questionnaire for the Measurement of Extroversion and Neuroticism," *Life Sciences,* **3**:1103–1109.

26. S. R. Garfield (1970), "The Delivery of Medical Care," *Scientific American,* **222**:15–23.

27. J. O. Jackson and M. Greenlick (1974), "The Worried-Well Revisited," *Medical Care,* **12**:659–667.

28. R. Hetherington, C. E. Hopkins, and M. I. Roemer (1975), op. cit.

29. Other differences were that, in the satisfaction study, more Blue Cross respondents than respondents in the prepaid practice plan were women and were unemployed.

30. Since many respondents gave several reasons for their choice, we aggregated the data to indicate what proportion of the sample mentioned each reason spontaneously.

31. As Table 7.4 shows, when the distribution of chronic illnesses among the two groups of respondents is tested for significance using X^2 rather than the F distribution, as was the case in the result presented in Table 7.3, the difference between prepaid practice and Blue Cross respondents does not achieve statistical significance.

32. Because of the small sample sizes on which these differences are based the results do not achieve statistical significance even though the percentage differences are relatively large.

33. In the satisfaction study sample the information concerning the health status of family members reflects the structure of the varying health care plans as well as patient characteristics and behavior.

34. D. Mechanic (1972), op. cit., pp. 102–111.

35. E. R. Weinerman (1964), "Patients' Perceptions of Group Medical Care," *American Journal of Public Health,* **54**:880–889.

36. A. Donabedian (1965), *A Review of Some Experiences with Prepaid Group Practice* (Ann Arbor: Bureau of Public Health Economics), The University of Michigan Research Series No. 12, pp. 7–47.

37. A. Donabedian (1969), op. cit.

38. M. I. Roemer and W. S. Shonick (1973), op. cit.

39. E. R. Weinerman (1964), op. cit., p. 885.

40. M. I. Roemer et al. (1973), *Health Insurance Effects: Services, Expenditures, and Attitudes Under Three Types of Plans* (Ann Arbor: University of Michigan School of Public Health).

41. O. W. Anderson and P. B. Sheatsley (1959), op. cit.

42. F. E. Gartside et al. (1973), *Medicaid Services in California Under Different Organizational Modes* (Los Angeles: University of California School of Public Health).

43. D. Mechanic (1972), op. cit.

44. N. M. Simon and S. E. Rabushka (1954), *A Trade Union and Its Medical Service Plan* (St. Louis: Labor Health Institute).

45. H. Schwartz (1972), *The Case for American Medicine: A Realistic Look at Our Health Care System* (New York: McKay), pp. 153–198.

46. In this and all subsequent tables, the two firms are treated as a single sample. When inserted as a dummy variable in a regression analysis, firm was found to be unrelated to either of the satisfaction indices. Furthermore, the interaction of firm and plan was not significant in relation to each of the satisfaction indices, suggesting that the effect of health care plan on satisfaction does not vary systematically depending on whether the analysis is carried out with respondents from one or the other firm.

47. Respondents with children over 12 only were also questioned about their satisfaction with medical care their children had received in the past year. These data are not reported here because they are viewed as more speculative than the data that are reported. Because respondents are probably less likely to accompany children over 12 to the doctor's office than children under 12, one would expect responses to satisfaction items dealing with child care to be more clearly anchored in personal observation for respondents with children under 12. Consistent with this expectation, relations between the index of satisfaction with child care and other variables are somewhat higher when respondents without children under 12 are excluded from the analysis.

48. In comparing the results obtained for the satisfaction indices, keep in mind that the samples are different since not all the respondents had children under 12 or used services for their children.

49. Married respondents whose spouses had received some medical services in the past year were questioned about their spouses' general level of satisfaction. In contrast to the use of multiple items in measuring satisfaction with own care and with child care, a single question was used to indicate spouses' satisfaction: "On the whole, is he very satisfied with the care he has received, somewhat satisfied, or is he not satisfied at all?" Blue Cross respondents attributed higher levels of satisfaction to their spouses than prepaid practice respondents ($p < .01$). Thus the proxy data for spouses' overall satisfaction is fully consistent with the previously presented satisfaction data.

50. The zero-order correlation between marital status and satisfaction with medical care ($r = .05$) was not statistically significant. Marital status only achieved significance when considered in conjunction with the respondent's employment status.

51. T. W. Bice and E. Kalimos (1971), "Comparisons of Health-Related Attitudes: A Cross-National, Factor Analytic Study," *Social Science and Medicine,* 5:283–318.

52. Significant zero-order correlations were observed between social desirability bias and satisfaction ($r = .08$), and between neuroticism and satisfaction ($r = .10$). However, neither social desirability bias nor neuroticism emerged significant when examined in conjunction with the other measured attitudinal variables.

53. The index of uncomfortable feelings and emotions and the index of worries were also significantly associated with satisfaction at the zero-order level ($r = .07$ and $r = .08$, respectively), though neither remained in the final equation.

54. D. P. Crowne and D. Marlow (1964), *The Approval Motive* (New York: Wiley).

55. Unstandardized rather than standardized regression coefficients are reported here because use of the latter statistic requires that the distribution of the independent variable in the sample approximate its true distribution in the population. This requirement was not met here. Prepaid practice participants are overrepresented relative to their actual proportions in the two firms from which the sample was drawn, and in the metropolitan area generally. These respondents were deliberately overrepresented to achieve adequate numbers in prepaid practice and Blue Cross. This allowed us to test for the effects of prepaid group practice in a way that would be maximally efficient and robust relative to the assumptions of multiple regression analysis. Unstandardized regression coefficients are appropriate to report because they are indifferent to marginal distributions on the independent variable. They are descriptive of differences between means, and may be interpreted as measures of effects.

56. R. L. Bashshur et al. (1967), "Consumer Satisfaction with Group Practice, The CHA Case," *American Journal of Public Health,* **57**:1991–1999.

57. E. Freidson (1960), "Client Control and Medical Practice," *American Journal of Sociology,* **65**:374–382.

58. E. Freidson (1961), *Patients' Views of Medical Practice* (New York: Russell Sage).

III
ILLNESS, ILLNESS
BEHAVIOR,
AND HELP-SEEKING:
IMPLICATIONS FOR
THE DESIGN OF
HEALTH SERVICES

Chapter 8

Illness, Illness Behavior, and Help-Seeking: Implications for Increasing the Responsiveness of Health Services

The effective design of medical care must take into account the complexity of motivation and behavior that affects how people define and respond to illness. Throughout this book I have maintained that the design of organizations for providing a personal service to clients, based on a set of special techniques but also on the use of the practitioner-client relationship as an instrument for change, requires detailed consideration of the varied needs of clients and their perceptions of services. In Part II we considered some of the structural factors that affect the behavior of physicians and the reactions of patients. In Part III we focus in much greater detail on the factors affecting the use of services and communication between practitioners and patients.

Although we usually conceive of medical care as a service sought by people experiencing significant disease and disability, we now know that the decision to seek medical care is based on a complex sociocultural process as well. In the following chapters we examine the processes of seeking help for psychological distress and for preventive medical services, the problems of communication that develop between physicians and patients, and some of the difficulties of achieving conformity with medical advice and changing people's behavior in a more healthful way. In this introduction I provide an overview of the problems related to patients' perceptions and responses.

In considering help-seeking processes, we should distinguish instances when an asymptomatic person seeks assistance, as in the case of most preventive and screening services, from those that involve some explicit complaint. Getting preventive care is in many ways like the consumption of other services—the consumer must weigh the benefits to be achieved against the costs expended. Although this may also characterize seeking care for acute complaints, processes involving the acutely ill are more complicated by complex psychological processes of attribution.

In the preventive health area the most commonly used model for research is the one developed by Rosenstock. The model is based on two classes of variables: the person's psychological readiness to take specific action, and the extent to which a specific course of action is believed to be beneficial. Thus, it involves a calculus of utility based on the perception of threat and the efficacy of the means to reduce it. Rosenstock suggests four variables that affect the process of decision: the person's perceived susceptibility to a particular threat, the perceived seriousness of the threat, and the benefits of, and barriers to, taking action. Since these variables do not theoretically account for the activation of behavior, Rosenstock adds a class of variables he calls "cues to action." These cues trigger behavior at a particular time. As Rosenstock explains:

It appears essential to include a factor that serves as a cue or a trigger to set off appropriate action. The level of readiness provides the energy to act and the perception of benefits (fewer barriers) provide a preferred path of action. However, the combination of these could reach quite considerable levels of intensity without resulting in overt action unless some instigating events set the process in motion. In the health area, such events or cues may be internal (e.g., perception of bodily states) or external (e.g., interpersonal interactions, the impact of media of communication, knowledge).[1]

From a practical standpoint, the model suggests that, by manipulating any combination of variables affecting action, the propensity to seek preventive care can be increased. Although the model has been useful for integrating various data on preventive health behavior,[2] its predictive power has been modest. In part this reflects the crudeness of measurement involved; in part, the complexity of many preventive health behaviors. Probably the most easily manipulated variable in the model is the "triggering forces," but these alone will only motivate persons who already have a propensity to seek a service. Most neglected in the model, and in action programs, are the environmental conditions facilitating a desired action. Does a person motivated to take some action know clearly how to do so? Are sites of service readily available and accessible? And are there facilities to assist persons who have difficulties with transportation, child care, or whatever? Too frequently preventive health programs activate desires for action, but do not provide adequate organizational arrangements to facilitate follow-up.

Much of the work on help-seeking has concentrated on persons who have symptoms of some kind, for which they either take or forego some action. Interest in illness behavior arises from an awareness that some patients with severe symptoms either do not seek help or delay for long periods before taking appropriate action. Much of the early work concentrated on the sociocultural characteristics of persons who sought help readily in comparison to those who delayed, but such work is of limited usefulness unless it further elaborates the social psychological processes that explain why there are differences in help-seeking in varying social classes, ethnic groups, and age and sex classifications.[3] Also, there is growing awareness of the extent to which the availability and organization of health services interact with sociocultural and psychological propensities to seek care. Although important differences in illness behavior among persons and social groups exist, overemphasizing them may lead to neglecting the extent to which such behavior is amenable to control by health care facilities and how they deliver services.

A major limitation of much research on illness behavior and help-seeking has been the failure to include the patient's symptoms or health status level as an important explanatory or control variable. In most circumstances the nature and quality of symptoms are a crucial determinant of the patient's attribution process and how it develops. Although much research indicates that symptoms that disrupt capacity to function and to follow usual routines are extremely important in decisions to take action, researchers have often conveniently ignored symptoms in their investigations because they are difficult to measure and may further involve practical problems of access to medical information.

An interesting development in illness behavior research is the growing concern with the processes of attribution, processes in which decisions are made about the meaning of symptoms and what to do about them. Attribution research attempts to locate the influences that affect how people interpret variations in their physical and psychological functioning. One theory of emotional behavior—the Schachter-Singer model[4] of the cognitive effects on emotional arousal—has been a valuable stimulus to this research. Briefly, this approach views emotion as a product of a state of arousal and the cognitive definition of it. It maintains that arousal is a general state, and is experienced differently depending on the meanings provided by social and environmental cues. Similar arousal, thus, may be experienced as happiness, anger, excitement, or whatever depending on the social context within which it occurs and the various meanings available to the persons who attempt to understand their experiences. The Schachter-Singer model has been usefully extended to the interpretation of drug effects[5] and the study of obesity[6] as well as to illness attributions. Although students of emotion differ in their views about the model's adequacy as a theory of emotions, it has served as a useful framework for research, and has stimulated a variety of interesting empirical inquiries.

One of the earliest attempts to apply attributional analysis to the study of illness behavior was Kadushin's description[7] of the stages of individual decision-making in seeking psychotherapy. He described these stages in a five-step model: (1) the person must decide that he or she has a problem and that it is an emotional problem; (2) he must decide whether and to what extent to discuss his problem with relatives and friends; (3) he must decide at some point that his present efforts to deal with the problem are inadequate and that some kind of professional help is needed; (4) he must choose an institutional sphere or profession that he feels can appropriately deal with the problem; and (5) he must select a particular practitioner.[8] Kadushin illustrates in his research how persons with varying sociocultural characteristics make different attributions and decisions, and he presents a theory of social circles in which he maintains that the probability of seeking psychotherapy is dependent on being part of a social network of persons who have either sought psychotherapy or know others who sought psychotherapy.

Although Kadushin focuses on "emotional" problems, the approach is amenable to the study of any type of symptom or problem, or the use of any type of service. For example, it is possible to study the factors leading to the initial recognition of symptoms, how the person explains the occurrence and cause of the symptoms, how causal attributions affect the types of remedies considered and adopted, how the person seeks information and chooses among various alternative search procedures, and how the person comes to seek a particular source of assistance.

As previously noted, the nature and quality of symptoms are important factors in at least directing the initial attributions. Some symptoms, such as a fractured leg, are so clear-cut and disabling that they allow very few socially acceptable attributions (or only one). Other symptoms are amenable to alternative meanings: myocardial pain may be perceived as indigestion; a severe headache as a manifestation of stress; and lack of energy may be defined as either a physical or psychological problem. The manner in which symptoms occur and their patterning provide varying opportunities for attributional creativity. Individuals are not entirely passive in response to symptoms. They engage in various exploratory and testing behaviors to assess the characteristics of their symptoms and the manner in which they respond to changes in personal behavior or in the environment. Unfortunately, although such testing behavior may appear to be psychologically rational, it may lead to severe consequences as in the case of the man with a myocardial infarction who tries to work off his pain with vigorous exercise.

The ordinary response to an unusual symptom is to engage in hypothesis testing that assists one in understanding its meaning. Symptoms occur very frequently. Most people, however, observe their symptoms over time, considering various possible explanations that might account for their occurrence. It is particularly when symptoms are acute, allow for few interpretations, involve indications where patients have been warned to seek care immediately, or are unusual or unfamiliar that persons more readily and quickly seek assistance. But the great majority of symptoms are explained away by easily available interpretations that allow their normalization. Sore muscles are explained by an unusual amount of recent exercise; a back pain by having sat in a particular chair too long; a headache by too much pressure on the job. In contrast, when individuals come to physicians alarmed about what appears to be a relatively innocuous complaint, the processes of attribution the person has engaged in, or the social context of the person that shapes the meanings he or she arrived at, may well have triggered a sense of threat. Physicians who work in emergency rooms often complain about the high proportion of patients with nonurgent complaints. But the doctor's idea of urgency may be very different from that of the patient who has attempted to make sense of particular symptoms and problems, and who has become alarmed.

When students first began using drugs like marijuana and LSD, for example, the untutored student experimenting with such drugs would occasionally appear at an emergency room in panic that was interpreted by physicians inexperienced with drug reactions as psychotic behavior. These students had not been adequately prepared for a "bad trip" and would become frightened, fearing that they were "going crazy." Such reactions were less likely among the experienced user or the student taking drugs in the company of experienced users.[9] As drug use has become more commonly a part of the general student culture, these reactions appear to be less frequent. Similarly, physicians who have had more experience with such problems are less likely to perceive the panic as a psychotic episode.

Any symptom can be attributed to either internal or external causes. Such attributions of causality may be influenced by the particular qualities of the symptoms, but may be influenced by other factors as well. Thus, anxiety may be perceived as a response to a forthcoming event, such as an examination or other situation in which a person's self-esteem may be under threat, or it may be seen as due to some inherent biological or psychological characteristic unrelated to any specific environmental threat. It is through such causal attributions that the significance of one's experience takes shape. For example, as I observe my colleagues at the Center for Advanced Study, each of whom has a year to pursue research work or writing without other obligations, I sense a certain common anxiety. We all know that when we are at our own universities an unproductive semester or year can be attributed to our teaching or committee obligations or other deterrents to research and writing. But an unproductive fellowship year cannot easily be attributed to external causes—failure to produce can only be attributed to oneself. Consistent with this is the observation that scientists are more likely to seek psychotherapeutic help when they are "hung up" in their scientific work.[10] Some individuals attribute being "hung up" to a basic failure of the self, not to the nature of their work or to external deterrents.

The processes of attribution change over time as different ideas are tested. If indigestion is attributable to having eaten rich and exotic foods, do the symptoms subside when one returns to a more bland diet? If the headaches have been caused by pressures on the job, do they persist when one goes on vacation? Many of these informal tests of hypotheses are rational and may be used by physicians, too. However, there may be also serious discrepancies between patients' attributional tendencies and their modes of hypothesis-testing, and the medical realities of their situation. For example, patients may minimize the importance of symptoms for considerable periods of time, thus delaying appropriate help. The symptoms that trigger alarm and activate the help-seeking process are not necessarily those of greatest medical significance. Chest pain or cancer symptoms that appear in a relatively innocuous form—interfering, at least initially, in no significant way with life routines—may be neglected. Public education may be particularly valuable in such cases. Education campaigns alert people to the importance of the symptoms, and thus short-circuit the attributional process, as seen in the public information campaigns on the major signs of cancer requiring a medical checkup. Devising appropriate public campaigns can be extremely difficult, however; in the case of chest pain, for example, the nature of the information provided could result in either far too many or far too few people seeking medical attention. Learning how to provide the optimal communication will require considerable communications research as well as a clear concept of what symptoms require evaluation and treatment.

Since health professionals commonly deal with problems that involve considerable uncertainty—either because it is difficult to assess the nature of the problem or because scientific knowledge about assessment or management is lacking or contradictory—they too must engage in various attributional processes that are more social in character than medical. Some professionals may come to emphasize an external cause for particular symptoms; others may pursue various hypotheses concerning internal biological or psychological processes. Such variations are particularly characteristic of schools of psychological and psychiatric treatment, which may give more or less emphasis to genetic and biological aspects, early development, environmental stressors, and social conditioning. The psychodynamic schools invariably encouraged their patients to adopt an internal causal framework for their problems; new schools based on social learning theory emphasize external causal sequences. Bandura states the distinction well from a social learning perspective:

The content of reconstruction is highly influenced by the interviewer's suggestive probing and selective reinforcement of content that is in accord with his theoretical orientation. Heine, for example, found that clients who were treated by client-centered, Adlerian, and psychodynamic therapists tended to account for changes in their behavior in terms of the explanations favored by their respective interviewers. Even a casual survey of interview protocols would reveal that psychotherapists of different theoretical affiliations tend to find evidence for their own preferred psychodynamic agents rather than those cited by other schools. Thus, Freudians are likely to unearth Oedipus complexes and castration anxieties, Adlerians discover inferiority feelings and compensatory power strivings, Rogerians find compelling evidence for inappropriate self-concepts, and existentialists are likely to diagnose existential crises and anxieties. It is equally true that Skinnerians, predictably, will discern defective conditions of reinforcement as important determinants of deviant behavior.[11]

The attributions patients make—and sometimes those health professionals make—are shaped by the climate of thinking and general theoretical conceptions dominant in the society at large. At the height of influence of psychodynamic theory, patients were more inclined to explain their difficulties in terms of developmental or sexual problems; similar problems are now more commonly conceived in terms of defective interpersonal relationships, distorted family structures, barriers to self-actualization, and even social and political repression. The meanings people use in arriving at attributions depend on their awareness and knowledge of alternative theories.

Changes in professional definitions of the causes for given problems can have enormous practical significance. For example, during World War II when soldiers showed evidence of personal disorganization under the stress of battle conditions, they were evacuated to psychiatric units where they were given psychodynamic treatment. The focus on early life events in this treatment as a means of explaining behavior in combat provided an internal cause to explain the soldier's performance, and considerable secondary gain in the form of exemption from further combat service. Such soldiers tended to focus on their "personal problems," and it became very difficult to return them to the front lines. In contrast, during the Korean War personal disorganization in combat was frequently defined as a common occurrence resulting from combat conditions. Soldiers were treated on the front lines, and personnel treated their reactions as normal responses to sustained stress. Using this treatment strategy, it became much easier to guide the soldier through the situation and return him to a functioning status.[12] Similar experience has now become commonplace in the ordinary practice of community psychiatry.[13]

In short, the way in which persons conceptualize their problems will affect the extent to which they experience secondary pain and distress. By secondary pain, I refer not to the distress caused by the symptom or problem, but to the painful meanings that may be associated with the definition of the problem. It is less painful, for example, to explain a student's failure as due to lack of interest or to a mode of studying than to stupidity. Similarly, social failures are less painful when the locus of control is seen outside the person than when they are attributed to personal defects or failures. It is more respectable to be unemployed because of structural unemployment than because of laziness or incompetence. Some students of suicide have suggested that the relatively low rates of suicide among blacks as compared to rates of homicide is a product of causal attributions. They argue, for example, that blacks are more likely to attribute failures to social constraints; persons with fewer social constraints on their achievement are more likely to blame themselves for their failures and distress. Thus, the theory argues, blacks are more likely to express aggression outwardly, and whites more typically engage in self-aggression.[14]

Much work remains in adequately describing the sequence of forces affecting how people come to conceptualize problems. The practicalities of research have resulted in an emphasis on cross-sectional investigation in contrast to longitudinal efforts, and thus it is exceedingly difficult to unravel the interaction of influences that trigger help-seeking. In the chapter that follows, James Greenley and I explore selective processes into care through an epidemiological study of the help-seeking process. Among the questions we address are: What is the role of the magnitude of symptoms on the decision to seek care and the type of care sought? To what extent do social and cultural factors affecting help-seeking have their influence through their effect on the occurrence of symptoms, on general inclinations to seeking help, or on specific types of help-seeking? Are social and cultural factors more powerful in affecting the decision to seek help, or in determining the type of help sought? We pay attention to the magnitude or intensity of symptoms rather than to their particular configuration. Increasingly, we will have to pay more attention to the specific aspects of varying problems. Traditional psychotherapeutic approaches, for example, have not defined rigorously the more specific components of patients' diffuse complaints. Since the form of therapy was approximately the same, regardless of the symptoms, and since the emphasis was on developmental processes, the careful classification of symptoms has not been a high priority. A useful corrective has been the growth of social learning approaches to psychotherapy that require clear specification of the patient's problems and specific goals for therapy. As Bandura notes:

> One of the major obstacles to the development of effective change programs arises from the failure to specify precisely what is to be accomplished, or the common practice of defining the intended goals in terms of hypothetical internal states.

When the aims remain ambiguous, learning experiences are haphazard, and whatever procedures are consistently applied tend to be determined more by personal preferences of change agents than by clients' needs.

The appropriate methods and learning conditions for any given program of behavioral change cannot be meaningfully selected until the desired goals have been clearly defined in terms of observable behavior. Rapid progress is further assured by designating intermediate objectives, which delineate optimal learning sequences for establishing the component behaviors of more complicated social performances. The necessity for behavioral specification of objectives is most clearly illustrated in the case of complex patterns of behavior which cannot be achieved with any degree of success until they are analyzed into essential constituent functions.[15]

The need to develop priorities in the ordinary treatment of problems in medicine, with both intermediate and long-range objectives, is reflected in the growing adoption of the problem-oriented record.

ALTERNATIVE APPROACHES TO THE PATIENT IN AMBULATORY MEDICAL CARE

Delineating problems and specifying goals is a particularly acute issue in ambulatory medical care where it is often difficult to untangle the forces motivating the patient to seek care from the symptoms and problems the patient presents. Although much has been written about the patient's "hidden agenda," it has been difficult for investigators interested in such problems to study underlying motivations in any rigorous way or to develop better techniques for their clinical recognition and management. The dilemma of the physician in managing such psychosocial problems within the context of a busy practice has already been described. Here I wish to suggest some preliminary thoughts about how the management of such problems is affected by the organization of care and the conceptual models that physicians typically use. The possible approaches can be illustrated by an example from the world of jurisprudence.

In Western legal systems, courts have an elaborate body of statutes that serve as guideposts for adjudicating disputes. When a case is brought before a court, the role of the judge is to settle the dispute through existing rules, and not to examine the motivation of the parties for bringing the issue to the court or to attempt to understand the hidden agenda (the real motivations that lead the litigants to focus on the manifest question before the judge). The judge may fully realize that the real dispute may not be what it appears to be: the patient may have brought a suit against a physician because he is furious at what he perceives to be the physician's lack of interest in his case, and not because he truly believes that the physician committed a legal fault; the district attorney may have arrested a group of prostitutes for political reasons or because they would not cooperate in providing the police with information, rather than because they violated the law; shoplifters may be prosecuted occasionally because the store wishes to make an example of them to deter others. Judges may be aware that very few of such disputes reach the court, but they see their role and responsibility as applying the relevant legal principle—not searching to understand the problems and conditions that resulted in the dispute coming to court.

Other legal systems operate differently. For example, let us look at the judicial process among the Barotse, a tribe in Northern Rhodesia, studied by Max Gluckman.[16] Judges in this context commonly perform their function by exploring in depth the nature of the dispute that brings the issue to the court, and by attempting to resolve the basic conflicts and disagreements among the parties involved. The judges seek a great deal of information beyond the basic dispute, allowing each contestant to tell his tale in full and encouraging the participation of other interested parties as well. Particularly in kinship disputes, the aim of the judge is to keep kin united and to maintain the integrity of the village; the judge sees his main role as reconciling the parties to the dispute and reaching a compromise judgment.

Our concern here, of course, is with modern medicine and not with the assumptions of our legal system. Like the typical Western judge, most physicians have limited concepts of problems and diseases that they feel are relevant to their sphere of action, and they tend to focus on the symptoms the patient presents, often ignoring the underlying motivations that have led the patient to visit the doctor. But increasingly, primary care physicians are being asked to give less attention to disease concepts and differential diagnosis, and more to understanding the patient's basic troubles. They are being asked to function more like a Barotse judge, and less like a modern Western judge.

Although there is widespread appreciation that illness, and even infectious disease, arises from complex interactions between agents, environment, and characteristics of the patient, physicians have not felt able to deal efficaciously with the sociocultural, environmental, and psychological concomitants of disease. Nor have many felt a legitimate right to move too far beyond the patient's specific complaint, in a way that would involve more intimate aspects of the patient's life style and personal associations. Thus, the pragmatic approach has been to search for "disease." Despite growing indications that this strategy has limited usefulness in ambulatory care and in coping with the growing proportion of chronic, degenerative, and psychosocial problems, it has been difficult to develop an effective strategy for dealing with these problems. Part of the problem arises from the traditions of medical practice, the sources of its dominant theories and approaches, its present organization, and its dominance over the work of other health professionals who might approach the patient's problem from other points of view. Part stems from the uneven knowledge we presently have and the intractability of many chronic and behavioral problems. And still another part stems from the view of many physicians that they lack a mandate to meddle in patients' life situations.

Yet the fact is that much of the work of the physician in ambulatory medical practice concerns psychosocial problems. First, there are those problems of generalized distress often associated with a variety of somatic and psychophysiological indications. Patients frequently complain of diffuse physical distress or lack of vitality concomitant with disruption in sleep, appetite, and the like. These symptoms are difficult to manage. Like fever, they may be indicative of a wide range of diseases or of life distress in general. Second, the possible etiological significance of psychological stress, and distress, in a variety of illnesses requires the physician to take such factors into account, although causal relationships between stress and illness remain hazy. Third, almost every major disease with which a physician deals has important psychosocial consequences for the patient and his or her family and may involve such issues as self-esteem, family role organization, interpersonal relationships, employment, and functional capacity. The course of these associated problems may have a crucial effect on the patient's physical functioning, and the degree to which the condition becomes disabling and disruptive. How these problems are handled may affect the degree of secondary pain and disability. Although physicians often recognize the presence of these problems, they frequently feel impotent in dealing with them, and thus may ignore them as a way of coping with their own sense of discomfort. Linda Aiken, in her study of the response to myocardial infarction, explores some of the difficulties inherent in the management of these patients, and suggests some alternative approaches (see Chapter 12).

In dealing with psychosocial dimensions of illness, physicians have lacked techniques in which they have confidence. Although some new ways of modifying behavior have proved to be effective in various instances, physicians have been slow to adopt them or to work with other professionals who can effectively use them. Although physicians may not be the most appropriate practitioners to use behavior modification techniques, many patients requiring such services come to physicians, and the system of care must be capable of either providing the necessary service or providing effective referral.

Neither the training of the physician nor the dominant mode of organizing care allows effective use of health professionals knowledgeable about social learning approaches and group techniques. Nor does the existing economic structure of medical practice facilitate the use of less expensive treatments applied by personnel other than physicians. The fee-for-service structure induces the provision of discrete services that consume minimal time, and physicians who spend a great deal of effort dealing with patients' problems are at an economic disadvantage. Similarly, salaried practice typical of prepaid groups, as presently organized, involves such heavy patient loads as to make psychosocial care relatively minimal. In recent years a variety of successful experiments have been carried out using nurse-practitioners, physician-assistants, family counselors, ombudsmen, and the like. If such innovations are to be implemented as part of the pattern of practice, the remuneration structure must in some fashion include payment for these functions. At the present time, for example, physicians and health units have little incentive to devote attention to the social care of the aged, although such care may contribute more to the health and functioning of the aged than far more expensive (and routinely provided) medical care.[17]

The economic structure of medicine and its organizational auspices do little to encourage the effective use of other helping resources in the community. Physicians do a poor job in coping with alcoholism, drug abuse, and obesity, but neither are they well informed about the potential group supports for such patients in the community such as Alcoholics Anonymous. Medical dominance, and the arrogance about treatment sometimes associated with it, leads to ineffective mobilization of community resources in responding to common problems of living. The effective mobilization of support networks would contribute a great deal to reducing the burden on primary medical care, leaving more time for dealing in greater depth with those problems requiring a physician's care.

THE CHARACTER OF DOCTOR-PATIENT TRANSACTIONS

Patients tend to have ambivalent attitudes about physicians. They feel extremely dependent on physicians when they anticipate or have serious illness; they also feel some resentment about their dependence and the authority of the physician. This is perhaps exemplified by the tendency to speak favorably about one's personal physician, but to be critical of physicians in general. Underlying this ambivalence are often very high and somewhat unrealistic expectations of the physician and excessive criticism of any failures to live up to this ideal image. Physicians are expected to be technically skilled, highly competent, dedicated, compassionate, interested in patients, available whenever needed—in short, godlike. To be moody, distracted, critical, hurried, or to behave in typically human ways leads to severe criticism, even condemnation. More educated and sophisticated patients appear to feel especially ambivalent about their dependency and the authority of the physician, knowing that physicians, like other professionals, have only a narrow expertise, but wanting at some level to believe in the mystique of the physician.

The doctor-patient relationship, to a larger degree than most other formal relationships, includes important irrational components. Of course, all human relationships, and particularly those involving love, marriage, and the family, steer some course between rationality and unconscious forces. But among more formally structured relationships in society, doctor-patient relationships display enormous richness and complexity in emotions and behavior.

Although interesting for their own sake, social psychological investigations of doctor-patient interactions are particularly important because of the strong tendency of economists, industrial engineers, systems analysts, and many others working on health policy issues to view medical relationships narrowly. They tend to approach the doctor-patient relationship as a highly rational transaction, and give little attention to the processes that affect patient and physician motivations, communications, and mutual influence. Policy solutions that lack sensitivity to the psychological dimensions of doctor-patient interaction may be highly destructive to the more intangible aspects of the physician's role and to the physician's usefulness to the patient.

Psychological factors affect the behavior of the physician as well as the patient. It would be a mistake to assume that physicians are not drawn to patients who have certain characteristics: attractiveness as persons, social status, the ability to make physicians feel valued for the services they provide, and having an interesting and challenging medical problem. Although the values of medicine prescribe universalistic behavior, and thus help minimize their consequences, such preferences still operate in subtle ways. Physicians are not unaffected by their background and experience. What they value will inevitably affect how they carry out their tasks, and may even affect such important decisions as willingness to resuscitate patients.[18, 19]

Personal authority and the structure of the clinical situation enhance the physician's influence. Many of the supportive and treatment effects of medical care depend on the physician's suggestive powers and credibility.[20] We know a great deal, for example, about the power of placebos, and about how placebo effects may be enhanced or eroded in different practice circumstances.[21] As the physician's function becomes more technical and less holistic, the possibilities to make use of these suggestive powers become more limited.

One of the key issues in doctor-patient relationships is the ability of the physician to achieve the patient's cooperation in adhering to advice. As the chapters by Bonnie Svarstad and Linda Aiken illustrate, physician-patient communication can become complex, and the problem in communicating advice often stems from the physician's inadequacies, the assumptions the physician makes, or the structure of the clinic situation. As Svarstad points out, much of the literature has dealt with failures to adhere to advice in terms of deficiencies in the understandings and characteristics of patients, but the difficulty often resides in the communication process itself and in the inconsistent ways in which physicians address themselves to the task. Physicians, as Svarstad points out, are frequently unclear about what they expect the patient to do. This lack of clarity may result from physicians' assumptions that patients share their conceptual understanding of the situation, their feeling that the format in which their instructions are followed is not particularly important, or poor and confusing communication. Physicians give great attention to properly assessing and treating the patient's problem, but devote little effort to improving adherence to advice.[22]

THE DILEMMA OF THE PHYSICIAN'S AUTHORITY

As the movement toward public accountability gains momentum, and as people increasingly come to feel that they should have control over decisions affecting their bodies, challenges of the physician's authority and modes of practice become more common. The movement itself is ideological and is not attuned to the subtleties of medical interactions or the real complexities embodied in medical practice. It is implied that it is relatively easy for the physician to communicate to the patient the risks and benefits of various actions. Although physicians can surely do more than at present in educating patients and in facilitating their choice of treatments and risks, there are complex trade-offs involved that often get lost in rhetorical flourishes.

First, with the growth of medical knowledge and technology, the determinations involved may in fact be extremely complex and difficult to communicate. Second, communicating risks to persons not conversant with medicine may unduly alarm them, and lead them to irrational choices. Moreover, seriously ill patients are often anxious and upset and not in a position to weigh the pros and cons of various alternatives objectively. Also, physicians are very busy, and inordinate amounts of time spent in trying to help patients understand the risks and benefits of various alternatives may make it impossible to meet other needs of the patient, or to take care of other patients. Finally, to the extent that the physician's thinking process and uncertainties are made clear and explicit, the opportunities to achieve gains in the patient's morale—and even condition—from the suggestive influences of the medical situation may be seriously undermined.

To achieve beneficial outcomes for their patients, physicians may withhold information. For example, when they prescribe drugs that they feel the patient must take, doctors may say little about adverse effects either because they do not want to frighten the patient away from taking the drug, or because they feel the information may contribute toward these side effects. We know that the placebo effect can also produce adverse side effects[23]—patients given inert drugs report a variety of disturbing symptoms. In short, many physicians feel that acting in the interests of their patients involves managing information, not telling the patient everything there is to know or that can be communicated. They are aware that sharing information may have its own adverse side effect—patients may become alarmed, depressed, or irrational. It is no easy matter to weigh the benefits to the patient of full information against attempts to maximize possible therapeutic outcomes. Nevertheless, physicians usually trust their own intuition rather than seek hard evidence to evaluate under what conditions information is harmful. Perhaps it would be wiser to err on the side of fuller revelation since patients should, to the extent possible, make the decisions about undertaking risks.

Professionals characteristically believe in their autonomy in their work, and that in practice situations their judgment—not formal rules and regulations or bureaucratic procedures—is paramount. Physicians see themselves as having special knowledge and expertise derived from scientific training and clinical experience that make their judgments in matters of practice superior to those of the uninitiated. The practice of medicine extends well beyond its science, however, and encompasses broad social and ethical issues. Physicians often treat these as technical issues, but in fact have no special knowledge in these areas. Moreover, patients, regardless of physicians' claims of autonomy, retain certain legal rights of consent. Claims are increasingly made by patients and their attorneys that consent was violated, introducing significant strains in the practice of medicine.

In the rise to professional status, a profession must achieve the public's recognition and acceptance of its special claims. Until recently the claims of the physician had wide acceptance. Acceptance is still widespread, but the legitimacy of these claims has been eroded by public criticisms of the profession, by the increased sophistication of consumers, by the growing organization and militancy of other health professions that are increasingly challenging the special position of the physician, and by the changing character of medical care itself, which is undermining the very special ties between patients and individual physicians. As these new political conditions arise, the opportunity for physicians alone to define the limits of their autonomy is increasingly challenged, and although the fall of the high standing does not appear imminent, physicians in the future will no doubt have to give up part of their autonomy to other health workers. The changing nature of medical organization will require it, as will the growing political forces working to restrict the dominance of medicine.

NOTES

1. I. Rosenstock (1969), "Prevention of Illness and Maintenance of Health," in J. Kosa et al., eds., *Poverty and Health: A Sociological Analysis* (Cambridge: Harvard University Press), p. 178.
2. M. Becker, ed. (1974), "The Health Belief Model and Personal Health Behavior," *Health Education Monographs*, **2**:entire issue.

3. D. Mechanic (1969), "Illness and Cure," in J. Kosa et al., eds., op. cit.

4. S. Schachter and J. Singer (1962), "Cognitive, Social and Physiological Determinants of Emotional State," *Psychological Review,* **69**:379–399.

5. H. Becker (1974), "Consciousness, Power and Drug Effects," *Journal of Psychedelic Drugs,* **6**:67–76.

6. S. Schachter (1968), "Obesity and Eating," *Science,* **161**:751–762.

7. C. Kadushin (1958), "Individual Decisions to Undertake Psychotherapy," *Administrative Science Quarterly,* **3**:379–411; and (1969), *Why People Go to Psychiatrists* (New York: Atherton).

8. C. Kadushin (1958), op. cit., pp. 386–387.

9. H. Becker (1967), "History, Culture and Subjective Experience: An Exploration of the Social Basis of Drug-Induced Experiences," *Journal of Health and Social Behavior,* **8**:163–177.

10. P. L. Giovacchini (1960), "On Scientific Creativity," *Journal of the American Psychoanalytic Association,* **8**:407–426.

11. A. Bandura (1969), *Principles of Behavior Modification* (New York: Holt, Rinehart and Winston), p. 9.

12. A. J. Glass (1958), "Observations upon the Epidemiology of Mental Illness in Troops During Warfare," *Symposium on Preventive and Social Psychiatry* (Washington, D.C.: Walter Reed Army Institute of Research).

13. G. Caplan (1964), *Principles of Preventive Psychiatry* (New York: Basic Books).

14. A. F. Henry and J. F. Short, Jr. (1954), *Suicide and Homicide* (New York: Free Press).

15. A. Bandura (1969), op. cit., pp. 111–112.

16. M. Gluckman (1965), *The Ideas in Barotse Jurisprudence* (New Haven: Yale University Press).

17. See H. Smits and P. Draper (1974), "Care of the Aged: An English Lesson?" *Annals of Internal Medicine,* **80**:747–753.

18. D. Sudnow (1967), *Passing On: The Social Organization of Dying* (Englewood Cliffs, N.J.: Prentice-Hall).

19. L. Lasagna (1970), "Physicians' Behavior Toward the Dying Patient," in O. Brim, Jr. et al., eds., *The Dying Patient* (New York: Russell Sage).

20. J. Frank (1961), *Persuasion and Healing* (Baltimore: Johns Hopkins Press).

21. D. Mechanic (1968), *Medical Sociology: A Selective View* (New York: Free Press), pp. 185–189.

22. P. Ley and M. S. Spelman (1967), *Communicating with the Patient* (London: Trinity Press).

23. G. Honigfeld (1964), "Non-Specific Factors in Treatment: In Review of Placebo Reactions and Placebo Reactors," *Diseases of the Nervous System,* **25**:145–156.

Chapter 9

Patterns of Seeking Care for Psychological Problems

James R. Greenley and
David Mechanic

We have explored how patients come to seek care from ambulatory medical care facilities and the degree to which the design of medical services facilitates responsive care. Primary care physicians are, of course, only one of many sources of help for psychosocial difficulties, and a large variety of agencies and self-help groups have emerged to assist people with personal problems. In recent years sociologists and other social scientists have explored the processes through which persons in distress define themselves as having problems, interpret the nature of these problems, decide to seek assistance, and identify and choose among the available alternatives. As was suggested in the previous chapter, such decisions generally depend on the quality and nature of symptoms, on people's interpretations of symptoms and attributions of cause, on sociocultural characteristics and their effect on defining and encouraging appropriate uses of varying sources of assistance, and on the availability and accessibility of various kinds of help.

Those seeking help from agencies offering psychological services have repeatedly been found to have social and cultural characteristics different from those who do not seek assistance.[1-3] The basis of these relationships is not fully clear, since there may be several alternative ways in which social and cultural characteristics can come to be associated with the use of particular sources of assistance. Persons with certain characteristics may be more likely to experience personal problems, and thus more commonly seek assistance. Or these sociocultural characteristics may be indicative of differing propensities to use helping services or different attitudes toward problems and seeking assistance. Further, it is not clear if sociocultural propensities are related to help-seeking because they reflect a generalized dependency syndrome, or because they come to be linked to very specific kinds of services. Since most studies of help-seeking for personal problems have been restricted to a single source of help, such as psychiatric services, they are not particularly helpful in clarifying which of these varying possibilities most closely fits the facts. Also, since most studies fail to measure need for service explicitly (as reflected in symptoms or health level), they provide no opportunity to examine the role of varying levels of problems and distress in help-seeking.

Kadushin[4] and Gurin et al.[5] attempt to deal with some of these issues and present similar models of help-seeking behavior. Both models include the process of identifying the problem, the decision to seek help, and the choice of a particular therapeutic resource. Along with other descriptive studies of both community and national samples, the Kadushin[6] and Gurin et al.[7] studies have found that individuals who can be classified as follows are overrepresented among users of outpatient psychiatric and counseling services: higher educational level, higher income level, urban or suburban background, Jewish identification, low religious participation, and female. University student populations have been studied with similar results. In general, the following types of students are overrepresented among psychiatric clinic users: women,[8-10] older students,[11-12] students with fathers of higher status backgrounds,[13-14] urban or suburban residence,[15-16] Jewish identification,[17-18] lack of religious affiliation,[19-21] lack of religious activity,[22-24] and study concentration in the humanities or social sciences.[25-27] Although the types of differences reported vary, some of the findings are impressively consistent.

A variety of explicit and implicit interpretations have been suggested to account for the pattern described above. One view is that sociocultural differences encompass underlying factors affecting the overall tendency to seek assistance. Srole et al.,[28] for example, maintain that women use more services than men for psychological problems because they are more willing to accept a dependent position. Henry and associates[29] view the overrepresentation of persons with Jewish backgrounds as resulting from a particular inclination toward introspection in the Jewish culture. Other interpretations focus on sociocultural factors as determinants of the type of help sought. For example, Kadushin[30] suggests that different social circles encourage the use of diverse types of professionals. He found that higher status persons and those who were not religious were more likely to use psychotherapists in analytic clinics, and that lower status persons and those with greater religious affiliations were more likely to be drawn to religious-based counseling clinics. Gurin and his colleagues[31] suggest that, while the more educated tend to seek help for personal problems from psychiatrists, the less educated more commonly visit lawyers and welfare agencies with their problems. Overall, Gurin et al. present the most complex discussion concerning these sociocultural effects, concluding that certain factors such as sex and age largely affect the decision to seek help; others such as religiosity and income influence the choice of a professional; and still others such as education and urban background influence both decisions.[32]

An alternative view is that sociocultural differences in seeking help reflect the occurrence of psychological distress and personal problems among different subgroups in the population. Snyder and his associates,[33] for example, consider this alternative and suggest, somewhat inconclusively, that sociocultural differences cannot be explained in terms of varying levels of pathology among relevant subgroups. One of the more suggestive studies to date compares users and nonusers of a university psychiatric clinic in terms of sociocultural characteristics, controlling for the number of personal problems reported.[34] Although Scheff's data are crude, they provide substantial support for the contention that sociocultural determinants of the use of a psychiatric clinic are particularly strong among students with lower levels of distress. Since Scheff's study was confined to a single helping agency it does not allow exploration of the sociocultural determinants of seeking different types of help, and thus provides no further illumination of the hypotheses suggested by Gurin and associates and Kadushin. In this chapter, we expand the analysis of these issues by examining the sociocultural determinants of help-seeking; the sociocultural determinants of choice of particular sources of help; the role of psychological distress in help-seeking and choice of practitioner; the occurrence of distress in varying sociocultural subgroups; and the relevance of sociocultural determinants controlling for distress.

PROCEDURES

The data reported here come from the first wave of a panel study of university students. Although the data are taken from a cross-sectional analysis, the issues we examine involve a process that occurs over time. Our ideal would have been to study a very large population over time to identify persons in the population who have varying kinds of problems and those who seek different types of care. But the effort and cost of such a study, particularly if it included objective independent data and respondent reports, are prohibitive. Thus, it seemed more reasonable to employ a compromise methodology that allowed comparison of the characteristics of a random sample of a defined population with those in this defined population who sought care for personal problems and psychiatric distress. Detailed data were gathered from a random sample of a university student population.[35] In addition, data were also gathered from samples of students seeking assistance at a university psychiatric outpatient service and at a university counseling service.[36]

A self-administered questionnaire was mailed to a random sample of the university population, and with repeated follow-ups we attained an 82 per cent response rate including 1502 respondents. Students applying for help at the university psychiatric and counseling services were given the identical questionnaire. Of the psychiatric outpatient service applicants, 63 per cent or 156 applicants returned the questionnaire. Of applicants to the university counseling service, approximately 50 per cent or 58 applicants returned the questionnaire.[37]

Respondents were asked whether they had discussed personal problems with any of a wide variety of professional and nonprofessional agencies or individuals within the last three months. Using these responses, five subgroups of the random sample were distinguished, each representing users of one of the following sources of help: (1) psychiatric services, including the university outpatient psychiatric service, a local community mental health center, and private psychiatrists; (2) the university counseling service; (3) clergymen; (4) medical services, including the student health service and private physicians (nonpsychiatrists); (5) other formal agencies such as women's counseling center and a telephone suicide prevention center.[38] These subgroups of the random sample are not mutually exclusive. A student, for example, may report having seen both a psychiatrist and a religious counselor; approximately 18 per cent of help-seeking students appear in more than one of these user groups.[39]

Several indicators of psychological distress and personal problems were used. Two such indices will be reported on here, although the others yielded comparable results. First, we used a 52-item problem checklist taken in large part from Scheff's[40] 58-item student problem inventory. The items cover academic problems, physical and psychophysiological symptoms, and family, religious, financial, and other personal problems. The inventory was developed on the basis of presenting complaints of patients coming to the student psychiatric clinic.[41] Second, we used Langner's[42] 22-item screening scale of psychiatric symptoms with minor modifications in wording and response categories. This list of primarily psychobiological symptoms to some extent confounds symptoms characteristic of physical and psychiatric illness, but it is the scale most frequently used in community epidemiological surveys. Since the group involved in this study is young and has a low prevalence of physical illness, such confounding is probably limited in this sample. Studies by Langner[43] and Manis[44] provide data validating the ability of this scale to distinguish between treated and community populations, but the Dohrenwends,[45] Phillips and

Clancy,[46] and Seiler[47] have all properly noted certain biases in the scale. We use the scale, therefore, with full awareness of its problems, and with the belief that it is a crude measure of level of psychological distress. None of the measures used take into account symptoms characteristic of acute psychoses or behavior disorders. Such items were included in the questionnaire but occur with low prevalence in both the general population and the psychiatric sample. Such items were incorporated in one of the scales we developed, but this scale did not yield results that significantly varied from those on which we report.

RESULTS

In Table 9.1 we compare the sociocultural attributes of applicants to the psychiatric and counseling service with the attributes of those in the random sample. Substantial differences emerge between the sociocultural characteristics of the help-seeking samples and the random sample. The largest differences are found with respect to the two measures of psychological distress.[48] In addition, compared to the random sample, applicants to the psychiatric service are more likely to be women, of Eastern European ancestry, and from the northeastern part of the United States. Their families have higher social and educational backgrounds and less involvement in a religion. Students in the psychiatric sample are more likely to be Jewish or to have no religious affiliation, less likely to be Catholic, and are less likely to engage in religious activity. They are also less likely to be lower classmen and most likely to be studying in the humanities, social sciences, or fine arts. There were no evident differences by age within the limited age range of the sample, by marital status, or by urban background.

When applicants to the counseling center are contrasted with students in the random sample on these sociocultural characteristics, a somewhat different picture emerges. Although applicants to the counseling center are more likely to be women, to be lower classmen, and to be in the younger age group, they are less likely to be married. In short, we find systematic differences in the two help-seeking samples, with the exception of sex.

Since the sociocultural factors are themselves intercorrelated, some may be spuriously associated with help-seeking. Therefore, we examined this issue using Goodman's[49,50] suggested analysis of multivariate contingency tables. For example, father's religious activity may be related to the use of psychiatric services due to its association with the student's religious activity. Multivariate models examining both variables relative to the use of psychiatric services allow an assessment of whether father's religious activity remains important when the student's activity is controlled. Controlling for student's religious activity, father's activity is not associated with seeking psychiatric help. Similarly, none

Table 9.1. Social Characteristics and Symptom Scores of the Psychiatric, Counseling, and Random Samples

Social and Demographic Characteristics	Student Group				
	Random Student Sample	Outpatient Psychiatry Sample	Difference (%)	Student Counseling Sample	Difference (%)
Sex (% female)	38.1[a]	48.7	10.6*	67.2	29.0***
Age (% 19 or under)	26.3	19.9	− 6.4	39.7	13.4*
Marital status (% married)	20.4	18.7	− 1.7	8.8	−11.6*
College year (% freshmen, sophomores, or juniors)	53.7	43.0	−10.7*	72.4	18.7**
Religion:					
(% Jewish)	7.9	18.3	10.4***	14.8	6.9
(% Catholic)	29.6	12.0	−17.6***	29.6	0.0
(% none, agnostic, or atheist, i.e., nonaffiliated)	22.4	45.7	23.3***	29.6	7.2
Respondent's religious activity (% never participate)	20.3	39.1	18.8***	20.7	.4
Father's religious activity (% never participate)	14.5	27.1	12.6***	16.3	1.8
Birthplace (% from northeastern U.S.)	9.8	23.9	14.1***	13.0	3.1

Ancestry (% Eastern European)	9.7	22.3	12.6***	19.6	10.0
Father's education (% postgraduate)	22.3	34.1	11.8***	15.8	6.5
Father's occupation (% with Duncan occupational score of 80 or more)	20.5	30.7	10.2**	20.7	.2
Major field of study (% humanities, social sciences, and fine arts)	39.5	57.8	18.3***	47.9	8.3
Problem and symptom scores					
Life problem count (% reporting 27 or more problems)	23.8	51.9	32.1***	43.1	19.4**
Langner 22-item screening score (% with score of 9 or more)	21.8	54.4	32.6***	39.7	17.9**

[a] Sample sizes are 1502 for the random, 156 for the psychiatry sample, and 58 for the counseling sample except where, due to missing data, they may be slightly smaller. Significance levels are based on chi-square analyses with $df = 1$.

* $p < .05$.
** $p < .01$.
*** $p < .001$.

of the following variables was found to be significantly related to seeking psychiatric care when controlling for the variables in parentheses: Jewish identification (birthplace in Northeast, Eastern European ancestry); father's education (no religious affiliation, student's religious activity); father's occupational status (birthplace in Northeast); majoring in the social sciences, humanities, and fine arts (birthplace in Northeast). The following variables were not found to be spuriously related to application for psychiatric assistance: sex, college year, having no religious affiliation; non-Catholic identification; student's religious activity, birthplace in Northeast, and Eastern European ancestry. A similar analysis regarding applicants to the counseling center found that women were not significantly overrepresented among those seeking help when age or marital status was controlled. Age, marital status, and year in college were factors remaining significantly related to counseling center use when sex was controlled. Since these variables may be related to help-seeking through a common relationship to various attitudes and behavioral orientations, these findings are difficult to interpret. Without a clearer causal model than is presently available, it is difficult to offer an obvious explanation.

The size of the random sample allows further comparisons of students who sought different types of assistance. Within the random sample, those who report seeking psychiatric assistance are significantly more likely to be women, in the older age groups, and to have fathers with higher educational status. Those who used psychiatric services were also more likely to report majors in the social sciences, fine arts, and humanities. Students in the random sample who reported using the counseling center were significantly more likely to be of Eastern European ancestry and to have fathers of higher educational status. Those who sought help from religious counselors, as might be expected, were significantly more likely to be Catholic, to be more religious, and to have more religious fathers, and were significantly less likely to have no religious affiliation. Users of other formal help agencies were significantly more likely to be Catholic and were older (see Table 9.2).

As we noted earlier, those who seek help report higher levels of psychological distress than are evident in the random sample (see Table 9.1). Yet the differences between the random sample and the populations of those who sought help are smaller than one might anticipate. For example, 22 per cent of the students in the random sample have a score of 9 or more on the Langner scale, but only 54 per cent of the psychiatric applicants have a comparably high score. Thus, approximately one-fifth of the random sample reports greater distress than approximately half of the psychiatric applicants. Applicants to the counseling center also report more symptoms and problems than the general population. Although the levels of distress reported are somewhat higher among the psychiatric applicants, differences between this group and applicants to the counseling center are not statistically significant. Within the random sample, those who report seeking help from psychiatry or counseling have levels of distress very similar to those characteristic of the samples of applicants to those facilities (see Table 9.2). As before, those who seek assistance from the counseling center report somewhat lower levels of distress relative to those seeking assistance from psychiatry. Students consulting religious counselors have distress scores closely resembling students going to the counseling center. Those who report seeking assistance from nonpsychiatric physicians or other formal sources of help have distress levels that are not significantly different from the random sample as a whole.

Since levels of distress are of great importance in the help-seeking process, we had to assess to what extent sociocultural predictors of help-seeking are spuriously related to seeking assistance due to their association with the occurrence of symptoms and problems. Thus we examined the factors related to help-seeking that might differentiate students with high and low distress levels and problem scores. These analyses were carried out within the psychiatric sample, the counseling sample, and the random sample.

We found no statistically significant differences in distress and problem levels in any of the three samples with respect to Jewish or Catholic origins, having a religious affiliation, religious activity, father's religious activity, father's education or occupation, or ancestry. Students in the psychiatric sample who were born in areas other than the Northeast (largely from Wisconsin) reported more problems than those from the Northeast, but this difference was not apparent in the other two samples. There were no statistically significant differences in the counseling sample, due in part to the smaller size of the sample.

In the random sample there was a statistically significant tendency for students in the humanities, social sciences, and fine arts to report more psychological distress than those in other fields; younger students, those who were unmarried, and lower classmen also reported more problems. These differences, however, are generally small and of limited practical significance. However, women both in the random sample and in the psychiatry sample were significantly more likely to report psychological distress, regardless of the measure used, although there were no significant sex differences in the counseling center sample. In short, only the sex variable yielded statistically significant differences in more than one sample. Thus it seems unlikely, except for this single exception, that the sociocultural influences on help-seeking can be explained by the occurrence of distress in varying sociocultural subgroups.

Nevertheless, further analyses regarding these possibly spurious relationships were undertaken using Goodman's multivariate contingency table analysis. The models examined include use of a particular helping service, a sociocultural factor, and the Langner measure of psychological distress.[51] Hold-

Table 9.2. Sociocultural Factors and Psychological Distress in Help-Seeking Subgroups of the Random Sample

Sociocultural Variables	Total Random Sample	Help-Seeking Subgroups of the Random Sample					
		Psychiatric	Counseling	Religious	Medical	Other Formal Agencies	All
Sex (% female)	38.1	67.7***	33.3	42.5	54.6**	38.1	42.2
Age (% 19 or under)	26.3	8.8*	43.3	37.5	26.1	23.0	24.9
College year (% freshmen, sophomores, or juniors)	53.7	41.2	70.0	52.3	58.6	45.3*	49.9
Religion (% nonaffiliated)	22.4	15.2	17.2	5.0*	14.1	23.4	18.0**
(% Catholic)	29.6	36.4	27.6	52.5**	28.2	35.7*	34.6*
Religious activity (% never participate)	20.3	29.4	16.7	0.0***	18.2	20.9	18.4
Father's religious activity (% never participate)	14.5	18.6	13.8	2.6**	13.8	16.1	15.0

Ancestry (% Eastern European)	9.7	17.2	25.0*	6.1	11.5	12.8	13.0
Father's education (% postgraduate)	22.3	47.1*	46.7*	12.5	21.6	27.4	27.3
Major field (% humanities, social science, and fine arts)	39.5	63.6**	51.7	44.7	48.3	41.5	45.0
Problem and symptom scores							
Life problem count (% ≤27)	23.8	50.0***	36.7	47.5***	29.6	21.3	26.0
Langner 22-item screening score (% 9 or more)	21.8	55.9***	40.0*	35.0	22.7	24.7	26.3*
N^a	1502	34	30	40	88	239	365

[a] Significance levels for tables are based on chi-square analyses ($df = 1$) with Ns varying slightly from those given due to small amounts of missing data.

* $p < .05$.
** $p < .01$.
*** $p < .001$.

ing the Langner index values constant, the relationships between all but one of the sociocultural predictors of help-seeking at either the psychiatric service or the counseling center remain statistically significant.[52]

The only exception in the above analysis concerned the influence of sex in relation to the psychiatric help-seeking sample. Holding distress constant, sex is no longer significantly related to applying for psychiatric care ($X^2 = 2.05$, df = 1, $p > .05$). The sex differences remain, however, in comparison of the counseling center sample with the random sample and between the users and nonusers of psychiatric services within the random sample.[53] In short, sociocultural differences between help seekers and nonhelp seekers persist when symptom levels are held constant.

As a further step, we examined the data for interaction effects such as the observation by Scheff[54] that sociocultural selection in help-seeking is greatest among those with lesser as compared with more severe symptoms. For the most part, we could find no statistically significant interactions.[55] However, examining the data as a whole, there is evidence that selection on certain sociocultural factors is somewhat smaller among persons with more severe problems. But the picture that emerges is not consistent from one sample to another; at best, these data provide only very weak support for the interaction hypothesis.

Since the overrepresentation of women among those seeking help is one of the most consistent findings in the literature, the relationship of sex, distress, and use of services is particularly interesting. Within the psychiatric applicant sample, women are more likely to be overrepresented among those with more symptoms and problems. Careful reading of Scheff's[56] study indicates that, although his data generally support the hypothesis that sociocultural selectivity is greatest among those with fewer problems, he has a statistically significant reversal on the sex variable. Scheff reports, consistent with our observations, that women are overselected into psychiatric care particularly in the higher distress groups. Although neither Scheff nor we have a plausible interpretation for this reversal, the consistency of the finding is intriguing. Examination of students who sought other types of assistance does not reveal the same pattern.

The data obtained from our random sample of students allow us to ask whether selection into helping relationships on the basis of sociocultural factors is a generalized response or if it is more specific to particular types of helping agencies. Table 9.2 provides comparisons of the total random sample with subgroups within the random sample seeking various types of assistance in relation to sociocultural factors. Although the number of students seeking each type of assistance is relatively small within the random sample, it is encouraging to find such consistency between this analysis and the one dealing with the special psychiatry and counseling center samples. The final column in the table includes all students who appear in any of the help-seeking subgroups of the random sample. A comparison of this subgroup with the total sample shows relatively little difference. Only three characteristics yield statistically significant differences, and the magnitude of these relationships is small and of little practical significance.

However, the table shows much larger selectivity for seeking particular types of assistance. Those seeking psychiatric assistance include disproportionate numbers of women; older students; those whose fathers have had postgraduate education; those majoring in the social sciences, fine arts, and humanities; and those with more distress and problems. Those who sought assistance from the counseling center include disproportionate numbers of students of Eastern European ancestry, having fathers with postgraduate education, and having high levels of distress. As noted earlier, those attracted to religious counseling have more significant religious affiliations and also more problems. Those reporting seeking help for personal problems from nonpsychiatric physicians are disproportionately women, a finding that is consistent with almost every study on medical utilization. Finally, those seeking help from other formal agencies show only small variations from the random sample as a whole, although two of these differences achieve statistical significance.

It is worthy of note that degree of psychological distress and life problems can affect the type of assistance people seek. The highest levels of distress are reported by those seeking psychiatric care, followed by those seeking help from clergymen and counselors. Lower levels of distress are found among those seeking other types of formal assistance. We should keep in mind that many formal help-giving agencies are organized around specific problems—draft counseling, academic assistance, drug information, and the like. Students going to these sources might have very specific problems, but generally have levels of distress no greater than the population at large. In contrast, psychiatric and counseling agencies have rather diffuse therapeutic functions and attract students with a wide variety of troubles.

There are two cautions in attempting to generalize from these data. Students and student helping services might be quite different from community populations and their helping resources and, thus, generalized distress may bring nonstudents to available categorical helping agencies. Particularly in situations where there is more stigma associated with seeking psychological services than in a student group, one might anticipate that persons seeking categorical assistance on the average have higher levels of distress than in the population at large. Certainly it has been maintained, with some supporting data, that persons seeking assistance from lawyers, nonpsychiatric physicians, and the like generally have high levels of distress. A second caution is that we have aggregated a wide variety of agencies in the "all other formal agency" group, thus averaging the sociocultural differences that might exist among such agencies. Also, while most of these other formal agencies are probably sought out by persons with relatively lower levels of distress, users of certain categorical agencies may be highly distressed. A much larger sample would be required to examine the factors affecting the use of each of these agencies in a more specific and detailed way.

Lower levels of social and cultural selectivity found in the medical and other formal help-seeking groups may also be due to the way the question was asked. A major difficulty faced in a cross-sectional study is that one attempts to ask a simple question that characterizes a complex attribution process through which a person attempts to understand and define what he is feeling. Although we were fully aware of the problem, no very good solution was available. We anticipated that if we used the words "psychological" or "psychiatric," many students would not admit to having such problems or seeking help for them. Thus, we compromised and asked students whom they had consulted concerning "personal problems." The difficulty, of course, is that this designation, like the others, is open to a variety of interpretations and possibilities for denial and rationalization. The meaning of the word is perhaps less ambiguous for the student with a frank psychiatric difficulty, but it is not clear what types of help-seeking from a nonpsychiatric physician would and would not be considered personal problems. Thus, students might not consider a viral respiratory condition a personal problem, but might include such problems as venereal disease, birth control advice, or an allergy within this designation. To the extent that students defined the concept of "personal problem" very broadly, they would tend to approximate the random sample in their social characteristics. We know, however, that students were quite selective in indicating that they talked with nonpsychiatric physicians about personal problems since such reports were much less common than the actual use of medical facilities.

DISCUSSION

Several conclusions appear to be warranted on the basis of our data. First, our findings are consistent with those of many other studies—people from a defined population seeking assistance for personal or psychological problems have social and cultural characteristics that differ from those found in the population who do not seek comparable assistance. However, few studies have examined the possibility that such factors emerge because different social and cultural groups may experience different levels and types of distress. Our findings suggest that, for the most part, this possibility can be discarded.

Largely for convenience, most studies by sociologists ignore the magnitude of symptoms and distress, since such variables are difficult to measure and pose significant methodological problems. Nevertheless, it is foolhardy to neglect in any sophisticated model of the help-seeking process the variable that is the single most important predictor of seeking certain types of assistance. We have found that selectivity by reported distress and problems is strong both in the special help-seeking samples and in the comparable help-seeking subgroups of the random sample. Despite this, however, we can confirm what other studies have reported; many more people reporting high levels of psychological distress choose not to seek help than do so.

It is unlikely that our findings result merely from limitations in our measures of personal or psychological distress. The findings are consistent across a range of psychological distress measures incorporating various levels of severity and modes of expression of distress, such as those linked with psychophysiological reactivity, mood disorders, and common life problems. Somewhat unexpectedly, we found that levels of distress were related not only to help-seeking but the particular types of assistance sought. Students seeking psychiatric assistance reported higher levels of distress than those consulting counseling services or clergymen, and in turn these students were higher on distress than students consulting other formal helpers. It would be useful to attempt to replicate this finding in various contexts before attributing too much significance to it. If sustained, this finding would suggest that distress is not only a trigger toward seeking help, but also contributes to shaping the nature of the decision process. On an intuitive level, it is obvious that persons in difficulty attempt to match their specific difficulty with an appropriate helper. In this case, however, the students seeking assistance from different agencies are expressing similar types of distress, and the differences observed relate to the magnitude of the reported distress.

We have also examined students' reported propensities to seek assistance from physicians and from professionals dealing with psychological problems.[57] Those students who sought help both in the special samples and in the random samples reported considerably higher levels of help-seeking inclination. Because of the cross-sectional nature of these data it is impossible to ascertain whether these are preexisting tendencies or whether students report higher inclinations to seek help because they have actually done so. This problem exists despite our attempts to obtain information from help-seeking respondents at the time of their application for service and before they might have received care or been otherwise influenced by the agency.

There are some curious aspects to these various help-seeking inclination measures. In general, regardless of the measure of help-seeking inclination or the type of practitioner mentioned (physician versus professional dealing with psychological problems), those who sought psychiatric assistance report higher help-seeking tendencies in both the special samples and in the random sample. In every instance, students who did not seek formal assistance are lower on the inclination to seek care measures. These data suggest that there might be a generalized dependency attitude related to seeking help for psychological problems. We have not been able to find any strong predictors of these generalized attitudes toward seeking assistance for psychological problems. Once again, the most consistent predictor is sex; as anticipated, women report higher inclinations to seek help, but these sex differences are relatively modest. It may be that the type of generalized dependency encompassed by such measures is developed in early socialization and requires different types of predictors than ones included in our study.

Our data are consistent with the following interpretation. Although persons may have varying thresholds to perceive personal problems, the probability of perceiving a problem and the desire to take some action increases as psychological distress increases. Distress triggers a decision-making process that is conditioned by the person's socialization and sociocultural context. Sociocultural factors reflect various attitudes, orientations, family and peer pressures, and social circles that may contribute to orienting persons who perceive problems toward an appropriate and acceptable source of help. To a large extent the distress component and the sociocultural influences operate independently of one another. Although we carefully examined the data for interaction effects on the assumption that sociocultural selectivity would probably be greatest when the symptom levels were more modest, the evidence of this was weak. This may be because we studied reasonably competent young adults with some history of success in coping as evidenced by admission to the university. As we noted, there was relatively little extreme psychotic symptomatology in this population; distress was mainly characterized by anxiety, depression, and psychophysiological discomfort. Other studies suggest that if we included more extreme and bizarre psychotic manifestations, interaction effects may have appeared. When a person is violent, hallucinating, and blatantly violates ordinary standards of behavior, processes of social control or help-seeking are likely to be initiated regardless of sociocultural context.[58] Although the source of care used appears to be largely conditioned by sociocultural processes, and levels of distress, perhaps a more generalized dependency orientation may play some part in the selection of a helping practitioner.

In short, the model fitting these data is very similar to those suggested by Kadushin and Gurin and associates. Although most sociological studies have only focused on the sociocultural aspects, a more sophisticated understanding clearly requires consideration of level and type of distress as well as a richer view of the attribution processes by which persons come to perceive they have a problem, define the nature of the difficulty, and proceed on the pathway of finding appropriate assistance.[59]

NOTES

1. G. Gurin, J. Veroff, and S. Feld (1960), *Americans View Their Mental Health* (New York: Basic Books).
2. T. J. Scheff (1966), "Users and Non-Users of a Student Psychiatric Clinic," *Journal of Health and Social Behavior,* 7:114–121.
3. C. Kadushin (1969), *Why People Go to Psychiatrists* (New York: Atherton).
4. Ibid.
5. G. Gurin et al. (1960), op. cit.
6. C. Kadushin (1969), op. cit.
7. G. Gurin et al. (1960), op. cit. Cf. pp. 332–339.
8. C. B. Kidd and J. Caldbeck-Meenan (1966), "A Comparative Study of Psychiatric Morbidity Among Students at Two Different Universities," *British Journal of Psychiatry,* 112:57–64.
9. L. S. Linn (1967), "Social Characteristics and Social Interaction in the Utilization of a Psychiatric Outpatient Clinic," *Journal of Health and Social Behavior,* 8:3–14.
10. T. J. Scheff (1966), op. cit.
11. R. M. Boyce and D. S. Barnes (1966), "Psychiatric Problems of University Students," *Canadian Psychiatric Association Journal,* 11:49–56.
12. T. J. Scheff (1966), op. cit.
13. Ibid.
14. B. R. Snyder and M. J. Kahne (1969), "Stress in Higher Education and Student Use of University Psychiatrists," *American Journal of Orthopsychiatry,* 39:23–35.
15. L. S. Linn (1967), op. cit.
16. T. J. Scheff (1966), op. cit.
17. S. H. King (1968), "Characteristics of Students Seeking Psychiatric Help During College," *Journal of the American College Health Association,* 17:150–156.
18. T. J. Scheff (1966), op. cit.
19. R. M. Boyce and D. S. Barnes (1966), op. cit.
20. J. S. Davie (1958), "Who Uses a College Mental Hygiene Clinic?" in, B. M. Wedge, ed., *Psychosocial Problems of College Men* (New Haven: Yale University Press).
21. S. H. King (1968), op. cit.
22. Ibid.
23. L. S. Linn (1967), op. cit.
24. T. J. Scheff (1966), op. cit.
25. R. M. Boyce and D. S. Barnes (1966), op. cit.
26. M. A. Davidson and C. Hutt (1964), "A Study of 500 Oxford Student Psychiatric Patients," *British Journal of Social and Clinical Psychology,* 3:175–185.
27. T. J. Scheff (1966), op. cit.
28. L. Srole, T. S. Langner, S. T. Michael, M. K. Opler, and T. A. C. Rennie (1962), *Mental Health in the Metropolis: The Midtown Manhattan Study* (New York: McGraw-Hill).
29. W. E. Henry, J. H. Sims, and S. L. Spray (1968), *Public and Private Lives of Psychotherapists* (San Francisco: Jossey-Bass).

30. C. Kadushin (1969), op. cit.

31. G. Gurin et al. (1960), op. cit.

32. Investigators such as Linn (1967) op. cit. and Vailant who report sociocultural differences in seeking help are difficult to place in the context of this discussion because they focus on only one type of professional helper or incorporate no measure of psychological distress. See G. E. Vailant (1972), "Why Men Seek Psychotherapy: I. Results of a Survey of College Graduates," *American Journal of Psychiatry*, **129**:645–651.

33. B. R. Snyder and M. J. Kahne (1969), op. cit.

34. T. J. Scheff (1966), op. cit.

35. This population consisted of all students registered at the University of Wisconsin at Madison on November 20, 1971, including graduate and professional students.

36. These students were all from the population from which the random sample was drawn. They were applicants, but not necessarily recipients of service; for example, some students were referred elsewhere and others were told they did not need professional services. No student appears in more than one of these samples.

37. For each of these samples, available record sources were used to assess systematic differences between respondents and nonrespondents. Using university record sources, 156 nonrespondents in the random sample who were enrolled in the College of Letters and Sciences were compared with a random sample of 97 respondents. The nonrespondents were significantly older: 18.6 per cent of the respondents and 8.2 per cent of the nonrespondents were age 19 or under ($\chi^2 = 6.02$, df $= 1$, $p < .05$). Of the nonrespondents, 8.2 per cent were from the South, but only 1 per cent of the respondents were from that region (difference significant with $\chi^2 = 7.13$, df $= 1$, $p < .01$). After we developed acceptable intercoder reliability, each student was coded as either having no evidence of psychological problems or possibly having such problems. A larger percentage of nonrespondents (10.1 per cent) than of respondents (2.1 per cent) were rated as having psychological problems ($\chi^2 = 10.30$, df $= 1$, $p < .01$). Congruent with this finding, more nonrespondents (33.5 per cent) than respondents (20.6 per cent) had been placed on strict university probation ($\chi^2 = 4.91$, df $= 1$, $p < .05$). Similarly, 11.4 per cent of the nonrespondents had dropped out of the university, as compared to 4.1 per cent of the respondents ($\chi^2 = 4.02$, df $= 1$, $p < .05$). As might be expected, therefore, a tendency existed for nonrespondents to be referred to and to have had contact with psychological and counseling professionals more often. This suggests that the random sample underestimates the degree of psychological distress in the population.

Respondents and nonrespondents among applicants to the student outpatient psychiatric clinic were compared, using screening forms completed by applicants at the time of their initial visit to the clinic. Because several different forms were used by the clinic during the course of our study, we examined the one completed by most students (87 respondents and 49 nonrespondents). More respondents (34 per cent) than nonrespondents (15 per cent) had fathers with high status occupations as indicated by their having Duncan occupational scores of 80 or greater ($\chi^2 = 10.31$, df $= 2$, $p < .01$). All respondents had living mothers; the mothers of 8 per cent of the nonrespondents were dead ($\chi^2 = 4.73$, df $= 1$, $p < .05$). Respondents were somewhat more likely to report that their fathers were dead or that their parents were divorced. In no other instances were significant differences between respondents and nonrespondents found, including comparisons on treatment for emotional problems and a set of diverse symptom items.

Finally, using screening forms completed by applicants on their first visit, comparisons were made between the 58 respondents to the student counseling center and the total group of applicants from whom responses might have been obtained. While 25 per cent of the total sample were 19 years old or less, 40 per cent of respondents fell in this age range ($\chi^2 = 6.49$, df $= 1$, $p < .05$). No significant differences were found by sex, marital status, college year, or region of birth.

38. These other formal agencies or professionals were: school and private psychologists; social workers; T groups; a women's counseling service; a telephone suicide prevention center; vocational rehabilitation, family court, and draft counseling organizations; a veteran's hospital; a community law office and lawyers; university administrators.

39. From 23 to 29 per cent of each group seeking psychiatric, counseling, religious, or medical services for personal problems also reported having been to another formal agency, but only 16 per cent of the total sample reported using these formal agencies. Of users of counseling services, 30 per cent reported seeking medical help for personal problems, compared to 6 per cent of the total sample who reported similar use of medical service. In no other case were more than 12 per cent of one group also represented in another group.

40. T. J. Scheff (1966), op. cit.

41. A measure not reported here but giving consistent results was a sum of these reported problems weighted by the student's report of the seriousness of that problem.

42. T. S. Langner (1962), "A Twenty-Two Item Screening Score of Psychiatric Symptoms Indicating Impairment," *Journal of Health and Human Behavior*, 3:269–276.

43. Ibid.

44. J. Manis, M. Brawer, C. L. Hunt, and L. Kershner (1963), "Validating a Mental Health Scale," *American Sociological Review*, 28:108–116.

45. B. P. Dohrenwend and B. S. Dohrenwend (1969), *Social Status and Psychological Disorder* (New York Wiley-Interscience).

46. D. L. Phillips and K. J. Clancy (1970), "Response Biases in Field Studies of Mental Illness," *American Sociological Review*, 35:503–515.

47. L. H. Seiler (1973), "The 22-Item Scale Used in Field Studies of Mental Illness: A Question of Method, a Question of Substance, and a Question of Theory," *Journal of Health and Social Behavior*, 14:252–264.

48. Since checks on response biases within the random sample suggest that respondents underrepresent the magnitude of distress in the student population, symptom level differences between the random and help-seeking populations may be slightly smaller than those reported here. Yet given the relatively high response rate and the limited suspected distortion, such bias can account only for a small proportion of the differences between the two populations.

49. L. A. Goodman (1972), "A General Model for the Analysis of Surveys," *American Journal of Sociology*, 77:1035–1086.

50. L. A. Goodman (1973), "Causal Analysis of Data from Panel Studies and Other Kinds of Surveys," *American Journal of Sociology*, 78:1135–1191.

51. All variables were dichotomized as in Table 9.1. Chi-squares were examined for three variable models incorporating all two-way classifications in contrast to Chi-squares for models that incorporated as given only the Langner index-use of services classification and the Langner index-social variable classification [cf. L. A. Goodman (1972), op. cit.].

52. Within the random sample a multiple regression analysis of these questions leads us to the same conclusion, although in themselves these multiple regression analyses are inconclusive due to the skewed dependent variables (use of services) which make the results suspect.

53. Females remained significantly overrepresented in the counseling center user group ($\chi^2 = 16.59$, df $= 1$, $p < .001$) and the psychiatric services user group ($\chi^2 = 9.21$, df $= 1$, $p < .01$).

These results suggest that our finding regarding the special psychiatric outpatient sample should not lead us to conclusions based on it alone. Rather, it might more cautiously be interpreted as a random finding of little substance.

54. T. J. Scheff (1966), op. cit.

55. Following Goodman (1972, 1973), op. cit., models incorporating all two-way classifications as given were examined to see if they adequately fit the data in the case of each three-variable model. The one significant interaction occurs among year in college, the Langner index, and use of all other formal help sources by a sub-group of the random sample. A model incorporating all two-variable associations among these three variables does not fit the data ($\chi^2 = 32.48$, df = 1, $p < .001$). Since no other set of variables including these variables exhibited any significant interaction, this finding might most appropriately be attributed to chance.

56. T. J. Scheff (1966), op. cit.

57. D. Mechanic and J. R. Greenley (1974), "The Prevalence of Psychological Distress and Help-Seeking in a College Student Population," *Social Psychiatry*, in press.

58. D. Mechanic (1968), *Medical Sociology: A Selective View* (New York: Free Press).

59. D. Mechanic (1972), "Social Psychologic Factors Affecting the Presentation of Bodily Complaints," *New England Journal of Medicine*, **286**:1132–1139.

Chapter 10

The Utilization of Preventive Medical Services by Urban Black Mothers

Doris P. Slesinger

The success of preventive and curative health services depends on the ability of health care providers to reach persons who require services. Simply eliminating economic barriers is not enough. If services are not made accessible and easy to use, health care providers may still fail to reach the individuals and families most in need of them. The failure to use services often results from inhibitions related to personal and community patterns of behavior and association. Understanding these inhibitions can help us design programs that will effectively reach those who are most in need. The following study on the use of preventive medical services is one attempt to locate those factors that encourage the effective use of preventive services.

INTRODUCTION

The utilization of preventive medical services[1] has been studied from many different perspectives: the economic, the social psychological, the organizational, and the sociodemographic.[2] Most of these studies, however, are concerned with the separate effects of each of these factors. This research proposes one model that encompasses all of these elements. Specifically, this study explains differentials in preventive medical behavior in terms of the reiative strengths of four levels of behavioral influence—the individual's demographic characteristics, the features of the immediate social setting, the individual's health attitudes and orientations, and the characteristics of the delivery system used by the individual. Figure 10.1 shows the interrelationships among the concepts.

Socioeconomic characteristics are measured here by mother's education, family income, and family head's occupation. Social setting describes the relationships a person has with primary and secondary groups. Operational measures of primary relationships include household composition (e.g., husband-wife unit, mother living alone with children, or mother with children living in an extended family); number and spacing of children; and frequency of visiting friends and relatives. Ties with secondary groups are measured by membership in clubs and organizations, frequency of reading newspapers or watching television, frequency of church attendance, length of residence in city, and so on. Medical orientation[3] represents the individual's attitudes toward and knowledge of health and health institutions, as measured by an index of health knowledge, one of propensity to seek a doctor's care, and a measure of general attitudes toward preventive health care. In Figure 10.1, delivery system refers to the medical systems available to the public: outpatient hospital clinics or emergency rooms, group practices, private physicians, and nonhospital clinics.

The dependent variable is an index of preventive medical behavior that was constructed from items about use of medical services for prenatal and postpartum care of the mother, immunizations for the infant, and regular physical checkups for both the mother and child.[4]

Although Figure 10.1 shows relationships between background characteristics and utilization of services, there are ambiguities about the suggested direction of some of the relationships. For example, previous research on preventive

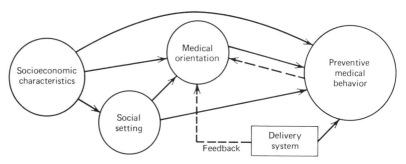

Figure 10.1.   Sociocultural model of preventive medical behavior.

health services utilization suggests that experiences in dealing with the medical system influence the attitudes persons have about that system. Such feedback sequences are shown by dotted lines in the diagram.

In general, then, the figure suggests that current socioeconomic characteristics such as income and education are a starting point for explaining utilization differentials. These characteristics affect what we call "social setting," which includes the type of family unit in which a mother lives as well as various ties to relatives, friends, social clubs, and more impersonal organizations. At the same time, the socioeconomic characteristics also help to determine values, attitudes, and beliefs. Of course these values, attitudes, and beliefs are also affected by the social contacts each mother has developed through the years. Thus, any patterns of behavior we examine will be affected by all three components—the socioeconomic status level, the social setting, and the medical orientations of the individual. In addition, society restricts the choice of institutions from which a mother may obtain the health care she desires. This choice of institution we include under "delivery system" and this, too, affects her utilization behavior.

Previous research has indicated some consistent direct relationships between income and preventive medical care.[5-8] Fewer data are available relevant to "social setting" variables. There is some evidence of a negative relationship between parity and prenatal care,[9-11] parity and infant immunizations,[12] and parity and routine physical checkups for children.[13-14] With respect to research on medical orientations, one study reports little relationship between health knowledge per se and utilization,[15] although a number of researchers have found a positive relationship between education (or social class) and health knowledge.[16-18]

Researchers have measured propensity to use the medical system by presenting respondents with a list of hypothetical conditions and asking them to note the likelihood of consulting a doctor.[19-21] In these studies there appears to be a weak but positive relationship between expressed opinions and actual behavior. The literature also indicates positive attitudes toward use of preventive care by varying populations. Anderson[22] reports that when people are asked whether they should see a doctor once a year for a checkup, around 70 per cent say yes. In another study of attitudes toward preventive care such as hearing and vision screening tests, DPT shots, and a tuberculosis screening test for children, more than 95 per cent of the mothers, regardless of social class, ethnicity, or educational level replied that they thought such procedures were "very important."[23]

Various researchers suggest that disadvantaged populations have stronger feelings of powerlessness and hopelessness with respect to controlling their lives. In addition, they are more likely to feel isolated from the mainstream of middle class society, its material benefits, and its social institutions.[24] These attitudes combine to give the disadvantaged a general feeling of being excluded from equal access to social institutions, including medical ones. Morris et al.[25] note that mothers who feel socially isolated and powerless are less likely to obtain innoculations for their babies than are mothers of comparable socioeconomic levels who are not alienated. Bullough[26] found that social isolation was negatively related to obtaining prenatal and postnatal care, well-baby checkups, and immunizations. Thus, a measure of alienation was included in this analysis.

SOURCE OF DATA AND METHODOLOGY

Data are from "Contrasts in Health Status: A Comparative Inquiry into the Health Needs, Barriers and Resources of Selected Population Groups," by the Institute of Medicine of the National Academy of Sciences.[27] As part of this investigation, a household survey was conducted from December 1970 through April 1971 in two sections of Washington, D.C.: Shephard Park–Tacoma, a middle income residential area, and Congress Heights, a low income area.

A total of 1436 interviews was completed in both areas from a total of 1609 eligible families, a response rate of 89.3 per cent. For this analysis, a subsample of 1274 families was chosen which consisted of native born, black mothers of children ages 6 months through 11 years.

A comparison of this sample with the black families in the 1970 Census of Washington, D.C. indicates that the sample mothers are on the average slightly better educated, are more likely to be working, and have higher status jobs. However, 36 per cent of the sample mothers are heads of families compared with 28 per cent in the District, and 27 per cent are receiving some form of public assistance, compared with 8 per cent of the total black Washington families.

The method of analysis chosen for these data is Multiple Classification Analysis (MCA).[28] In the analysis that follows, each variable will have values expressed as gross deviations from the grand mean of the total group, which are category specific values of the Preventive Medical Behavior Index. The net deviations from the grand mean illustrate the category-specific index values when the effects of the other specified variables in the model are statistically controlled.

RESULTS

Scores on six items of preventive medical behavior pertaining to the mother and her youngest child were added together to form a Preventive Medical Behavior Index. These scores were grouped into a 5-point scale. Table 10.1 shows the distribution of the mothers on this index.

Table 10.1   Percent Distribution of Preventive Medical Behavior Index

1 Low	10
2	17
3	24
4	25
5 High	23
Not ascertained	1
Total (%)	100
(N)	(1274)
Mean score	3.27
Standard deviation	1.29

Socioeconomic Factors

To measure socioeconomic status, three variables proved to be as powerful as any combined index or other possible measures. They are mother's education, family income, and head's occupation. Table 10.2 shows the MCA performed on the Preventive Medical Behavior Index using the three variables.[29] We see a direct, linear relationship between education and preventive medical utilization. College graduates have almost a full point higher score than the average, while mothers with no more than elementary school training have about two-thirds of a point less than average. High school graduates comprise almost half of the sample population, and have index scores just about at the mean of the total group.

There is also a direct, linear relationship with family income, although the extreme categories differ less from the average score compared to the education categories. Families with incomes of less than $4000 have a score of .58 less than average, while those earning $15,000 are .75 above the mean. Families with incomes between $6000 and $10,000 have scores identical to the grand mean.

In families where the head is employed as professional or manager the preventive medical score is about .50 of a point higher than the mean. The two middle groupings of occupations are about .10 above the mean, while service workers and laborers have about .12 less than average. The one group that falls well below the average contains the housewives and other nonemployed heads. Their score is .77 below the group mean. We note that the only groups

Table 10.2   Multiple Classification Analysis and Correlations of
Preventive Medical Behavior Index and Selected Socioeconomic
Variables

Variable	Per Cent	Gross Deviation from Grand Mean of 3.27
Mother's education		
elementary	4	$-.64^a$
some high school	28	$-.51^a$
high school graduate	43	.01
some college	16	$.50^a$
college graduate	9	$.91^a$
Total	100	$R = .348$
Family income		
<$4,000	17	$-.58^a$
$4,000–5,999	16	$-.38^a$
$6,000–7,999	18	.00
$8,000–10,999	17	.00
$11,000–14,999	15	$.46^a$
$15,000+	13	$.75^a$
not ascertained	4	.02
Total	100	$R = .332$
Head's occupation		
professional, managers, officials, proprietors	17	$.50^a$
clerical, sales	24	.07
craftsmen, operatives	21	.10
service, laborers	22	$-.12$
housewife, student, retired	13	$-.77^a$
not ascertained	3	.15
Total	100	$R = .274$
Total SES		$R = .408$

^{a} Deviation from the mean is significant at $<.05$ level, t-test.

that are significantly different from the mean are the professionals and the non-employed; there appears to be no significant difference among the occupational levels below professionals.

Table 10.2 also shows the correlations of each of the variables and combinations of them with preventive medical behavior. We note that by combining mother's education, family income, and head's occupation, we reach a multiple correlation of .408, or explain about 17 per cent of the variance in preventive medical behavior.

Social Setting Variables

Basic to the social setting concept is the idea of "social isolation" from or "social integration" into primary or secondary groups. It is hypothesized that the greater the degree of integration, the higher the utilization.

Two sets of variables are employed here, the first pertaining to primary group relationships, the second to secondary relationships.[30] Table 10.3 shows the MCA for each of these variables. Column 2 indicates the deviations of preventive medical behavior scores from the grand mean for each variable separately. We see first of all when we examine household composition that nearly 60 per cent of the families lived in units of mother, husband, and children. This group had the highest preventive medical score, .24 above the mean. Another 30 per cent are mothers living alone with their children. These mothers have the lowest Preventive Medical Behavior Index score, .40 units below the mean.

When we examine mothers living in an extended family, we would expect them to fall between these extremes. Table 10.3 illustrates this, with the presence or absence of a husband affecting the score. Mothers living without a husband, but with other adult relatives, are .31 below the mean; if their husband is present in the extended household, their score is .12 above the mean. Clearly, mothers living in households with no husband present use preventive medical measures less than mothers in a husband-wife unit. This relationship also holds when a control for socioeconomic status is imposed (see column 3).

Next we suggest that mothers with larger numbers of children are less likely to seek preventive care than mothers with a smaller number of children.[31] Table 10.3 basically supports this. As the number of children in the household increases, the preventive medical behavior score consistently decreases, with a slight reversal in the three and four child categories. The data support both Watkins's[32] and McKinlay's[33] findings that utilization of preventive medical services declines as number of children increases.

In addition, another aspect of the effect of number of children can be examined with respect to the spacing of children. Underlying this relationship,

Table 10.3 Multiple Classification Analysis and Correlations of Preventive Medical Behavior Index and Selected Socioeconomic and Social Setting Variables

		Deviations from Grand Mean	
Variable	Per Cent (1)	Gross (2)	Net of SES (3)
Primary Group Relationships			
Household composition			
mother alone with child(ren)	30	$-.40^a$	$-.14^a$
extended family without husband	7	$-.31^a$	$-.13$
extended family with husband	5	$.12$	$.09$
mother, husband, and child(ren)	58	$.24^a$	$.08^a$
Total	100	$R = .241$	$R = .413$
Number and spacing			
one	26	$.26^a$	$.18^a$
two, widely spaced	18	$.14$	$-.01$
two, closely spaced	15	$.08$	$.04$
three, widely spaced	10	$.08$	$.07$
three, closely spaced	8	$-.51^a$	$-.41^a$
four +, widely spaced	11	$-.21$	$.01$
four +, closely spaced	11	$-.36^a$	$-.15$
Total	100	$R = .200$	$R = .428$
Visiting friends and relatives			
sometimes	78	$.10^b$	$.05^b$
rarely	22	$-.34^b$	$-.16^b$
not ascertained	c	d	d
Total	100	$R = .148$	$R = .414$
Total primary		$R = .321$	$R = .439$
Secondary Group Relationships			
Television			
sometimes	96	$.02^b$	$.01^b$
rarely	4	$-.54^b$	$-.45^b$
not ascertained	c	d	d
Total	100	$R = .156$	$R = .417$

Table 10.3 (Continued)

Variable	Per Cent (1)	Deviations from Grand Mean Gross (2)	Net of SES (3)
Clubs			
yes	25	.46[b]	.19[b]
no	75	−.15[b]	−.06[b]
not ascertained	c	d	d
Total	100	$R = .205$	$R = .416$
PTA			
yes	51	.21[b]	.09[b]
no	45	−.27[b]	−.13[b]
not ascertained	4	.26	.21
Total	100	$R = .187$	$R = .417$
Church attendance			
1/week or more	24	.26[a,b]	.13[b]
1/month	32	.14[a]	.08
few times/year	36	−.21[a]	−.10
never; no religious affiliation	8	−.38[a,b]	−.29[a,b]
not ascertained	c	d	d
Total	100	$R = .175$	$R = .420$
Region of birth			
Washington, D.C.	38	−.15[a]	−.06
other South Atlantic	51	.01	.00
South Central	5	.53[a]	.36[a]
rest of U.S.	6	.33[a]	.03
not ascertained	c	d	d
Total	100	$R = .138$	$R = .414$
Total secondary		$R = .301$	$R = .441$
Total social setting		$R = .410$	$R = .470$

[a] Deviation from the mean is significant at $<.05$ level, t-test.
[b] Difference between two category means is significant at the $<.05$ level, t-test.
[c] Less than 1 per cent.
[d] Deviation from the mean not shown when category cell size is less than 20.

we believe, is that mothers with children born close together are more likely to be tied to the home and less likely to make use of preventive medical services. Those mothers with the two youngest children closely spaced[34] are considerably less likely to have used medical services than those mothers with children spaced three or more years apart. This relationship remains when socioeconomic status is controlled (see column 3).

The final variable in the primary group section concerns visiting patterns. We suggest that the more frequently mothers visit friends and/or relatives, the lower their social isolation, and thus the higher their preventive medical utilization. Table 10.3 basically shows that for the group that rarely[35] visits friends and/or relatives the preventive medical behavior scores are significantly different from those of persons who visit more frequently. When socioeconomic status is controlled, the same relationship holds.

In summary, primary group relationships are related to preventive medical behavior; when socioeconomic status is controlled, the range of differences is reduced in every case (for example, the score of mother and children living alone changed from −.40 to −.14), but the direction of the deviations remained the same.

Thus, these data show that when we remove the effect of high or low socioeconomic status, mothers living alone with their children, mothers with large numbers of children, mothers with two or more children closely spaced, and mothers who rarely visit friends and/or relatives have a lower score on the preventive medical behavior index than mothers not in those categories.

Now let us turn to variables that tap mothers' contacts with the larger society. We suggest that respondents who are exposed more to the wider norms of society through the mass media are more likely to use preventive medical services. In addition to exposure to society's norms, we agree with Mellinger and colleagues, who state:

> we regarded frequency of exposure to the various mass media as one indicator of social isolation from or participation in the community. Our assumption is that people who have little contact with community life through the mass media are thereby cut off from important sources of information concerning public health needs and resources and, to this extent, are less likely to avail themselves of preventive medical services . . . .[36]

Table 10.3 indicates that mothers who rarely watch television, who do not belong to clubs or organizations, and who rarely or never attend church are all below the mean in their preventive medical behavior and are significantly different from those who do participate in these activities. If we remove the effect of socioeconomic status, the range of the deviations is slightly reduced in each case, but little change in any relationship is noted.

The final social setting variable is the effect of migration on the mothers' preventive medical behavior. We hypothesized that mothers from a southern background are less likely to seek preventive care than mothers born in other regions. This was based on data often found in national statistics that the South as a region usually had lower rates of health utilization than other regions of the United States. Table 10.3 shows just the opposite: the highest preventive medical score was exhibited by those mothers born in the South Central states. Those born in the Washington, D.C. area had the lowest index score, followed by those from the neighboring South Atlantic states. When socioeconomic status is controlled, the South Central area still has a fairly high index value, .36 above the mean. All other regions approach the norm.

Looking at the correlations in Table 10.3 we note that the primary group relationships taken together explain about 10 per cent of the variance (R = .321), as do the variables characterizing secondary relationships. When these groups are added together, the social setting grouping explains 17 per cent of the variance (R = .410). When added to the socioeconomic variables they reach a correlation of .470 or explain 22 per cent of the variance.

The largest contributor to explaining additional variance is the combined variable, number and spacing of children. Membership in organizations and watching television add an additional amount, as does frequency of visiting and region.[37] Region requires some additional analysis to see why mothers who migrated from the South Central states are more likely than others to have higher preventive medical scores.[38]

Medical and Life Orientations

The next set of variables examined are not social structural ones, but rather those dependent on the individual's attitudes and orientations toward health and life in general. Table 10.4 shows the MCA results for four variables used here: health knowledge, propensity to seek care, attitudes toward preventive care, and an anomie measure.[39]

The table indicates that for all four measures, as the index value increases, the preventive medical behavior score of mothers also increases. Regarding health knowledge, mothers correctly answering all four questions have an index score .17 above the mean, while mothers who are ill-informed are .90 below the grand mean. Controlling for socioeconomic status (column 3) reduces this range somewhat, but there is still a positive effect as knowledge score increases. The same is true of propensity to seek care and responses toward preventive health care.

The three questions that measure the degree of alienation[40] show the predicted inverse relationship. As anomie scores rise, the utilization of preven-

Table 10.4 Multiple Classification Analysis and Correlations of Preventive Medical Behavior Index for Orientation Variables

| | | Deviation from Grand Mean of 3.27 | | |
| | Per Cent | Gross | Net of SES | Net of SES and Social Setting |
Variable	(1)	(2)	(3)	(4)
Medical Orientations				
Health knowledge				
(1) low	3	$-.90^a$	$-.61^a$	$-.56^a$
(2)	17	$-.19$	$-.03$	$-.04$
(3)	27	$-.09$	$-.03$	$-.02$
(4) high	53	$.17^a$	$.07^a$	$.06^a$
not ascertained	b	c	c	c
Total	100	$R = .178$	$R = .419$	$R = .478$
Propensity				
(1) low	14	$-.55^a$	$-.45^a$	$-.39^a$
(2)	26	$-.09$	$-.10$	$-.07$
(3)	34	$.10$	$.09$	$.08$
(4) high	25	$.25^a$	$.22^a$	$.18^a$
not ascertained	1			
Total	100	$R = .271$	$R = .451$	$R = .504$
Health attitudes				
(1) negative	6	$-.83^a$	$-.57^a$	$-.53^a$
(2)	24	$-.37$	$-.28$	$-.27$
(3)	34	$.08$	$.05$	$.06$
(4) positive	35	$.34^a$	$.26^a$	$.24^a$
not ascertained	1	c	c	c
Total	100	$R = .198$	$R = .441$	$R = .489$
Total medical orientation		$R = .338$	$R = .474$	$R = .518$
Anomie				
(1) low	14	$.24^a$	$.08$	$.04$
(2)	20	$.10$	$-.07$	$.08$
(3)	30	$.00$	$-.02$	$-.02$
(4) high	31	$-.21^a$	$-.09$	$-.08$
not ascertained	5	$.22$	$.24$	$.24$
Total	100	$R = .126$	$R = .413$	$R = .474$
Total orientation		$R = .348$	$R = .477$	$R = .521$

^{a} Difference between two category means is significant at the $<.05$ level, t-test.
^{b} Less than 1 per cent.
^{c} Deviation from the mean not shown when category cell size is less than 20.

208

tive medical behavior scores decline, from .24 above the grand mean for mothers with low anomie scores to .21 below the mean for mothers with high anomie scores. At the same time we note that a considerable portion of the range is eliminated by controlling for socioeconomic status. The difference in scores between the two extreme groups is no longer statistically significant. This is not surprising in that the poor usually have higher alienation scores than those economically better off.

A close examination of column 4 in Table 10.4, which represents the net deviations of the orientation variables when the effects of both socioeconomic status and social setting are controlled, indicates that there is little change in the deviations as a result of such controls. In other words, the differences in preventive medical utilization we observe in the medical orientation variables still hold when both socioeconomic status and social setting variables are controlled.

We noted above that with socioeconomic status variables alone we were able to explain 16.6 per cent of the variance in preventive medical scores. Adding social setting variables increased this to 22.1 per cent, and adding the medical orientation items to the model increased the multiple correlation to .518 or explained 26.8 per cent of the variance. Anomie did not add a significant additional increment. Therefore, in the remaining analysis only medical orientation variables will be included in the model.

Type of Delivery System

We turn now to the final item in the model, the type of medical system mothers use.[41] Table 10.5 shows that most families use more than one type of delivery system. One-fifth use all three types, 24 per cent use a combination of private physician and an outpatient clinic or emergency room of a hospital, and an additional 21 per cent use combinations including nonhospital clinics.

The largest group using a single system consists of 18 per cent who use private physicians only. This group has the highest mean preventive medical behavior score (.32 above the mean), followed by those who use other services in addition to private physicians. Not unexpected is the finding that those who claim no regular source of care have the lowest preventive medical behavior score (.74 below the mean), closely followed by families that use only the outpatient department or emergency room of hospitals.

Looking at column 3, which shows the preventive medical behavior scores controlling for socioeconomic status, we see that virtually all differences among groups are eliminated except for two groups whose scores remain well below the mean—those with no regular source of care, and mothers who use only outpatient departments or emergency rooms of hospitals. If social setting variables

Table 10.5   Multiple Classification Analysis and Correlations of
Preventive Medical Behavior Index by Type of Delivery System

| | | Deviations from the Grand Mean | | |
| | | | | Net of SES, Social Setting, and Medical |
Delivery System	Per Cent (1)	Gross (2)	Net of SES (3)	Orientation (4)
Outpatient department or emergency room of hospital only (OPD/ER)	6	$-.68^a$	$-.43^a$	$-.39^a$
Nonhospital clinic only	8	.03	.06	.10
Private physician only	18	$.32^a$	.08	$-.01$
OPD/ER and nonhospital clinic	11	$-.25^a$	$-.01$	.06
OPD/ER and private physician	24	.11	.05	.04
Nonhospital clinic and private physician	10	.06	.02	$-.03$
All three types	20	.01	.06	.07
No regular provider	3	$-.74^a$	$-.55^a$	$-.35^a$
Total	100	$R = .211$	$R = .424$	$R = .526$

^{a} Deviation from the mean is significant at $<.05$ level, t-test.

and medical orientation measures are controlled in addition to socioeconomic status (column 4), the same pattern is repeated.

Table 10.5 also shows that adding the type of delivery system used by the family increases the multiple correlation for our final model to .526, or in all we are able to explain 27.7 per cent of the variance.

Table 10.6 gives the results of the Multiple Classification Analysis for each variable included in the total model. Here we are able to compare the gross deviation from the grand mean for each category with the deviation remaining after all other variables in the model have been statistically controlled.

The categories that are significantly different from the grand mean can be summarized as follows:

1. Mother's education and family income both appear to provide evidence that preventive medical behavior increases with socioeconomic status.

Table 10.6 Multiple Classification Analysis of Preventive Medical Behavior Index: Total Model

	Deviations from Grand Mean	
Variable	Gross (1)	Net[a] (2)
Socioeconomic Variables		
Mother's education		
elementary	−.64[b]	−.07
some high school	−.51[b]	−.22[b]
high school graduate	.01	−.02
some college	.50[b]	.27[b]
college graduate	.91[b]	.34[b]
Family income		
<$4,000	−.58[b]	−.04
$4,000–5,999	−.38[b]	−.17[b]
$6,000–7,999	.00	−.03
$8,000–10,999	.00	−.10
$11,000–14,999	.46[b]	.18[b]
$15,000+	.75[b]	.18
not ascertained	.02	.24
Head's occupation		
professional, managers, officials, proprietors	.50[b]	.00
clerical, sales	.07	.08
craftsmen, operatives	.10	.01
service, laborers	−.12	.01
housewife, student, retired	−.77[b]	−.26[b]
not ascertained	.15	.37
Social Setting		
Household composition		
mother alone with child(ren)	−.40[b]	−.10
extended family without husband	−.31[b]	−.15
extended family with husband	.12	−.03
mother, husband and child(ren)	.24[b]	.07

211

Table 10.6 (Continued)

	Deviations from Grand Mean	
Variable	Gross (1)	Net[a] (2)
Number and spacing		
one	.26[b]	.24[b]
two, widely spaced	.14	−.05
two, closely spaced	.08	.10
three, widely spaced	.08	−.03
three, closely spaced	−.51[b]	−.40[b]
four +, widely spaced	−.21[b]	−.05
four +, closely spaced	−.36[b]	−.18
Visiting friends and relatives		
sometimes	.10[c]	.03 ns
rarely	−.34[c]	−.11 ns
not ascertained	[d]	[d]
Television		
sometimes	.02[c]	.01[c]
rarely	−.54[c]	−.46[c]
not ascertained	[d]	[d]
Clubs		
yes	.46[c]	.13[c]
no	−.15[c]	−.04[c]
not ascertained	[d]	[d]
PTA		
yes	.21[c]	.10[c]
no	−.27[c]	−.12[c]
not ascertained	.26	.09
Church attendance		
1/week or more	.26[b,c]	.08
1/month	.14	.03
few times/year	−.21[b]	−.06
never; no religious affiliation	−.38[b,c]	−.12
Region of birth		
South Central	.53[b]	.33[c]
Washington, D.C.	−.15[b]	
other South Atlantic	.01	−.02[c]
rest of U.S.	.33[b]	
not ascertained	[d]	[d]

Table 10.6   (Continued)

	Deviations from Grand Mean	
Variable	Gross (1)	Net[a] (2)
Medical Orientations		
Health knowledge		
(1) low	− .90[c]	− .54[c]
(2)	− .19	− .04
(3)	− .09	− .01
(4) high	.17[c]	.05[c]
not ascertained	[d]	[d]
Propensity		
(1) low	− .55[c]	− .54[c]
(2)	− .09	− .04
(3)	.10	− .01
(4) high	.25[c]	.05[c]
not ascertained	[d]	[d]
Health attitudes		
(1) negative	− .83[c]	− .41[c]
(2)	− .37	− .22
(3)	.08	.06
(4) positive	.34[c]	.10[c]
not ascertained	[d]	[d]
Type of Delivery		
OPD/ER	− .68[b]	− .39[b]
nonhospital clinic	.03	.10
private physician	.32[b]	− .01
OPD/ER and nonhospital clinic	− .25[b]	.06
OPD/ER and private physician	.11	.04
nonhospital clinic and private physician	.06	− .03
all three types	.01	.07
no regular provider	− .74[b]	− .35[b]

[a] Net of the effect of all other variables in the model.
[b] Deviation from the mean is significant at <.05 level, *t*-test.
[c] Difference between two category means is significant at the <.05 level, *t*-test.
[d] Deviation from the mean not shown when category cell size is less than 20.

2. Mothers who are not employed have a preventive medical behavior score significantly below the mean of the total group (even when income and education are controlled).
3. Mothers with one child have significantly higher preventive medical behavior scores than does the total group. Mothers of three children, with the two youngest closely spaced (i.e., born within two years of each other), have significantly lower scores.
4. The measures of secondary group involvements, such as watching television and belonging to clubs and the PTA, indicate that those who participate are significantly different and have higher scores than those who do not participate.
5. All of the measures of medical orientation consistently indicate significant differences between the high and low ends of the index scales. Those high on health knowledge, propensity to consult doctors, and those who have positive health attitudes are more likely to have higher preventive medical behavior scores. We also note that those variables change very little when the effects of socioeconomic status or social setting variables are controlled.
6. Finally, mothers who use the outpatient department or emergency rooms of hospitals have scores significantly below the mean of the group, as do mothers who report having no regular provider for their medical needs. Again, this relationship holds when other variables in the model, including socioeconomic status, are controlled.

Two of the social setting variables show no deviations statistically significant from the mean: household composition and church attendance. In the former, however, the unit composed of husband, wife, and child or children did have a score statistically different from the mean at the .10 level. And in both variables the values of the scores on the Preventive Medical Behavior Index are consistently in the predicted direction, when all the other variables in the model are controlled.

Medical "Tracers"

An important aspect of the National Academy of Sciences study design was the attempt to measure the quality of care provided to children by different types of delivery systems. For this purpose, specific medical conditions or "tracers" were chosen.[42] When mothers were interviewed in their homes, permission was requested to examine children between 6 months and 12 years of age at a clinic. Ninety per cent of the mothers gave permission.

In the group of mothers analyzed here, of a total of 1262 families, tracer data are available for 909 children on all of the applicable tracers. The tracer conditions used on the study children were iron-deficiency anemia, middle ear infection and associated hearing loss, and visual disorders.

Kessner and Kalk[43] review the epidemiology of the tracers in detail and conclude that although there may be a genetic component to these conditions, all are usually amenable to medical treatment and are correctable. In other words, these conditions reflect behavioral and environmental factors to some degree. This being the case, it is reasonable to relate past preventive medical behavior to the current health status of the child, keeping in mind that these tracer conditions are very specific. We do not mean to say that a child without the tracer criteria is "healthy." We are saying that a child who fails a tracer criterion is *not* "healthy."

A gross summary score of number of tracers failed was constructed; the number failed ranged from 0 to 3. Each child was rated on two ear conditions (infection and hearing loss) and either anemia (if the child was under 4) or visual disorders (if the child was between 4 and 12).

Table 10.7 shows the deviations from the grand mean for mothers by the

Table 10.7   Multiple Classification Analysis of Preventive Medical Behavior Index for Tracer Conditions Failed

			Deviations from Grand Mean			
Number Failed	Per Cent (1)	Gross (2)	Net[a] (3)	Net[b] (4)	Net[c] (5)	Net[d] (6)
None	37	.07	.03	.06	.06	.06
One	28	−.10	−.04	−.07	−.07	−.06
Two	6	−.26	−.19	−.15	−.13	−.13
Three	1	−.77	−.60	−.51	−.51	−.51
Not ascertained on one or more tracers	2	−.09	−.07	−.11	−.09	−.06
No information (child not examined)	26	.10	.07	.05	.05	.04
Total	100					

[a] Net of socioeconomic status.
[b] Net of socioeconomic status and social setting.
[c] Net of socioeconomic status, social setting, and medical orientation.
[d] Net of socioeconomic status, social setting, medical orientation, and type of delivery system.
[e] Difference between two category means is significant at the <.05 level, *t*-test.

number of tracer conditions her child failed. The striking feature of the table is the consistent decrease in mean preventive medical behavior score with each increase in the number of tracers failed. This finding suggests that there is some relationship between our measure of preventive medical behavior of the mother and the health condition of her child with respect to the tracers. When controls for socioeconomic status, social setting, and medical orientation are imposed, we see that the range is somewhat restricted, but the inverse relationship between preventive medical behavior and number of tracers failed still holds. However, no differences are statistically significant when any of the controls are imposed. Nevertheless, the fact that the number of tracers failed and preventive medical behavior score are inversely related is nonetheless suggestive: the children of mothers who rate high on preventive behavior are less likely to fail specific tests of health status.

CONCLUSIONS

This model of preventive medical utilization is conceived of as being affected by three basic components: the socioeconomic status of the mother, her social setting, and her attitudes and values toward the medical system. We found that 17 per cent of the variance in a 5-point index of utilization of preventive medical services was explained by socioeconomic status alone, an equal amount by social setting variables alone, and 11 per cent by medical orientations alone. When all three were combined into one model, the total multiple correlation was .518, or 26.8 per cent of the variance was explained. Adding the type of medical delivery system the mother and her family used completed the suggested model, and yielded a multiple correlation of .526.

Our attempt to delineate mothers who are "socially isolated" as inferred from their social activity with friends, relatives, membership in clubs, church attendance, and the like did significantly identify low users of preventive medical services. In addition, we have evidence that mothers' expressed attitudes about using medical services are quite consistent with the actual use made of them. These relationships remain when the effect of socioeconomic status is controlled.

Because the study was conducted at one point in time, and respondents were asked during the interview for data pertaining to previous actions, we cannot address the "feedback" aspect of the model. That is, we cannot untangle the causal web of people's behavior being affected by their attitudes, or their attitudes affecting their behavior. In addition, although we have found an association between certain characteristics of the mothers' life style and her preventive medical behavior, we cannot say that the former affects the latter. The associations we detect may be due to other factors not examined here. For example, there may be other factors causing both a mother's social isolation and her lack of utilization of medical services, or her use of medical services and her child's health status. Personality or other individual characteristics or family patterns passed down through a heritage may also affect both the specific life style and the pattern of medical utilization. Researchers in this area, therefore, must be careful not to imply causality to evidence of associations between demographic and social characteristics of the mother and her medical behavior.

NOTES

1. By preventive medical services we mean services obtained by the conscious action of a person while in a state of perceived good health to seek out and receive some medical attention for maintaining health or preventing illness.

2. J. B. McKinlay (1972), "Some Approaches and Problems in the Study of the Use of Services—An Overview," *Journal of Health and Social Behavior*, **13**:115–152.

3. The term "medical orientation" is borrowed from E. A. Suchman (1964), "Sociomedical Variations Among Ethnic Groups," *American Journal of Sociology*, **70**:319–331, and is employed here in the sense he uses it.

4. The index included the following medical services, as reported by the mother:

   a physical checkup within the last 12 months
   a physical checkup within two years before the last one
   first prenatal visit in first trimester of last pregnancy
   postpartum checkup obtained after last pregnancy
   infant given diphtheria, whooping cough, and tetanus shots
   child taken for general physical checkup at least once every two years

5. B. Bullough and V. L. Bullough (1972), *Poverty, Ethnic Identity and Health Care* (New York: Appleton-Century-Crofts).

6. A. Yankauer, W. E. Boek, E. D. Lawson, and F. A. J. Ianni (1958), "Social Stratification and Health Practices in Child Bearing and Child Rearing," *American Journal of Public Health*, **48**:732–741.

7. N. M. Morris, M. H. Hatch, and S. S. Chipman (1966), "Alienation as a Deterrent to Well-Child Supervision," *American Journal of Public Health*, **56**:1874–1882.

8. National Center for Health Statistics (1965), *Physician Visits: Interval of Visits and Children's Routine Checkup. U.S. July 1963–June 1964*, Series 10, No. 19 (Washington, D.C.: Government Printing Office).

9. J. B. McKinlay (1970), "The New Latecomers for Antenatal Care," *British Journal of Preventive Social Medicine*, **24**:52–57.

10. E. L. Watkins (1968), "Low Income Negro Mothers—Their Decisions to Seek Prenatal Care," *American Journal of Public Health*, **58**:655–667.

11. P. B. Cornely and S. K. Bigman (1963), "Some Considerations in Changing Health Attitudes," *Children*, **10**:23–28.

12. N. M. Morris et al. (1966), op. cit.

13. National Center for Health Statistics (1969), *Family Use of Health Services,* Series 10, No. 55 (Washington, D.C.: Government Printing Office).

14. National Center for Health Statistics (1964), *Medical Care, Health Status and Family Income,* Series 10, No. 9 (Washington, D.C.: Government Printing Office).

15. L. Pratt (1971), "The Relationship of Socio-Economic Status to Health," *American Journal of Public Health,* **61**:281-291.

16. D. Rosenblatt and E. A. Suchman (1964), "Blue Collar Attitudes and Information Toward Health and Illness," in A. Shostak and W. Gomberg, eds., *Blue Collar World* (Englewood Cliffs, N.J.: Prentice-Hall), pp. 324-333.

17. D. Dennison (1972), "Social Class Variables Related to Health Instruction," *American Journal of Public Health,* **62**:814-820.

18. S. King (1962), *Perceptions of Illness and Medical Practice* (New York: Russell Sage).

19. D. Mechanic and E. H. Volkart (1961), "Stress, Illness Behavior, and the Sick Role," *American Sociological Review,* **26**:51-58.

20. T. W. Bice and E. Kalimo (1971), "Comparisons of Health-Related Attitudes: A Cross-National Factor Analytic Study," *Social Science and Medicine,* **5**:283-318.

21. National Center for Health Statistics (1969), *International Comparisons of Medical Care Utilization: A Feasibility Study* by K. L. White and J. Murnaghan, Series 2, No. 33 (Washington, D.C.: Government Printing Office).

22. O. W. Anderson (1963), "The Utilization of Health Services," in H. E. Freeman et al, eds., *Handbook of Medical Sociology* (Englewood Cliffs, N.J.: Prentice-Hall).

23. W. F. Dodge et al. (1970), "Patterns of Maternal Desires for Child Health Care," *American Journal of Public Health,* **60**:1421-1429.

24. D. Rosenblatt and E. A. Suchman (1964), op. cit.

25. N. M. Morris et al. (1966), op. cit.

26. B. Bullough (1972), "Poverty, Ethnic Identity and Preventive Health Care," *Journal of Health and Social Behavior,* **13**:347-359.

27. D. M. Kessner, C. K. Snow, and J. Singer (1974), "Assessment of Medical Care for Children," in *Contrasts in Health Status,* Volume 3 (Washington, D.C.: Institute of Medicine, National Academy of Sciences), pp. 9-24.

28. MCA is a dummy variable regression technique where the dependent variable may be either dichotomous or an interval scale, but the independent variables may be any combination of nominal, ordinal, or interval scales because all variables are dichotomized within categories. See F. Andrews, J. Morgan, and J. Sonquist (1967), *Multiple Classification Analysis: A Report on a Computer Program for Multiple Regression Using Categorical Predictors* (Ann Arbor: University of Michigan, Institute for Social Research). This is a regression technique that provides the analyst with a multiple correlation for a model as well as the proportion of variance explained in the dependent variable. This method also allows computation of category values (Melecharized beta coefficients) that show deviations from the grand mean. One can also determine net effects by controlling for selected independent variables in a model.

29. In addition to these variables, the following were carefully examined: own/rent home; on public assistance; has health insurance; poverty status. None had the explanatory power of the above three.

30. Additional measures of social setting were examined, but dropped from the model because the categories within them showed no significant differences when socioeconomic status was controlled. They are: mother's work status; frequency of reading newspapers; and frequency of going out to movies, restaurants, and so forth. Two variables exhibited no clear pattern

among the categories, and were also dropped: length of residence in Washington, D.C., and size of place of mother's birth. One additional variable, stage of childbearing, was examined and omitted from the model because of no additional explanatory power in the additive model. This variable was a combination of mother's age, number of children, and the ages of those children.

31. In this study the number of children the mother had was not asked in the questionnaire. What is available is the number of children the mother had who are currently living in the household. Thus we do not know whether a mother with one child is at the beginning of her childbearing, or if the one child is the youngest child, and the last one at home.

32. E. L. Watkins (1968), op. cit.

33. J. B. McKinlay (1970), op. cit.

34. Defined here as the two youngest children born two or fewer years apart.

35. Defined as once a month or less.

36. G. Mellinger, D. I. Manheimer, and M. T. Kleman (1967), *Deterrents to Adequate Immunization of Preschool Children* (Berkeley: Survey Research Center, University of California), p. 22.

37. A stepwise regression analysis was performed and the order of contribution to explaining additional variance was as follows: number-spacing, PTA, region, clubs, TV, visiting, household composition, and church attendance.

38. A simple crosstabulation analysis reveals that mothers born in the South Central states are more likely to (1) have lived in Washington, D.C. from 3 to 12 years (61 per cent compared to 31 per cent of the total sample); (2) come from a medium large city (31 per cent come from a birthplace of 100,000–499,999 compared to 10 per cent of the sample); (3) live in a household composed of husband and children only (76 per cent compared to 58 per cent); and (4) have their children widely spaced (47 per cent compared to 39 per cent of the total group). Other variables examined show few differences.

39. The wording of the questions, as well as the method of scoring, from which these indices were constructed are in Appendix A of D. Slesinger (1973), "The Utilization of Preventive Medical Services by Urban Black Mothers: A Sociocultural Approach," unpublished Ph.D. dissertation, University of Wisconsin.

40. L. Srole (1956), "Social Integration and Certain Corollaries," *American Sociological Review*, **21**:709–716.

41. This distribution is based on the responses mothers gave when asked whether they or any members of their family used an outpatient department or emergency room of a hospital, a nonhospital clinic, or a private physician for their usual source of care.

42. The tracer methodology is described in detail in D. M. Kessner, and C. E. Kalk (1973), "A Strategy for Evaluating Health Services," in *Contrasts in Health Status*, Volume 2 (Washington, D.C.: Institute of Medicine, National Academy of Sciences).

43. Ibid.

Chapter 11

Physician-Patient Communication and Patient Conformity with Medical Advice

Bonnie L. Svarstad

Although many studies have tried to determine why patients do not follow medical advice, they have led to so many inconsistent findings that a more meaningful conceptual framework must be developed. This chapter reviews methods already tried and suggests an alternative approach to the study of patient conformity with medical advice. Previous approaches have placed too much emphasis on the patient and too little on the processes by which physicians transmit their expectations and attempt to motivate their patients. If it is true that patients lack high levels of knowledge and motivation, we sorely need to understand better how reasonable conformity with medical advice can be achieved.

THE INDIVIDUALISTIC MODELS

The most common approach to the study of nonconformity is to identify the "cooperative" and "uncooperative" patients and to search for the variables that

This study was conducted under the auspices of a neighborhood health center funded by the Office of Economic Opportunity. To preserve the anonymity of the participating physicians and patients, I do not name the health center.

differentiate them. The assumption is that the nonconforming patient has unique characteristics. This assumption and therefore the adequacy of various individualistic models, can be questioned on several grounds.

First, the findings have been inconsistent. Researchers who have compared patients' abilities and personality traits have reported inconsistent results regarding the role of each of the following factors in adhering to medical advice: intelligence,[1-2] anxiety,[3-4] defensiveness,[5] internalization,[6] authoritarianism,[7-8] Rorschach scores,[9-10] MMPI scores, [11-12] and psychopathy.[13] Those who have used the Barron Ego Strength Scale,[14] the Stroop Color Word Test,[15] a scale measuring use of conversion defenses,[16] and a scale measuring dependent-submissiveness[17] have reported results that were not significant. Investigators who have compared demographic characteristics have not been much more successful. There have been contradictory findings regarding the following sociocultural characteristics: sex,[18-20] age,[21-23] income,[24-27] occupation,[28-29] education,[30-33] race,[34-36] number of siblings,[37-38] family structure,[39-40] and family stability.[41-42] Similarly, little predictability is achieved when various attitudinal orientations have been examined: future orientation,[43] ethnocentrism,[44] anomie,[45-46] attitudes toward science,[47] and attitudes toward illness-dependency.[48]

Second, there is evidence that patients do not behave consistently across situations. For example, it is known that patient behavior varies from one time to another[49] and that patient behavior varies by the type of advice,[50-52] the number of physician instructions,[53-54] and the degree of medical supervision.[55] These data suggest that focusing on the *process* by which nonconformity is prevented and reduced may be more productive than concentrating on individual characteristics.

THE HEALTH BELIEF MODEL

Another approach to the study of nonconformity is to explore patients' beliefs about their illness and the advised actions.[56-59] Generally speaking, the "health belief model" postulates that patients' behavior is a function of the amount of threat perceived by patients and patients' perception of the value or attractiveness of the advised actions. Like the individualistic models, the health belief model places primary emphasis on patients and their motivations, predispositions, or level of "psychological readiness."

Although there is empirical support for the idea that behavior is associated with people's beliefs about their illnesses and treatments, the health belief model is limited. First, it tends to neglect the possibility that nonconformity can be unintentional. Patients may be motivated but, for various reasons, may not recall and understand what they are supposed to do. We know, for example, that patients do not recall many of the physicians' statements,[60] that they are often unaware of the fact that they have been misusing medications,[61] and that they have difficulty understanding other complex regimens.[62] Further, the model does not clearly specify the determinants of patient motivation. Proponents of the model hypothesize that various social agents (e.g., doctor, family, boss, friends) affect patients' motivation, but they do not specify how such social influence occurs or why it might fail.[63]

THE INTERACTION MODELS

Although many social scientists and health professionals have written about the importance of physician-patient interaction, few empirical studies have probed the relationship between physician-patient interaction and patient conformity with medical advice.

Utilizing Bales's Interaction Process Analysis and factor analytic techniques, Milton Davis examined the structure and process of physician-patient communication in a general medical clinic.[64-65] When he examined the relationship between patient compliance and certain types of physician-patient activities that occurred during the patients' subsequent visits, some significant findings were obtained.[66] Patients were more apt to comply if the physician had given suggestions and information and if the patients had asked for the physician's suggestions and opinions, expressed agreement, and expressed tension release. Noncompliance was more apt to occur if patients gave their own opinions or showed tension and if the physician engaged in certain activities (i.e., passive acceptance of the patient's active participation, asking for information without giving feedback, and expressing disagreement).

In a similarly designed study, Barbara Korsch and her associates examined the relationship between pediatrician-parent communication and the parents' subsequent conformity with advice.[67-70] Although these investigators also used a conceptual model based on Bales's system of classifying interaction, their results were not consistent with those of Davis. Instead, they found that physician friendliness and antagonism were significantly related to the parents' subsequent behavior.[71] Davis concluded that the passive patient was more compliant;[72] Korsch and her colleagues concluded that the active parent was more compliant.[73] The latter also concluded that parent expression of agreement or tension made no difference in parents' later behavior.[74] Although Davis suggested that compliance was higher when patients asked for suggestions and opinions, Korsch and her colleagues reported that the parents' level of questioning made no difference. Contrary to Davis's conclusions,[75] they found that the permissiveness of the pediatrician made no difference.[76] One of the few consistent findings was that noncompliance was higher when physicians asked for information without giving any feedback.

It is difficult to account for these contradictions. They might partially be explained by the different populations studied, but I suspect that the Bales system for analyzing interaction is simply inadequate for the purposes being discussed. As others have noted, the 12 categories in Bales's system are too broad to be meaningful. For example, the extent to which the physician gives instruction or suggestion can be measured, but the content, clarity, or salience of the suggestions or instructions cannot be explored. The extent to which the physician expresses positive or negative affect can be measured, but the other ways in which the physician might try to motivate the patient (e.g., discussing the rationale for a given prescription) cannot be isolated. The latter communication would be included in broad categories such as "giving orientation" or "giving opinions."

In short, a more meaningful conceptual model for studying physician-patient communication as it relates to patient conformity is needed.

THE RESEARCH PROJECT

The data on which this report is based were collected as part of an exploratory study that was conducted in a neighborhood health center located in an urban ghetto. Unlike other studies that have focused on patient failure to conform with medical advice, we began by asking, "Why do physicians sometimes fail to achieve the patients' conformity with medication advice?" The design of our study, which began in 1969, included systematic observation of physician-patient interaction, review of medical records and pharmacy files, follow-up interviews with the patients about a week after their clinic visits, and validation of the patients' reported behavior by means of a "bottle check." I observed 8 full-time physicians and was able to obtain a complete series of data on 153 adult patients, most of whom were black and Puerto Rican. Of this group, 131 patients were expected to follow medication advice. The sample included new and old patients, walk-in patients, patients with appointments, and patients with or without language difficulties. The patients were being treated for a variety of acute and chronic conditions. The most common diagnosis was essential hypertension.

All of the participating physicians were fully trained. Two physicians were board certified internists; four were board eligible internists; and two were general practitioners. The health center was funded by the Office of Economic Opportunity and was designed to provide high quality, comprehensive, and continuous health care. Many independent observers considered the center one of the most successful in the country.

THE INSTRUCTION PROCESS

My project began with some of the same unwarranted assumptions that have characterized previous research. I assumed that the physicians' expectations regarding medication use would be, for the most part, simple and unambiguous and that the patients—after receiving verbal advice and printed instructions on their medication containers—would know what the physicians expected them to do. The pilot study led me to question these assumptions. First, patients did not always leave the clinic with an accurate perception of what the physicians expected them to do. As illustrated in the following excerpt, the physicians sometimes had to clarify earlier instructions during the follow-up visits:

DOCTOR: Have you been taking the medicine for the gout?

PATIENT: No, I stopped that after the pains went away.

DOCTOR: You shouldn't have done that. I wanted you to continue taking it as that medicine prevents gout attacks.

PATIENT: (in a tone of surprise) Oh, I didn't know that! You didn't tell me that last time.

Second, I also had difficulty when I tried to identify what the physicians expected. Even though I had observed the clinic visit, reviewed the record, and examined carbon copies of the prescription forms, I was often confused. Before interviewing the patients, I often had to seek clarification from the physicians, pharmacists, and the *Physicians' Desk Reference* (a reference book that provides information about pharmaceutical products).

These experiences indicated that it might be fruitful to begin by examining the nature and outcome of physician instruction. The physician-patient encounter was viewed as a situation in which the patient must learn a very specific patient role or set of expectations about (1) which drugs should be taken, (2) how long each drug should be taken, (3) the dosage schedules that should be followed, and (4) how regularly the drugs should be taken. The working hypotheses were:

1. The patient cannot conform with the physician's expectations without having an accurate perception of the physician's expectations.
2. The patient's perception of the physician's expectations will be more accurate if (a) the physician transmits the expectations in an explicit manner; (b) the physician provides a written record of the expectations (e.g., medication label); (c) the medication label is consistent with what the physician requested; and (d) the physician informs the patient about the name and/or purpose of the drug.

The Nature of Physician Instruction

Examining the physicians' verbal instructions and the instructions attached to the patients' medication containers led to some interesting findings. First, it was evident that the physicians frequently did not discuss their expectations in an explicit manner. Of the 347 drugs prescribed or proscribed, 60 were never discussed during the observed visits. The physicians gave explicit, verbal advice about how long to take the drug in only 10 per cent of the 347 drug cases. How regularly the drug should be used was made explicit in about 17 per cent of the cases. In addition, several physicians discussed certain dosage schedules ambiguously. For example, when discussing antibiotics, several physicians gave the dosage schedule in hourly terms (e.g., "Take two capsules every 6 hours") without specifying how many should be taken during a 24-hour period. Apparently, the physicians assumed that their patients would be able to infer how long their drugs should be taken, how regularly they should be used, and what certain types of dosage schedules mean.

Second, patients did not always receive printed instructions or written reminders of what the physician expected regarding medication use. When the patient received no written instructions, it was usually because the physicians assumed that the patient still had a supply of the medication at home. But sometimes the physicians changed the previously prescribed dosage schedule and gave the patient no written record of the schedule now in effect. When the patient did receive a container of medication on the day of the visit (239 of 347 drugs), we examined the attached instructions. How long the drug should be taken was noted on only 10 medication containers. Of the 97 drugs dispensed for symptomatic relief, only 42 were dispensed with labels that noted that the drug should be taken "as necessary" or "as needed." As one physician later explained, "I don't always write that, but that's what I *mean*."

A third communication problem was discovered when we compared the medication labels (the labels that are typed and attached by the pharmacist) with the physicians' prescription request forms (the forms that indicate how the physician wants the medication to be labeled). Of the 179 drugs for which both types of data were available, we found an inconsistency in 20 per cent of the cases. In those cases where the physician wanted the label to include a statement about the symptom or condition being treated, the pharmacist sometimes omitted or incorrectly specified the symptom or condition. In other cases, the pharmacist did not translate the instructions into Spanish, as requested by the physician. Sometimes the containers were dispensed without the individualized labels that would have instructed the patient to take larger amounts on a more frequent basis than indicated on commercial labels (e.g., antacids for patients with peptic ulcers).

Fourth, an examination of the verbal and written instructions showed that in 29 per cent of the cases the physicians gave no information about the purpose and/or names of the drug. Several physicians were more apt to give this type of information; others typically referred to the drugs by their form, color, and/or size (e.g., "Continue taking the little white tablets"). I suspected that the latter type of instruction would be less effective, because patients often have several drugs that fit the same physical description. I also suspected that if the patient learned why the physician was giving the drug, the patient might be more able to infer what the physician expected regarding its use.

After preliminary analysis, a Physician Instruction Index was developed. This composite index was used to score the verbal and written instructions received by each patient. Verbal instructions were scored as follows: how long to take the drug (+1), how regularly to take the drug (+1), the dosage schedule (+1), and the purposes or name of the drug (+1). When written instructions were provided, the following scores were added: how long to take the drug (+2), how regularly to take the drug (+2), the dosage schedule (+2), and the purpose of the drug (+2). If the labeled instructions were not consistent with the physician's prescription request form, then a score of −2 was given. The composite instruction score could range from +12 to −2.

The 131 patients studied were classified into two groups: patients receiving high instruction (a composite instruction score of +4 or more) or low instruction (a composite score of less than +4). Forty-eight patients received high instruction; 83 patients received low instruction.

The Outcomes of Physician Instruction

When we asked patients which drugs the physicians wanted them to take and how each drug was supposed to be taken, we found many misconceptions. Of the 131 patients, 68 patients made at least one error when describing what the physician expected. The patients did not recall 6 per cent of the 347 drugs. They overestimated or underestimated how long 8 per cent of the drugs were supposed to be taken. They had an inaccurate perception of the dosage schedule in 11 per cent of the cases. They overestimated or underestimated how regularly they were supposed to take the drug in 17 per cent of the cases. In addition, patients misunderstood the purpose of 23 per cent of the drugs. For example, patients who had been given medication for hypertension sometimes thought that the drugs were for relief of asthma symptoms, palpitations, low back pain, and other problems.

Consistent with the working hypothesis, the patients who had a completely accurate perception of what the physician expected (n = 63) were more apt to conform with the physician's expectations; 60 per cent of these patients conformed with the physician's treatment plan. Of the patients who made at least one error when describing what the physician expected ($n = 68$), 17 per cent conformed. More importantly, there was a positive association between the amount of physician instruction, the accuracy of the patient's perceptions, and the rate of behavioral conformity. The patients who had received high instruction were more likely to have an accurate perception of the treatment plan than were the patients who had received low instruction (62 per cent and 40 per cent, respectively). Under the condition of high instruction, 52 per cent of the patients conformed. Of the patients who had received low instruction, 29 per cent conformed.

Modifying Conditions

Although many conditions might facilitate or inhibit the effectiveness of physician instruction, at least two sets of conditions should be considered. First are those affecting patient's attention, comprehension, and retention of the physician's "message." Patients' ability to learn was more limited when they were not familiar with the physician's language, be that English or medical terminology. For example, the terms "antibiotic" and "decongestant" may have different meanings or no meaning to patients who have difficulty with English or a low level of education. The patients sometimes referred to both kinds of medication as "cold pills," which were believed to serve the same purpose—the relief of cold symptoms. If any difference was attributed, it was that the antibiotic was a "stronger cold pill" which could relieve symptoms more quickly and effectively and which was given for a "bad cold." The patients' abilities to comprehend and retain information were also affected by how many drugs they had been given and whether they had prior experience with the drugs.

The second set of conditions relates to patients' willingness to ask for clarification or to make explicit statements that indicate their confusion or uncertainty about what the physician expects. These types of feedback seem to facilitate the instruction process by alerting the physician to the patient's particular need for additional instruction, interpretation, or clarification. Patients who provided such feedback received more instruction from the physician. The following excerpt illustrates how the patient can foster explicitness on the part of the physician:

PATIENT: Do I have to keep taking the medicine I got from Dr. _____ last month?

DOCTOR: (looks in chart) You mean the medicine for the gas?

PATIENT: Yes.

DOCTOR: Are you still taking that?
PATIENT: Well, yes. I thought I was supposed to.
DOCTOR: No, you can stop that. You only have to take that when you have
           gas.

Unfortunately, few patients (n = 27) provided feedback, and even then only limited feedback. As a result, it is difficult to say how our findings might have been affected if the patients had been more actively involved during the instruction process.

THE PROCESS OF MOTIVATING THE PATIENT

It has been suggested that patients' attitudes about taking medication might be affected by physician's attitudes about the medication,[77-78] but we know very little about the nature and outcome of physicians' efforts to motivate their patients. Physicians and patients often disagree with one another,[79] but it is not clear how physicians try to resolve these conflicts. It is useful to consider what social psychologists have suggested about the nature of social influence processes.[80-83] Physicians can be said to have at least three types of power that can be exerted in an effort to gain patients' motivation and behavioral conformity: (1) interpersonal power (i.e., appealing to patients' desire for social approval); (2) expert power (i.e., appealing to reason by justifying medication use); and (3) legitimate power or the power of medical authority (i.e., appealing to the norm that patients "should" or "ought to" comply with their physician's orders). In addition, physicians might be more apt to influence their patients if they emphasize what they expect.

With this in mind, I proceeded to the second phase of the inductive study. The physician-patient encounter was viewed as a situation in which the physician can motivate a patient by using a variety of influence strategies or appeals. We began with the following working hypotheses:

1. Patients will be more likely to conform if they have a high evaluation of the treatment plan.
2. Patients' evaluation of and conformity with the treatment plan will be higher if the physician makes a greater effort to motivate patients.

Friendliness, Justification, Authority, and Emphasis

The first strategy the physician might use is to express friendliness and receptivity toward the patient. Presumably, this is an appeal to the patient's desire for social approval, or an effort to get the patient to like the physician so that the patient will be more receptive to the physician's advice. This strategy involves greeting the patient in a courteous manner, showing interest in the patient's questions and remarks, expressing positive affect toward the patient, and extending a courteous farewell. A content analysis of transcripts showed that this was the most commonly used influence strategy; the physicians were friendly and receptive toward 42 per cent of the patients. Patient conformity was somewhat higher in those cases where the physician had been friendly, but the strategy by itself was not very effective. Further analysis indicated that friendliness was more effective if the patient also received high instruction. When there was both high instruction and friendliness, 78 per cent of the patients conformed. Under high instruction and low friendliness, 42 per cent conformed with the physician's treatment plan.

The second type of influence strategy is what can be called "justification"—an appeal to the patient's reason. Although the physicians in this clinic rarely gave the patients detailed explanations of the nature of their illness or of the long-term benefits that might be gained by using the prescribed medications, there was evidence that the physicians tried to justify why they were advising the use of drugs. In other words, they sometimes reported on the current status of the patient's condition before giving instructions, mentioned that the drug was important, or mentioned some other reason for taking the medication as advised. For example, one physician justified his advice by telling the patient, "Your second blood pressure (measurement) is still high so I would like to change the blood pressure medicine."

The strategy of high justification was evident in 40 per cent of the cases and was one of the more effective influence strategies. Under the condition of high justification, 55 per cent of the patients conformed with medical advice. Patients who received low justification conformed in only 27 per cent of the cases.

To determine whether the physicians exerted their medical authority, we did a content analysis of the language they used when advising the patient about medication. Physicians were regarded as having exerted their authority if they gave instructions in a demanding or authoritative manner (e.g., "You *must* take three pills a day") or if they appealed to the norm that patients have an obligation to comply with medical orders (e.g., "You should take the medicine every day"). To our surprise, the physicians exerted their authority with only 18 per cent of the patients. As in the case of physician friendliness, the strategy of exerting medical authority—by itself—was not highly effective. However, when the amount of physician instruction was controlled, the difference was more evident. When there was high instruction and high authority, 71 per cent of the patients conformed with the treatment plan. Under the condition of high instruction and low authority, 51 per cent of the patients conformed.

The fourth influence strategy—emphasis on what was expected—involved making two or more statements about the need to refill and continue taking the prescribed medications. Although it was not used often—there was emphasis in 12 per cent of the cases—this strategy seemed effective. When physicians placed emphasis on their expectations, 65 per cent of the patients subsequently conformed with advice. In comparison, low emphasis was associated with 34 per cent conformity.

Monitoring Patients' Use of Previously Prescribed Drugs

One of the most notable differences among the eight physicians was that some engaged in more extensive monitoring (or follow-up) of how their patients had taken previously prescribed medications. These doctors asked the patients whether they had taken each drug, how many tablets they were taking a day, how much medication was left in the container, and other probing questions. Other physicians asked global questions without asking for details (e.g., "Are you taking your medicines?"). Some physicians did not ask any questions and seemed to assume, sometimes mistakenly, that the patient had been conforming with advice.

Extensive monitoring or follow-up seemed to be important in several respects. First, patients who were advised to follow instructions regarding previously prescribed drugs ($n = 81$) may have made certain assumptions, depending on whether the physician questioned them about their behavior. If the physician did not always question them and did not ask probing questions, they may have assumed that the physician did not attach much importance to the drug or their use of it.

Second, high monitoring seemed to be an integral aspect of the physician's efforts to maintain effective control over the patient and to resolve any conflicts between them. More specifically, monitoring was a means of eliciting more accurate feedback about which patients had a low evaluation of the previously prescribed treatment and which patients were not conforming with previous advice. It was anticipated that when physicians received such feedback they would make a greater effort to motivate patients and, as a result, would be more successful in achieving the desired pattern of behavior.

In general, these anticipations were confirmed. When physicians engaged in high monitoring ($n = 31$), 52 per cent of the patients subsequently conformed with advice. Under low monitoring ($n = 50$), only 26 per cent of the patients conformed. Several important findings emerged on the dynamics of the monitoring. First, physicians who engaged in more extensive follow-up received more *accurate* feedback from the patients; their patients were more apt to express their complaints and to admit that they had not been conforming with previous advice.[84] When physicians did not engage in extensive follow-up or monitoring, patients were less apt to express complaints about their medication and more apt to conceal the fact that they were not taking the medication as prescribed at the previous visit. Second, we found that the physicians made a greater effort to motivate the patient when patients admitted nonconformity and/or complained that the medicine was not necessary, did not seem to help, or caused side effects. Under these circumstances, physicians were more apt to express friendliness, provide justification, exert authority, emphasize what was expected, or engage in other influence tactics (e.g., reassure the patient about side effects or suggest ways in which the patient could cope with the negative features of the drug).

Physicians occasionally tolerated or ignored patient deviation from previous advice and, in some instances, changed the treatment plan (i.e., lowered the dosage, gave a different drug, or temporarily stopped all treatment). In addition to the strictly medical reasons for changing a treatment plan, several additional explanations might account for such physician adaptations. Some physicians may believe that it is not essential or desirable to take the previously prescribed dosage or to take certain drugs (such as tranquilizers) on a regular basis. As one of the physicians explained:

> I rarely start a patient on a tranquilizer. If someone else has given it to them and they [patients] request it again, I am more likely to give it. But I feel funny starting it myself, and I refill it only if the patient brings it up again. Otherwise, I just wait until they mention it . . . . I don't care if they take it.

Such an adaptation may also be a strategy for maintaining the patients' commitment to at least some degree of long-term treatment and follow-up care, particularly where the patient is being treated for a chronic disease such as essential hypertension. Some physicians weigh the benefits and risks of *demanding* that patients follow the "ideal" treatment plan and decide that there are too many risks involved in pursuing a particular issue.

A Note on the Limitations of Medical Authority

Some evidence in this study suggests that physicians risk losing their power to influence patients if they frequently demand that patients follow "ideal" treatment plans and if they do not respond to patients' complaints about such plans. Two of the eight physicians frequently gave their instructions in a demanding or authoritative manner and frequently did not respond to patients' complaints about their medications. Their patients were more likely to conceal their nonconformity when the physician questioned them and were also less likely to conform even when the physician attempted to motivate them. On the basis of in-depth case analysis, it appeared that ignoring patients' complaints and demanding compliance eventually led to a breakdown in physician-patient communication, errors in clinical judgment, and patient mistrust of the physician's claims and appeals for conformity.

When physicians ignore patients' complaints and demand compliance, patients are faced with a dilemma. On the one hand, they may be afraid to take the medicine as prescribed. On the other, they may be reluctant to terminate their association with the clinic, believing that they need some type of treatment and follow-up for a chronic condition. Rather than follow the physician's plan of treatment, patients then decide to "test" the validity of an alternate plan—their own plan of treatment. For example, a patient may try taking less than the prescribed dosage or number of drugs. Since the patient may consider the physician intolerant and unresponsive, the patient will probably conceal his or her nonconformity on return visits to the physician. In effect, the physician begins to receive inaccurate information from the patient. In some cases, the physician may assume that the patient's condition improved or remained under control because the patient was taking the medicine as prescribed. By telling the patient that his or her condition is improved, the physician unwittingly confirms the patient's belief that it may not be necessary to take as much medicine as the physician claimed. This leads the patient to begin doubting the credibility and/or legitimacy of the physician's claims and appeals.

Consider the cases of Ms. A and Ms. B. According to Ms. A, her medication for hypertension did not help. When asked why, she told the interviewer:

> sometimes I don't take the medicine and the pressure goes down by itself. And when I go back to the doctor, he would say, "Yeah, it has come down good." And I haven't even taken any medicine for quite awhile.

Next, consider the case of Ms. B, a patient who had been seeing one of the two physicians who frequently demanded that his patients follow advice and who frequently ignored complaints. Ms. B had hypertension and had not been following medication advice for about six months before the observed physician-patient visit. She was supposed to be taking three medications: (1) "water pills" (hydrochlorothiazide), (2) "kidney pills" (hydralazine), and (3) "artery pills" (guanethidine). However, before the observed visit, she had been only taking the "water pills," some of the "kidney pills," and none of the "artery pills." The medical record indicated that the physician was probably unaware of her nonconformity until the observed visit, despite the fact that the patient had made several other visits to the clinic. The following is an excerpt of the observed physician-patient interaction. The discussion about hypertension was initiated by the patient, who seemed surprised that her blood pressure had gone up on the day of the visit.

PATIENT: Why did my pressure go up?

DOCTOR: I don't know.

PATIENT: Maybe she [assistant] didn't take it right?

DOCTOR: (laughs) Yes. You've done very well. The least it could do is go down. You taking the water pills?

PATIENT: Yes.

DOCTOR: How many?

PATIENT: Morning and evening.

DOCTOR: That's two a day?

PATIENT: Yes.

DOCTOR: The artery pill?

PATIENT: Which one is it?

DOCTOR: For the blood vessels.

PATIENT: The blue one?

DOCTOR: No, that's the kidney pill. Are you taking the kidney pill?

PATIENT: Yes.

DOCTOR: How many?

PATIENT: (responds slowly) Twice a day—or four times a day.

DOCTOR: Maybe it is up because you're not taking enough. You should take it at least three times a day, sometimes four.

PATIENT: I take two instead of four. It never went up *before* when I didn't take it four times! (said very assertively)

DOCTOR: (laughs) Caught you now! (reads chart) 150 over 98. It's up a little.

PATIENT: Maybe I'm nervous. Comin' to the clinic and waiting makes me nervous.

DOCTOR: Take them a little more—right on the nose, the kidney pills. At least three a day, preferably four a day. Do you need any more?

PATIENT: No. It was like I was drunk. I stopped taking so many.

DOCTOR: Oh, that was it, huh. [Physician dropped the subject. There was no further discussion about this condition, the medications, or the patient's complaint that the medicine made her feel "drunk."]

Although the physician expressed friendliness, exerted authority, and justified medication use by reporting on the patient's condition, this patient did not modify her behavior after the observed visit. She continued to take less than prescribed. To the patient, it appeared quite logical to challenge the physician's claim that she should take the medicine as prescribed.

Although the physician takes certain risks when exerting authority, this influence strategy may be effective, particularly if it is used sparingly and if the physician does not, at the same time, ignore the patient's point of view. The more successful physicians are probably those who realize that their authority is limited.

The Physician's Total Effort
To Motivate the Patient

Since physicians sometimes used a combination of influence strategies, it seemed useful to consider whether the *total* effort to motivate the patient was associated with the patient's subsequent evaluation of the treatment plan and behavioral conformity. A composite index was developed and useu .o score the physician's total efforts to influence the patient. The items were (1) friendliness, (2) justification, (3) exertion of authority, (4) emphasis, (5) monitoring, (6) responding to complaints, and (7) responding to admissions of nonconformity. The 131 patients studied were classified into groups where the physician made a high effort to motivate the patient ($n = 20$), a moderate effort ($n = 71$), and a low effort ($n = 40$).

There was a positive association between the physician's total effort to motivate and the patient's subsequent evaluation of the treatment plan. In the high effort group, 50 per cent of the patients had a high evaluation of the treatment plan. They tended to believe that their medications were efficacious and important, that the drugs were not causing side effects or harm, and that they would suffer various negative consequences if they stopped the medications (e.g., risk of having a stroke or heart attack). In the moderate and low effort groups, patients were less apt to have a high evaluation of their drugs (19 per cent and 11 per cent, respectively). The relationship between physician effort and patient's subsequent behavior was even more considerable. Under the conditions of high, moderate, and low effort to motivate, the rates of behavioral conformity were 80 per cent, 41 per cent, and 13 per cent, respectively. The relationship between physician effort to motivate and patient behavior was even more evident when the amount of physician instruction was taken into account. Under high instruction, patient conformity ranged from 100 per cent (high effort) to 11 per cent (low effort). In contrast, patient conformity ranged from 60 per cent (high effort) to 13 per cent (low effort) under the condition of low physician instruction.

RECAPITULATION

I do not pretend to have developed a refined theory of physician-patient communication as it relates to patient conformity with medication advice. But the approach described in this paper suggests a meaningful way of conceptualizing the problem. Two major dimensions of physician communication have been identified: (1) the physician's effort to instruct the patient, and (2) the physician's effort to motivate the patient. Complementary dimensions of the patient's attitudes and behavior have also been noted: (1) the patient's perception of what the physician expects, (2) the patient's evaluation of the treatment plan, and (3) the patient's behavioral conformity. At least two major dimensions of patient communication must be recognized by physicians: (1) patient feedback, which indicates the patient's need for clarification, instruction, or interpretation, and (2) patient complaints about the treatment plan and information about whether previous advice has been followed. Other conditions that might facilitate or inhibit the processes by which physicians instruct and influence their patients are those that limit the patient's ability to learn the instructions, and those that lead the patient to mistrust the physician's claims and appeals.

NOTES

1. S. P. Rosenszweig and R. Folman (1974), "Patient and Therapist Variables Affecting Premature Termination in Group Psychotherapy," *Psychotherapy: Theory, Research and Practice*, **11**:76–79.

2. E. A. Rubinstein and M. Lorr (1956), "A Comparison of Terminators and Remainers in Outpatient Psychotherapy," *Journal of Clinical Psychology*, **12**:345–349.

3. J. D. Frank et al. (1957), "Why Patients Leave Psychotherapy," *Archives of Neurology and Psychiatry*, **77**:283–299.

4. G. A. Hellmuth et al. (1966), "Psychological Factors in Cardiac Patients: Distortion of Clinical Recommendations," *Archives of Environmental Health*, **12**:771–775.

5. Ibid.

6. Ibid.

7. E. A. Rubenstein and M. Lorr (1956), op. cit.

8. M. S. Davis (1968a), "Physiologic, Psychological and Demographic Factors in Patient Compliance with Doctors' Orders," *Medical Care*, **6**:115.

9. F. Auld, Jr. and L. D. Eron (1953), "The Use of Rorschach Scores To Predict Whether Patients Will Continue Psychotherapy," *Journal of Consulting Psychology*, **17**:104–109.

10. R. G. Gibby et al. (1954), "Validation of Rorschach Criteria for Predicting Duration of Therapy," *Journal of Consulting Psychology*, **18**:185–191.

11. G. Calden et al. (1955), "The Use of the MMPI in Predicting Irregular Discharge Among Tuberculosis Patients," *Journal of Clinical Psychology*, **11**:374–377.

12. M. E. Rorabaugh and G. Guthrie (1953), "The Personality Characteristics of Tuberculosis Patients Who Leave the Tuberculosis Hospital Against Medical Advice," *American Review of Tuberculosis,* **67**:432–439.

13. G. Calden et al. (1955), op. cit.

14. S. P. Rosenszweig and R. Folman (1974), op. cit.

15. Ibid.

16. G. A. Hellmuth et al. (1966), op. cit.

17. M. S. Davis (1968a), op. cit.

18. W. M. Dixon et al. (1957), "Outpatient P.A.S. Therapy," *Lancet,* **273**:871–873.

19. L. Gordis et al (1969), "Why Patients Don't Follow Medical Advice: A Study of Children on Long Term Antistreptococcal Prophylaxis," *Journal of Pediatrics,* **75**:957–968.

20. T. Moulding et al. (1970), "Supervision of Outpatient Drug Therapy with the Medication Monitor," *Annals of Internal Medicine,* **73**:559–564.

21. L. Gordis et al. (1969), op. cit.

22. T. Moulding et al. (1970), op. cit.

23. V. Francis et al. (1969), "Gaps in Doctor-Patient Communication: Patients' Response to Medical Advice," *New England Journal of Medicine,* **280**:535–540.

24. L. Gordis et al. (1969), op. cit.

25. T. Moulding et al. (1970), op. cit.

26. D. K. Fink et al. (1969a), "The Management Specialist in Effective Pediatric Ambulatory Care," *American Journal of Public Health,* **59**:527.

27. R. Elling et al. (1960), "Patient Participation in a Pediatric Program," *Journal of Health and Human Behavior,* **1**:183–191.

28. L. Gordis et al. (1969), op. cit.

29. L. J. Moran et al. (1956), "Some Determinants of Successful and Unsuccessful Adaptations to Hospital Treatment of Tuberculosis," *Journal of Consulting Psychology,* **20**:125–131.

30. T. Moulding et al. (1970), op. cit.

31. V. Francis et al. (1969), op. cit.

32. D. K. Fink et al. (1969a), op. cit.

33. M. S. Davis and R. Eichorn (1963), "Compliance with Medical Regimes: A Panel Study," *Journal of Health and Human Behavior,* **4**:240–249.

34. V. Francis et al. (1969), op. cit.

35. R. Elling et al. (1969), op. cit.

36. N. W. Shelton and P. J. Sparer (1956), "Recidivism: The Basic Problem of Self-Discharge Among Hospitalized Tuberculosis Patients," in P. J. Sparer, ed., *Personality, Stress and Tuberculosis* (New York: International Universities Press), pp. 477–489.

37. L. Gordis et al. (1969), op. cit.

38. V. Francis et al. (1969), op. cit.

39. D. K. Fink et al. (1969a), op. cit.

40. L. Gordis et al. (1969), op. cit.

41. Ibid.

42. R. Elling et al. (1960), op. cit.

43. L. Gordis et al. (1969), op. cit.

44. Ibid.

45. Ibid.
46. M. S. Davis (1968a), op. cit.
47. Ibid.
48. Ibid.
49. M. S. Davis and R. Eichorn (1963), op. cit.
50. Ibid.
51. D. Fink et al. (1969b), "Effective Patient Care in the Pediatric Ambulatory Setting: A Study of the Acute Care Clinic," *Journal of Pediatrics*, **43**:927–935.
52. N. Berkowitz et al. (1963), "Patient Follow-Through in the Outpatient Department," *Nursing Research*, **12**:16–22.
53. V. Francis et al. (1969), op. cit.
54. C. Latiolais and C. Berry (1969), "Misuse of Prescription Medication by Outpatients," *Drug Intelligence and Clinical Pharmacy*, **3**:270–277.
55. D. S. Irwin et al. (1971), "Phenothiazine Intake and Staff Attitudes," *American Journal of Psychiatry*, **127**:1631–1635.
56. I. Rosenstock (1960), "What Research in Motivation Suggests for Public Health," *American Journal of Public Health*, **50**:295–302.
57. S. Kasl and S. Cobb (1966a), "Health Behavior, Illness Behavior and Sick Role Behavior: I," *Archives of Environmental Health*, **12**:246–266.
58. S. Kasl and S. Cobb (1966b), "Health Behavior, Illness Behavior and Sick Role Behavior: II," *Archives of Environmental Health*, **12**:531–541.
59. M. Becker et al. (1972), "Predicting Mothers' Compliance with Medical Regimens," *Journal of Pediatrics*, **81**:843–854.
60. P. Ley and M. S. Spelman (1967), *Communicating with the Patient* (London: The Trinity Press).
61. C. Latiolais and C. Berry (1969), op. cit.
62. V. Francis et al. (1969), op. cit.
63. S. Kasl and S. Cobb (1966a), op. cit.
64. M. S. Davis (1968b), "Variation in Patients' Compliance with Doctors' Advice: An Empirical Analysis of Patterns of Communication," *American Journal of Public Health*, **58**:274–288.
65. M. S. Davis (1971), "Variation in Patients' Compliance with Doctors' Orders: Medical Practice and Doctor-Patient Interaction," *Psychiatry in Medicine*, **2**:31–54.
66. Ibid.
67. V. Francis et al. (1969), op. cit.
68. B. Korsch et al. (1968), "Gaps in Doctor-Patient Communication: Doctor-Patient Interaction and Patient Satisfaction," *Pediatrics*, **42**:855–871.
69. B. Korsch and V. Negrete (1972), "Doctor-Patient Communication," *Scientific American*, **227**:66–74.
70. B. Freeman et al. (1971), "Gaps in Doctor-Patient Communication: Doctor-Patient Interaction Analysis," *Pediatric Research*, **5**:298–311.
71. Ibid.
72. M. S. Davis (1971), op. cit.
73. B. Korsch and V. Negrete (1972), op. cit.

74. B. Freeman et al. (1971), op. cit.

75. M. S. Davis (1968b), op. cit.

76. B. Freeman et al. (1971), op. cit.

77. D. S. Irwin et al. (1971), op. cit.

78. E. Reynolds et al. (1965), "Psychological and Clinical Investigation of the Treatment of Anxious Outpatients with Three Barbiturates and a Placebo," *British Journal of Psychiatry*, **111**:84–95.

79. M. S. Davis (1968b), op. cit.

80. J. R. P. French and B. Raven (1959), "The Bases of Social Power," in D. Cartright, ed., *Studies in Social Power* (Ann Arbor: University of Michigan Press).

81. B. Collins and B. Raven (1969), "Group Structure: Attraction, Coalitions, Communication, and Power," in G. Lindzey and E. Aronson, eds., *The Handbook of Social Psychology*, 2d ed. (Reading, Mass.: Addison-Wesley), pp. 102–204.

82. H. Kelman (1958), "Compliance, Identification, and Internalization: Three Processes of Attitude Change," *Journal of Conflict Resolution*, **2**:51–60.

83. P. Blau (1967), *Exchange and Power in Social Life* (New York: Wiley).

84. Pharmacy files, medical records, and patient interview data indicated that at least 40 patients had not been following advice *before* the observed clinic visit. Thus, we could determine which patients admitted or concealed the fact that they had not been conforming with previous advice.

Chapter 12

Chronic Illness and Responsive Ambulatory Care

Linda H. Aiken

Ambulatory medical care services are designed primarily to treat acute episodic illness despite increasing demand for care for chronic illness. Approximately half the population suffers from at least one chronic illness, and a significant proportion has multiple chronic problems.[1] Physicians, traditionally trained in acute care hospitals, tend to organize ambulatory care practice with an emphasis on episodic treatment and specialty care. Whether in hospital specialty outpatient clinics, or in office-based practice, physicians focus on patients' immediate symptoms and give less attention to long-term care and adjustment needs.

Chronic illness differs from acute conditions in fundamental ways that require a different approach to managing patients. First, patients with such illnesses fluctuate from a relatively normal state of health to serious relapses that may be life threatening. Second, the absence of cures and often only partial palliation of symptoms for chronic illness adversely affects the motivation of patients to follow consistently the medical regimen and the motivation of health professionals to stay involved in patients' care. Third, acutely ill patients are generally passive, accepting the physician's dominant role in diagnosis and treatment. Effective care for chronic illness requires more active participation from the patient. The role of health professionals in "applying technology," thus, may be less important in achieving effective outcomes than the patient's

239

acceptance of major changes in life patterns. Much of the care of the chronically ill requires long-term health maintenance activities and assistance in learning to live effectively with disabilities. But numerous studies[2-3] have shown that many patients—one-third to two-thirds—fail to follow physicians' recommendations. Thus, to be effective, practitioners must learn how to influence patients to modify their behavior.

Because the needs of the acute and chronic patient are different, it is not surprising that medical services designed for acute care are unresponsive to the needs of patients with chronic illness. This chapter examines the lack of responsiveness of ambulatory care to patients with one type of chronic illness—heart disease—and explores the nature of the problems faced by these patients and their families, and their impact on adjustment and disability. Many of the types of problems discussed pertain as well to other chronic diseases.

THE UNRESPONSIVENESS OF AMBULATORY CARE

There is a general awareness that chronic illness is handled poorly within the existing framework of medical services. Strickland,[4] for example, in surveying a national sample of physicians, found marked concern about the present capacity of our health care system to cope with long-term illness. Various reasons are given for this lack of responsiveness. First, our current system is geared to short, intensive patient interactions. Many chronically ill patients, however, require longer encounters in which an effective educational dialogue develops between health professional and patient. Second, much chronic illness management is handled by specialty clinics. Institution-based clinics traditionally set aside a limited number of hours a week for outpatient clinics. The bulk of the specialist's time is spent on the more acute problems of inpatients; this is what specialists have been trained to do, and it is here that their basic interests lie. Ambulatory patients are seen in clinics where physicians feel pressed to move patients along rapidly, and patients who are aware of others waiting feel obligated to limit the extent to which they ask questions or take the physician's time. Thus, the manner in which ambulatory care is organized in institutional settings where physicians' major responsibilities are to hospital patients results in patient load bottlenecks and insufficient time to provide responsive care.

The medical management of conditions such as heart disease is believed to require at least periodic supervision and assessment by specialists. But the vast majority of care involves long-term monitoring, relatively minor modifications in the therapeutic regimen, and counseling regarding adjustment to disability. Medical specialists provide much of the care for patients with heart disease, and since they are oriented toward the problems of physical assessment and management, the long-term monitoring and counseling functions are not carried out with equal enthusiasm and competence. Frequently, the physician's definition of the patient's problem is quite different from the patient's view, which tends to focus on adjustment problems to a much larger degree. The importance of adjustment is suggested by Wynn's[5] study of 400 patients recovering from myocardial infarction. Wynn found that disability due to fear and poor adjustment was greater than that due to the disease itself in about one-third of the patients.

Another significant deterrent to responsive ambulatory care for chronic patients is lack of continuity. Most institution-based ambulatory care clinics have rapid turnover of personnel either through attrition[6-7] or as a result of the system of physician rotation[8] practiced in most training institutions. Thus, patients either do not establish a relationship with a specific physician, or they are confronted at intervals with establishing new relationships. This may be a crucial issue since physicians must rely heavily on rapport with the patient to influence compliance with the medical regimen.

In addition to organizational problems within the medical care delivery system, there are serious inadequacies in the articulation of medical care services with other community support systems[9] vital to patients with chronic illnesses. Although many large medical centers employ a social worker or vocational rehabilitation counselor, in general these workers are completely overwhelmed by the numbers of patients needing their services. Furthermore, there is often less than desirable communication between institutionally based personnel and community agencies that provide medically related services. The problem of providing community support services is even greater in private office-based practice. Patients are left largely to their own resources to find employment, to negotiate with social security for disability status, or to obtain psychological counseling.

Inadequate communication between physicians, patients, and families also characterizes existing ambulatory services. In part, this results from organizational problems already described. In addition, physicians are both poorly trained and poorly motivated to manage social, psychological, and communicative problems with the same systematic rigor they bring to physiological problems. Despite the obvious potential of families for playing an integral role in patients' long-term adherence to medical advice and general adjustment, there is little evidence that wives or other family members have reasonable access to physicians in the ambulatory setting. Physicians do not give high priority to providing patients and families with information[10] and have a tendency to underestimate the patients' knowledge,[11] providing cryptic, oversimplistic explanations for conditions that patients know are complex. Such inadequate explanations probably have a negative effect on compliance since patients cannot operationalize the instructions. Advice to "use in moderation," "take it easy," and not to "overdo" can only be interpreted in a very personal way.

Therefore, physicians lose an opportunity to increase the patient's knowledge, and patients often feel hostile and resentful. Of course, not all communication problems can be blamed solely on physicians. Patients may not readily reveal their problems and concerns, either because they feel they are being rushed, because they feel less important vis-à-vis the physician, or because of inability to articulate concerns. These patient characteristics must be taken into account in the organization of ambulatory care and in the training of physicians.

MYOCARDIAL INFARCTION: THE PROBLEMS

For many persons, the original diagnosis of coronary heart disease or myocardial infarction is made as a result of chest pain. Thus, the onset is likely to be sudden, frightening, and followed by a highly stressful period of hospitalization. Discharge from the hospital is, in a very real sense, only the beginning of a long process of both physiological and psychological adjustment.

In the initial months after the myocardial infarction, many of the symptoms are both physiological and psychological in origin. For instance, the depression and irritability that so commonly characterize the early months[12-14] may be a physiological response to reduced cardiac function, long periods of inactivity, and drugs, and may also be due to fear of death, threat to self-image, and boredom. Return to work appears to be a benchmark in the recovery process. It represents adequate physiological recovery, and also reduces anxiety by offering a return to a former life style. Most men who will ever return to work do so within the first 6 to 10 months following the myocardial infarction.[15] Only a small proportion who have not returned to work within a year ever return. Those who are unable to return to work face the prospect of having to define new ways to structure their time. Further, all persons who have had one myocardial infarction face the possibility of a second attack leading to sudden death or greater residual disability. Many live with inadequate circulation that may contribute, along with psychological factors, to long-term irritability and restlessness, "personality changes," and sexual impotence. Thus, problems that may be manifested in classic psychological symptomatology may in fact be physiological in nature and vice versa.

The treatment of coronary heart disease may involve the use of drugs to enhance cardiac function, to control hypertension, or to reduce irritability and depression. Surgery is sometimes performed, depending on the orientation of the physician, to enhance coronary circulation. But the most commonly used treatment regimen involves basic modifications in habits such as smoking, diet, and activities. Many aspects of such a regimen are difficult to adhere to over long periods of time because they may significantly erode the quality of one's life, and the quality of life of others in the family.

In a study[16] of men recovering from myocardial infarctions we also studied wives' reactions and found that such families face many problems that appear to be related to adaptation to life with a chronic disease. Such problems should concern us all from a humanistic point of view. However, for those not convinced that social-psychological aspects of illness are within the sphere of medical responsibility, I will attempt to specify the implications of such problems for compliance and disability.

Of the husbands and wives interviewed, 80 per cent reported moderate to great change in their lives since the heart attack. Since most changes were perceived to be negative, there was a high prevalence of unhappiness and depression among the patients; 52 per cent of the men and 42 per cent of the wives reported that they had been unhappy since the heart attack. These figures are considerably higher than estimates of unhappiness[17] in a random sample indicating that 16 per cent of men and 17 per cent of women are "not too happy." The incidence of depression in the postmyocardial infarction group was also striking—73 per cent of the men reported that they were frequently depressed.

The specific changes occurring following the heart attack that were perceived to be problems are outlined in Table 12.1.[18] The most frequently cited problems were those relating to health restrictions. Three-fourths of the men reported that dietary and activity restrictions were problems of considerable concern. More than 50 per cent had either stopped smoking or were trying to stop. Many said that all of the things that made life worth living had now been restricted or eliminated.

More than half of the men were overweight at the time of the heart attack, and at the time of the interview 34 per cent were still overweight. On the whole, both the patients and their wives felt hostile toward the medical staff for the role they played in imposing restrictions. The hostility was not so much directed toward the restrictions themselves but toward those who imposed them without giving specific instructions or assistance to help them comply. Eighty-eight per cent of the patients believed they had some control over how serious their heart disease became, and 74 per cent felt that following a strict diet would help at least maintain current health levels. Hence, patients were at least intellectually ready to try to modify their behavior. However, the extent of instruction on diet consisted of a visit by the dietician at the time of hospitalization. The wife was included if she happened to be there. The consultation revolved around types of foods to be avoided. No assistance was given to anticipate such problems as how to cope with boredom without eating, how to prepare an interesting diet, and how a working man used to eating large meals could now feel satisfied by eating much less. On subsequent visits to the doctor, the patient was either admonished or praised for weight gain or loss, but rarely did physicians have anything more specific to say than "cut down."

Table 12.1   Husbands' and Wives' Reports of the Husband's Problems
Following Myocardial Infarction

Problem	Husband (%)	Wife (%)
Health restrictions		
having to restrict kinds of food eaten	78	78
having to restrict amount of food eaten	77	74
having to limit activities	74	73
having to stop smoking	58	55
Employment		
having to give up former work	66	54
has experienced financial problems	59	59
learning how to occupy himself in his leisure time	57	52
finding a job for which he is trained	48	26
Husband-wife relationship		
has experienced a change in sex life	62	55
wife is overprotective	55	55
wife nags him for not following the doctor's advice	41	54
husband-wife relationship has changed	30	25
feels resented by wife for being sick	22	24
Psychological response		
fears having another heart attack	60	74
knows he is sick but does not look sick to others	46	47
feels like less of a man	45	34
worries about dying suddenly	39	53

The restrictions on smoking produced similar problems. All patients were requested to stop, and some were even forced to stop by such threats as the withholding of heart surgery. However, less than half of those who had smoked prior to the heart attack stopped. The patient was given no assistance with how to stop, and not one patient was referred to any type of smoking clinic or consultant. To compound the problem, most of the men who tried to stop smoking either began to gain weight or became nervous and irritable, both contraindicated for coronary patients. There are two related points here. First, patients are required to change lifelong behavior patterns without professional help; and second, the resultant anxiety may be as detrimental[19–20] as the continuation of smoking and dietary habits.

The second major area of concern was related to employment. Although 78 per cent of the men studied were in at least their second year since the heart attack, 60 per cent were still unemployed. Most of the unemployed were not working due to doctors' advice, but many were looking for some type of part-time work, even without pay. About 10 per cent were actively seeking employment without success, usually due to poor training and advancing age.

The major problems relating to employment were financial in nature, or were due to a lowering of self-esteem resulting from loss of employment. Previous studies[21-24] of the meaning of work indicate that work is viewed as a source of gratifications in addition to earnings. Time becomes structured around work, one's friends and colleagues are often found through work, and one's status in society is partly a consequence of work. Thus, work often becomes an important part of one's self-identity. There is some evidence that white collar workers may identify with work more closely than blue collar workers because they are able to pursue more of their own goals and obtain more gratification through their work. We found that although blue collar workers tended not to identify with the content of the work itself, they were highly dependent on working time to structure their days. When unemployed, they had limited leisure time interests to pursue and few friends with whom to interact. The burden of this change in life pattern generally fell upon the wife.

Wives of blue collar workers have been described as isolated from their husbands' work interests and leisure time activities.[25] Great investments of time and energy are made in children at the expense of the husband-wife relationship. Komarovsky[26] noted that blue collar workers frequently have little of common interest to talk about with their wives. Over the years, this pattern of isolation leads the wife to associate with a group of family or friends who in some ways play a more significant supportive role than the husband. Thus, when a wife who has a well-established life pattern finds herself at home constantly with a husband with whom she has little in common, she becomes anxious and resentful. This adds to the husband's lack of self-esteem.[27]

Although physicians may view such problems as being neither feasible to treat nor within their sphere of influence, there is some evidence to the contrary. First, many of the problems hinge on the patient's unemployment. Physicians continue to advise patients not to work despite a lack of evidence that risk is increased by returning to work. In fact, we found that men who felt reasonably well but were discouraged from returning to previous employment undertook jobs at home that were more stressful than their usual work—shoveling snow, cutting grass, washing windows, and house painting. Perhaps the practice of encouraging men to give up their former work should be studied more thoroughly.

MYOCARDIAL INFARCTION: THE PROCESS OF ADJUSTMENT

Although a patient's eventual satisfactory posthospital adjustment is clearly associated with the degree of support he receives at home, relatively little is known about the mechanisms by which families facilitate or inhibit the adjustment process. There are indications, however, that spouses experience a crisis of major proportions due to feelings of insecurity, fear, and guilt; and that spouses assume an important role in the recovery process although that role has not been examined in detail.[28-31]

A major focus of our study was to begin to explore the role of the wife and family in the patients' social-psychological adjustment to disability. Wives appeared to adopt one of two roles: providing understanding and reassurance, or becoming the advocate for compliance and hence the adversary in some respects. For instance, half the patients perceived their wives as "the right hand of the doctor regarding restrictions," and one-third thought their wives supported the doctor's position on restrictions to the extent of ignoring their feelings. Regardless of the role the wife played, it was apparent that she had only secondhand information about the medical regimen. Wives essentially had no access to their husband's physician. Many accompanied their husbands on visits to the physician but were either asked to wait outside during the examination or were given only a superficial acknowledgment. As a result, wives felt that their information was inadequate, which increased their feelings of insecurity regarding their husband's condition, and also that they had no understanding of how to help their husbands comply.

One result of the wife's lack of information was a tendency to be overprotective.[32] Fifty-five per cent of the patients reported this to be a problem. Husbands perceived their wives' overprotectiveness as a way of controlling their behavior. Many husbands responded to this overprotection by becoming nervous and tense, or outwardly hostile. The stories differed from family to family but there was a consistent message: there existed a steadily eroding conflict over implications of the illness centering around activity, diet, smoking, and irritability even when the marriage and premorbid home life had been stable. Such conflict has negative implications not only for compliance but for the quality of life of all family members, and may also affect the patient's physical condition adversely.

A substantial part of this problem could be eliminated if wives were included as active participants in the treatment regimen and given accurate information. Organized groups for wives of men recovering from myocardial infarction and for the husbands themselves have been successfully used in various programs.[33-35] Here patients and their wives share experiences, and have a chance to test reality and to define what symptoms may be "normal" or expected. For instance, many wives were greatly concerned about what they described as "personality changes" in their husbands. They had no idea whether these changes were to be expected, whether they were permanent or temporary, and what could be done about them. An opportunity to learn that other wives had similar experiences and that the symptoms usually subsided in time would have been of considerable assistance. Young parents were particularly in need of help either from patients with similar problems or from health professionals regarding the impact of the husband's heart attack on the children. Approximately 20 per cent of the men studied had young children, and most were unclear as to necessary limits on their participation in children's activities. The literature on social-psychological adjustment following myocardial infarction does not deal adequately with parent-child relationships, and physicians rarely explore such issues with their patients.

IMPLICATIONS

Given that the chronically ill need consistent, long-term monitoring and social-psychological support in addition to access to specialty care, a feasible approach would be to use midlevel health practitioners, especially nurse practitioners, in their care. Demonstration projects have shown that nurses can effectively share a large and increasing responsibility in chronic disease care. Runyan[36] compared morbidity, hospitalization, and consumer acceptability between chronically ill patients receiving care in decentralized facilities staffed by specially trained nurses and those obtaining care in a more conventional manner in outpatient clinics. He found the nurse-run clinics superior to the outpatient clinic on all dimensions. Similarly, Lewis et al.[37] reported no differences in deaths or severity of disease between patients cared for in nurse clinics and those cared for by physicians. There were, however, significant differences in outcomes as measured by reduction of disability and relative decreases in discomfort and dissatisfaction of patients seen in the nurse clinic. The authors attribute these differences not to the abilities of the practitioners, but to the different processes of care emphasized by physicians and nurses. Physicians "are more concerned . . . with the biological and technical aspects of diagnosis and management of disease. Nurses, on the other hand, described their activities in terms of supporting role functions—more consistent with the majority of needs of the chronically ill."[38] Nurse practitioners could also play the role of ombudsman, helping consumers negotiate varying aspects of their care.

Several recommendations have emerged relevant to the doctor-patient relationship. The chronically ill have many problems that are not curable but that cause great unhappiness and discomfort. It was clear from our study that patients wanted to discuss these problems with their own physician even though they realized that there was little the physician might be able to do. For instance, 62 per cent of the patients studied had experienced a decrease in sexual activity. Many patients never discussed the issue with their wives but wanted to discuss it with someone, preferably their doctor. Although some cardiologists refer patients with "emotional" problems to psychiatrists for treatment, none of the patients studied had found psychiatric consultation fruitful. Both the husbands and their wives wanted their own physician to acknowledge their problems and to be supportive. Most psychological problems faced by the chronically ill could be handled as well by physicians and nurses within their own practices, and perhaps with better results, than by psychiatric consultations, which only adds to the fragmentation of care. The value of physicians consulting with both husband and wife has also been emphasized.

Our study showed that relatively few patients comply completely with medical advice, particularly if compliance means major behavioral change in several areas of living. This is consistent with Davis's[39] finding that there was a low rate of compliance for patients who were prescribed changes in three areas—work, diet, and personal habits—as compared to a high rate of compliance for patients whose prescriptions touched only one. A review of prescribed restrictions is needed to evaluate more scientifically the unintended consequences of too many restrictions. Employment is an area of special concern for reevaluation. The unintended consequences of unemployment in some cases seem clearly to outweigh the risks of employment.

In this chapter I have examined inadequacies in the current ambulatory care system as they relate to the care of the chronically ill. These inadequacies are due, in large part, to the acute-care orientation of health institutions and to the low priority placed on the continuing treatment of long-term chronic illness by health professionals. Incentives are needed to encourage physicians and other providers to give more attention to the needs of the chronically ill. Undergraduate and postgraduate medical education could be restructured to provide a more focused experience in ambulatory care in place of traditional rotations, which are of short duration and largely ancillary to inpatient care experiences. In addition, students must be exposed to the knowledge base and techniques for facilitating behavior change as well as the technical skills relevant to physiological problems. For such a change to occur, ambulatory care for the chronically ill must be perceived as a professionally rewarding activity within medicine with credible research and educational components. Thus, we need to develop medical and nursing educators with clinical and research skills in the long-term management of chronic illness who will be able to identify for students the challenges of such care. In addition, the financing of ambulatory care for the chronically ill does not provide incentives for institutional or provider change. Physicians consistently involved in long-term management and counseling activities must be reimbursed in a way similar to reimbursement for acute episodic illness. I have previously made a case for the use of new health practitioners to assume major responsibility for the basic care and management of the chronically ill. The two basic problems in the use of new health practitioners will be teaching physicians how to utilize their services most effectively, and influencing federal and private agencies to adopt a reimbursement mechanism to finance the services of new health practitioners.

NOTES

1. National Center for Health Statistics (1971), *Chronic Conditions and Limitations of Activity and Mobility: United States, July 1965–June 1967*, Public Health Service Publication 1000, Series 10, No. 61, Table E, p. 7.

2. M. H. Becker and R. A. Maiman (1975), "Sociobehavioral Determinants of Compliance with Health and Medical Care Recommendations," *Medical Care*, **13**:10–24.

3. M. S. Davis (1968), "Variations in Patients' Compliance with Doctors' Advice: An Empirical Analysis of Patterns of Communication," *American Journal of Public Health*, **58**:274.

4. S. Strickland (1972), *U.S. Health Care: What's Wrong and What's Right* (New York: Universe Books).

5. A. Wynn (1967), "Unwarranted Emotional Distress in Men with Ischaemic Heart Disease," *Medical Journal of Australia*, **2**:847–851.

6. M. Kramer and C. Baker (1971), "Nursing Exodus: Can We Prevent It?" *Journal of Nursing Administration*, **1**:15–30.

7. R. H. Pape (1967), "Touristry: A Type of Occupational Mobility," *Social Problems*, **11**:336–344.

8. A. L. Strauss (1971), "The Rotational System: Its Impact Upon Teaching, Learning, and the Medical Service," in *Professions, Work, and Careers* (San Francisco: Sociology Press).

9. S. Levine, P. E. White, and D. B. Paul (1963), "Community Interorganizational Problems in Providing Medical Care and Social Services," *American Journal of Public Health*, **53**:1183–1195.

10. B. M. Korsh, E. K. Gozzi, and V. Francis (1968), "Gaps in Doctor-Patient Communication," *Pediatrics*, **42**:855–871.

11. L. Pratt, A. Seligmann, and G. Reader (1957), "Physicians' Views on the Level of Medical Information Among Patients," *American Journal of Public Health*, **47**:1277–1283.

12. A. M. Mordkoff and O. A. Parsons (1967), "The Coronary Personality: A Critique," *Psychosomatic Medicine*, **29**:1–4.

13. H. A. Wishnie, T. P. Hackett, and N. H. Cassem (1971), "Psychological Hazards of Convalescence Following Myocardial Infarction," *Journal of the American Medical Association*, **215**:1292–1296.

14. A. Wynn (1967), op. cit.

15. E. Weinblatt, S. Shapiro, C. Frank, and R. Sager (1966), "Return to Work and Work Status Following First Myocardial Infarction," *American Journal of Public Health*, **56**:169.

16. Data reported here represent a study of 155 men recovering from myocardial infarctions. Their wives were included in the study. Husbands and wives were interviewed separately to elicit independent assessments of major problems and needs related to the heart disease, and to the process of learning to live with a chronic illness. Approximately half were being

treated in the outpatient cardiology clinic of a teaching institution; the remainder were patients of a private cardiologist practicing in a group setting.

17. N. Bradburn and D. Caplovitz (1965), *Reports on Happiness* (Chicago: Aldine).

18. The husband and wife were asked to assess independently the frequency and severity of the husband's major problems. The interviewer attempted to elicit only those problems that had evolved since the heart attack. However, any retrospective answer is subject to rationalization or forgetfulness. In addition, some problems such as decreased sexual activity were probably due in part to advancing age, although the interviewer tried to differentiate between age-related changes and illness-related changes.

19. W. I. Wardwell, M. Hyman, and C. B. Bahnson (1964), "Stress and Coronary Heart Disease in Three Field Studies," *Journal of Chronic Diseases*, 17:73–84.

20. R. Marks (1967), "A Review of Empirical Findings," *Milbank Memorial Fund Quarterly*, 45:51–108.

21. E. Lyman (1955), "Occupational Differences in the Value Attached to Work," *American Journal of Sociology*, 61:138–144.

22. F. Herzberg, B. Mausner, and B. Snyderman (1959), *The Motivation to Work* (New York: Wiley).

23. C. Safilios-Rothschild (1970), *The Sociology and Social Psychology of Disability and Rehabilitation* (New York: Random House).

24. L. A. Ferman (1964), "Sociological Perspectives in Unemployment Research," in A. B. Shostak and W. Gomberg, eds., *Blue-Collar World* (Englewood Cliffs, N.J.: Prentice-Hall).

25. L. Rainwater, R. P. Coleman, and G. Handel (1959), *Workingman's Wife* (New York: Oceana).

26. M. Komarovsky (1964), *Blue-Collar Marriage* (New York: Random House).

27. M. Komarovsky (1940), *The Unemployed Man and His Family* (New York: Holt, Rinehart and Winston).

28. S. H. Croog, S. Levine, and Z. Lurie (1968), "The Heart Patient and the Recovery Process," *Social Science and Medicine*, 2:121–123.

29. M. Skelton and J. Dominian (1973), "Psychological Stress in Wives of Patients with Myocardial Infarction," *British Medical Journal*, 2:101–103.

30. P. K. New et al. (1968), "The Support Structure of Heart and Stroke Patients: A Study of the Role of Significant Others in Patient Rehabilitation," *Social Science and Medicine*, 2:185–200.

31. S. H. Croog, A. Lipson, and S. Levine (1972), "Help Patterns in Severe Illness: The Roles of Kin Network, Non-Family Resources, and Institutions," *Journal of Marriage and the Family*, 34:32–41.

32. H. A. Wishnie, T. P. Hackett, and N. H. Cassem (1971), op. cit.

33. C. A. Adsett and J. G. Bruhn (1968), "Short Term Group Psychotherapy for Post-myocardial Infarction Patients and Their Wives," *Canadian Medical Association Journal*, 99:577–584.

34. R. H. Rahe, C. F. Tuffli, R. J. Sucher, and R. J. Arthur (1973), "Group Therapy in the Outpatient Management of Post-Myocardial Infarction Patients," *Psychiatry in Medicine*, 4:77–88.

35. C. B. Bilodeau and T. P. Hackett (1971), "Issues Raised in a Group Setting by Patients Recovering from Myocardial Infarction," *American Journal of Psychiatry*, 128:105–110.

36. J. W. Runyan (1975), "The Memphis Chronic Disease Program: Comparisons in Outcome and the Nurse's Extended Role," *Journal of the American Medical Association,* **231**:264–267.

37. C. E. Lewis, B. A. Resnik, G. Schmidt, and D. Waxman (1969), "Activities, Events, and Outcomes in Ambulatory Patient Care," *New England Journal of Medicine,* **280**:645–649.

38. Ibid., p. 648.

39. M. S. Davis and R. L. Eichhorn (1963), "Compliance with Medical Regimens: A Panel Study," *Journal of Health and Human Behavior,* **4**:240–249.

IV

TRENDS IN HEALTH POLICY, SOCIAL REGULATION, AND IN THE EVALUATION OF HEALTH PROGRAMS

Chapter 13

The Social Psychology
of Informed Consent
in Experimentation
and Therapy

Throughout this book it has been emphasized that the growing complexity of medical care and the varied functions of hospitals and other delivery systems result in increasingly complex expectations and frequent conflicts of values. As these problems become apparent, attempts are made to deal with them through administrative rules with the hope that appropriate regulations and new review procedures will prevent abuses. An excellent example, illustrating the conflicts and strains in dealing with conflicting goals and the difficulties of developing helpful rules, is the area of informed consent in research and therapy.[1]

There is a long-standing principle that a patient's agreement is necessary before subjecting him or her to a medical procedure, and such consent cannot be said to be meaningful unless the patient has reasonable information about the intervention and its risks and benefits. Although precise definitions of informed consent and their application to specific circumstances are difficult to formulate, these matters are taking on increasing importance in modern medical practice. The Department of Health, Education, and Welfare's definition of informed consent includes six elements: (1) fair explanation of the procedures to be followed and their purposes, including identification of any procedures that are experimental; (2) description of discomforts and risks reasonably to be expected; (3) description of benefits reasonably to be expected; (4) disclosure of any alternative procedures that might be advantageous for the subject; (5) an offer to answer inquiries concerning the procedures; and (6) an instruction that the subject is free to withdraw consent and to discontinue participation in the project or activity at any time.[2] Most commonly in experimentation, investigators are expected to obtain from the subject or from the subject's authorized representative a written consent embodying the points listed above.

The current controversy over consent and ethical experimentation illustrates how difficult it has become to balance the rights of individuals against the rights of institutions and the needs of society. Some argue that even more safeguards are necessary to protect patients against ambitious scientists who give higher priority to increased knowledge than to the interests of individual patients or subjects. Others maintain that the growing regulation of experimentation and the bureaucratic procedures developed to maintain it are hampering necessary research and substantially increasing the efforts and financial costs involved in investigation. Indeed, to the extent that definitions of risks are interpreted literally, even the research dealing with the topic of this book, which is relatively innocuous, could have been severely restricted. For example, the Policy and Procedures Governing the Protection of Human Subjects at the University of California–Berkeley defines social risk as follows:

> *Social risks* are related in the main to procedures that may place the reputation or status of a social group or an institution in jeopardy. Procedures designed to measure the characteristics of easily defined subgroups of a culture may entail risks if the qualities measured are ones which have positive or negative value in the eyes of the group. Even when research does not impinge directly on it, a group may be derogated or its reputation injured. Likewise, an institution, such as a church, a university, or a prison, must be guarded against derogation, for many people may be affiliated with, or employed by, the institution, and pejorative information about it would injure their reputations and self-esteem. In evaluating social risk, an investigator should ask himself how the findings will appear to persons belonging to any identifiable group—or affiliated with an institution—studied and reported on. These cautions are as equally warranted in the case of anthropological field research in distant cultures as in studies performed in domestic settings.

If we were to take the above statement literally, nothing but the most bland analysis would seem to be without risk. But what if the organization and procedures of the hospital encourage malpractice? Or university administrators are incompetent? Or prison administrators brutalize and dehumanize inmates?

The fact is that such broad and unrealistic statements of risk are viewed with skepticism, if not contempt, by those they are intended to regulate, and have little impact on their behavior. Perhaps more modest definitions, better fitted to the realities of research and the world we live in, might be more successful in achieving what is intended—a more sensitive consideration of the needs and interests of individual research subjects.

Recent concern about the use of human subjects is the result of highly publicized cases of abuse. In New York City, live cancer cells were injected into geriatric patients without their consent. The Tuskegee syphilis experiment funded by the Public Health Service is another example. A more general cause of concern is growing skepticism of the expert and professional dominance. As some of the negative consequences of science and technology have become more evident, so has distrust of research become more prevalent. American foreign policy, and particularly the war in Southeast Asia, contributed much to discrediting technology and expertise as forces for the good.

Linked with changing social attitudes and challenges to traditional authority are new claims for the individual's autonomy. Most people now receive much of their medical care in large institutions and often do not personally know the physicians and other providers of their health care. Thus, they have more reason to feel suspicious that the decisions made concerning them may not be the ones most in their interest. Although informed consent is an old issue, social change has made it more salient than ever before, and with increased education and sophistication among the public it is no longer an issue that can be resolved solely by professionals within their own terms.

Government has responded to increased public attention to experimentation by attempting to regulate research through new legislation and administrative guidelines. Recipients of federal funds for research from the Department of Health, Education, and Welfare and from the Food and Drug Administration must now receive informed consent from subjects, and also must submit their studies to peer review so that others can evaluate whether proper precautions are taken for the protection of human subjects. These efforts at first reflected a need on the part of public agencies funding research to respond to public pressures and to protect themselves from congressional criticism resulting from scandals involving the improper use of research subjects. Although the federal government establishes general policies for protection of subjects, the application of these policies is left to each of the research agencies involved. Each institution receiving federal research funds has been required to have a review committee to evaluate whether projects seeking funds are in conformity with federal guidelines on the use of human subjects.[3]

As problems have continued, federal guidelines have become more stringent and more numerous, creating an elaborate bureaucratic procedure that adds to the work and cost of completing a research project. But these mechanisms have not been particularly effective in dealing with many troublesome abuses because such problems are not easily handled by general rules or committee reviews of proposals.[4] No doubt the new rules and reviews have served as a deterrent to some, and have increased institutions' consciousness of ethical problems. But they may have achieved this at a relatively high cost, and some highly important investigations, when required to conform to these procedures, may become so tedious and costly that researchers are less likely to work in the area. The purpose of this chapter is not to discuss the advisability of one or another regulation, but rather to explore the problem of consent in its larger social and psychological context and why it is so difficult to govern it by bureaucratic regulation. In doing this we must consider the various interests involved in alternative concepts of consent and the implications of these concepts, not only for ethical behavior, but also in terms of social and cultural realities.

THE ASSUMPTIONS OF DOCTOR-PATIENT INTERACTION AND INFORMED CONSENT

Most medical practice is structured on the assumption that patients put themselves in a trusting relationship with a physician with the understanding that the doctor will serve as their agent. Many physicians assume that the ordinary patient has neither the knowledge nor the judgment to balance effectively the risks and benefits of various treatments, and in part enters the transaction to obtain such a judgment from the physician. As Paul Beeson, a distinguished physician, has noted:

> physicians are accustomed to the fact that everything they do has a risk; every treatment has a potentiality for harming the patient; consequently the physician is constantly making a judgment whether a thing is more likely to help than to hinder. As a matter of fact, we simply could not treat patients if we told them in advance every toxic effect of the treatment or diagnostic procedure we contemplated using in their case. We have to make that decision and we rely on the patient's trust and the fact that he cannot put himself in our place, and we make this decision.[5]

Problems of consent are particularly complex when the researcher acts in the dual role of therapist and investigator. Such investigation may involve patients in experimentation that has potential therapeutic benefit for them, or it may be completely unrelated to their treatment. But the close relationship patients may have with their physician may influence how patients respond when consent is requested—pressure or duress, however subtle, may be present. This has led Alexander Capron[6] to suggest that patients participating in medical experimentation require greater protection than normal volunteers who, he believes, are in a better position to evaluate risks and benefits. Duress, of course, is a far more obvious problem in research carried out in prisons and other involuntary institutions. Research on children and with others who lack competency to give consent also poses special difficulties. But our examination of the social psychology of consent will show that these are problems of degree that do not involve qualitatively different issues from those that apply to more conventional instances of seeking informed consent.

In dealing with patients, physicians are constrained by their own lack of knowledge and uncertainty about diagnosis, prognosis, and the likely effects of intervention. In addition, they are extremely busy and frequently under pressure. Careful disclosure to the extent possible is time consuming and, given the costs of medical care, expensive. Physicians must manage their time to meet the demands upon them, and literal conformity with consent doctrine would reduce their productivity. Despite such costs, physicians would probably conform more closely to consent principles if they felt that disclosure would significantly improve the patient's opportunity for a rational choice. But full and meaningful disclosure may require more knowledge and sophistication than the average patient has, more capacity of the physician to communicate risk in an understandable way than is commonly present, and more skill than is typical in managing the natural apprehensions of many patients.

Even under the best of circumstances, management of patient behavior can be difficult for physicians who have many patients. Most patients would prefer more time and discussion with the doctor than commonly takes place; and physicians, even under the best of circumstances, have difficulty dealing with the anxieties and apprehensions of patients and obtaining adherence to medical advice. Doctors are aware that, to the extent that they discuss possible side effects of drugs and other procedures, they lose some control over the patient's behavior, resulting in either less adherence to advice or the need to expend considerable time convincing patients of the wisdom of the prescribed course.[7] Doctors, thus, work on the assumption that they know what is in the interest of the patient, and they resent spending time on procedures that they feel will at worse undermine their therapy and at best waste a scarce resource—their time and energies. Many patients accept the physician's authority and judgment about the circumstances under which more specific consent should be sought. Attempts to formalize such informal understandings would, in the view of many physicians, be a deterrent to effective practice.

As we have seen, medical care has important psychological aspects, and the authority of the physician has considerable suggestive power. Research on placebos demonstrates the significant influence exerted by suggestibility in the doctor-patient relationship; placebos have been shown to lead also to complaints of various side effects, particularly when possible reactions are suggested by the physician.[8] Increased demands for technical consent not only may contribute to diluting the physician's influence on patients, but also may lead patients to fear and imagine side effects that they would not worry about in the absence of more detailed communication concerning risks. Particularly for the anxious or insecure patient, detailed technical consent can become a barrier to peace of mind and, under some circumstances, even to effective treatment. Although, intellectually, many patients would agree that fuller disclosure is valued and preferable, some find it difficult to manage psychologically. The fact is, however, that we have little empirical information on the consequences of disclosure, and such data would be far more valuable—particularly if obtained in controlled clinical trials—than much of the polemics that now characterize the literature. To weigh the costs and benefits of fuller disclosure, we must begin to learn what the real consequences are.

THE SOCIAL PSYCHOLOGY OF
INFORMED CONSENT AND RESEARCH

The social psychology of consent is more complex than the formal specification of rules would suggest. In ordinary discourse, communication is subtle in the phrasing of requests, the imposition of authority, and in influence attempts more generally. We influence others by how we structure communication, by the extent to which we invoke justification for our claims on the basis of social norms or reciprocity, and by the constraints of the situation itself. Even in the most mundane matters people do not ordinarily make choices free of social or psychological pressures. Much of what we do we undertake because we feel it is expected or demanded, and not as a translation of our innermost preferences.

Most social relationships have a transactional history in which certain implicit norms apply. Persons view relationships on the basis of fairness and reciprocity, and actions at any one time affect how future relationships evolve. Patients often feel dependent on and committed to their physicians, and reluctant to challenge them or to disagree with their decisions. As Gray[9] found, some patients participated in a medical experiment against their own wishes because they were fearful of weakening the doctor's sense of obligation to them should they need the doctor in the future. Whether in fact such obligation would be weakened is an interesting question, but what is important here is that patients chose to follow a course they found uncomfortable because they believed this to be true. And this is a belief that can be traced to common understandings of ordinary associations.

The willingness to consent is also associated with the character of phrases and words and the special meanings attributed to them. As Gray notes, patients differentiated between the words "new drug" and "experimental drug." Staff members quickly learned the appropriate and "more effective" vocabulary. We cannot, however, assume that the more frightening terms necessarily lead to the most rational consent decisions, although in the particular study reported by Gray the blander vocabulary resulted in misunderstandings by subjects. But certain vocabularies that imply "choice" may frighten patients into choices inconsistent with their best interests. Much of the early outcry concerning consent and experimentation followed media coverage of doctors who injected "live cancer cells" in chronically ill and debilitated patients. Although there was much to condemn in this study, public volatility on the issue probably resulted from fear of "live cancer cells." Anyone who deals with patients recognizes how modification of vocabulary, or even tone of voice or manner, can constrain or expand patients' willingness to make one or another decision. Obviously, patients vary; some are more aggressive, others more docile. But the impact of the authority of the physician and scientist is great, as suggested by the various experimental studies of Milgram[10] in which subjects were induced to harm others as a result of instructions by the experimenter.

The dual role of physician-researcher may at times pull the physician between two poles. In research centers particularly, pressures for research productivity and publication (which are related to gaining prestige and advancement) may push therapists in the direction of resolving conflicts in the interests of their research. Their ability to do so is enhanced by the faith patients may have in them and by the patients' dependence. As Moore, a noted surgeon, has written:

> There can be little question that personal ambition, usually for career advancement or public acclaim, underlies much intense motivation in research work and in the trial of new ideas, drugs, operations, or treatment. Such personal ambition is usually well hidden under the sophisticated affect of the dedicated clinical scientist and, far from being remiss, is the sign of a healthy society. . . . But ambition, no matter how praiseworthy, can certainly lead individuals astray.[11]

The typical medical position echoes the one stated by Beecher: "Security rests with the *responsible* investigator who will refer difficult decisions to his peers."[12] Unfortunately, reliance on individual responsibility in a sector as large and diversified as biomedical research provides patients little protection. The rewards for success in research are considerable, and the incentives to cut corners in obtaining consent can be seductive even for the ethical researcher who gives high priority to behaving in a principled fashion. Researchers are concerned about increased requirements for informed consent, not only because they are time consuming and costly, but also because they basically fear that if

subjects knew the truth about what was involved, they would not participate.
As Beeson has noted:

> the risk may be in our minds small, yet if we were to tell a person of all the possi-
> ble things that could go wrong in the course of the experiment he probably would
> not wish to submit to it. This despite the fact, and I think this ought to be pointed
> out, that it is surprising how willing people are to submit to clinical experiments,
> to having tests made upon themselves, even when they realize these are tests
> which are made purely for knowledge and not with the idea of benefiting them
> directly.[13]

Similarly, Beecher has commented that:

> The experienced clinician knows that if he has a good rapport with his patients
> they will often knowingly submit, for the sake of "science," to inconvenience and
> even to discomfort, if it doesn't last very long; but excepting the extremely rare
> individual, the reality is, patients will not knowingly seriously risk their health or
> their lives for a scientific experiment. It is ridiculous to assume otherwise. They
> will not do it.[14]

Yet, Beecher has shown by numerous examples from the medical literature that
it is not uncommon for patients to be subjected to risks in clinical research that
threaten their health.[15] Much resistance to more rigorously defined standards
of informed consent in experimentation and clinical research is based on a prevailing fear that subjects will exaggerate small probabilities of significant
damage and refuse to serve as subjects, thus retarding the development of scientific knowledge.

Although society must protect the patient as subject from the threat of research that is potentially damaging, it must also consider the allowable level of
risk in experimentation, given the benefits to be derived. All risks to subjects
from research can be removed only by excessively restricting research efforts
and by assuming a large price in terms of future benefits to mankind. But as
Titmuss[16] has noted, willingness to participate in research, particularly projects
where one obtains no direct benefits, is a gift to society, and something we have
no right to take involuntarily. What Beeson, who as a physician values basic
research, regards as "small risks" may be larger than the subject, who values
basic research less, may be willing to accept. It is insufficient to argue that
patients frequently take such risks in other spheres of their lives, and thus researchers can assume that they are allowable.

Yet, the difficulty in balancing benefits and risks for individuals and society
is a real one. Future patients reap important benefits from the development of
science and technology and from having well-trained physicians and researchers. But research and training also require that some patients take risks

and suffer inconveniences that may not benefit them. Even in teaching situations, doctors cannot learn and surgeons cannot develop their technical capacities without experience; but when these needs are explained, many patients would still prefer not to have medical students and young house officers gain their experience on them. This difficulty was managed most commonly by disproportionately using charity patients for research and teaching efforts, leaving the more affluent less disturbed. But as economic access to medical services increased for the population at large, medical educators and researchers were confronted with new difficulties. When patients are all on a par, it is clearly unethical disproportionately to use one segment of the population for research and training, particularly when these people have the least education, are least able to understand the way physicians communicate, and thus least able to give informed consent. A recent study[17] suggests that such disproportionate use of the poor continues in major teaching centers, and the ethical issues in this area are acute and will become even more so in the future.

One way of dealing with the researcher's fear—that more information will irrationally alarm the patient—is to spend sufficient time in educating patients so that they have a realistic appreciation of what is involved. Medical researchers who believe that such understanding is impossible among laypersons may really be suggesting that realistic appreciation of what is involved may be costly in time, staff, and other resources. At the same time that society demands that greater research resources be given to informed consent and patient education, it has cut back the resources available to the investigator. Thus, researchers are in a bind. They are expected to produce more for less, and want to allocate their limited resources in what they believe to be the best directions. Therefore, they feel that investments in subject education and consent drain the research budget and impair scientific productivity

Administrators who write guidelines must understand that rules have monetary as well as other costs. Informed consent in research requires communication, time, and effort; it requires better preparation of researchers for educating subjects and facilitating their ability to balance alternatives. Society cannot realistically impose new obligations on researchers without providing the means for their implementation or making clear what other priorities are to be sacrificed.

For the most part, the assertions about the unwillingness of persons to assume risks is conjectural. It would be useful to have hard data on the consequences of more complete information and understanding on the part of prospective subjects. Research on altruism suggests that people readily take risks for society if they are truly convinced that others will be benefited by their acts; indeed, such participation often gives subjects a feeling of sacrifice and self-worth that enhances their feelings of vitality and morality.[18]

PROCEDURES IN RESEARCH AND
IN ORDINARY MEDICAL PRACTICE

Although attention has focused on the institutional researcher, the problem of informed consent is important to the practice of medicine more generally. Many of the consent problems characteristic of research may be even more acute in ordinary medical practice. Researchers' judgments may be affected by their desire for prestige and promotion; practicing physicians, however, may have financial incentives to pursue certain clinical practices that may pose unnecessary threats to patients, or they may not take the time to explain procedures because "time is money." Although research activity is very limited in private medical practice, practitioners do use "experimental therapies" where efficacy and dangers remain unknown, as in the practice of psychosurgery. It is ironic that in such situations only very weak controls are imposed.

Whatever risks patients as research participants face in research institutions because of deviations from ethical requirements, they are likely to be at even greater risk in private practice, where physicians have no formal designation or training as researchers and function outside a scientific peer structure. The behavior of private practitioners is relatively invisible to colleagues, and risks may be taken in "research" having no scientific value. Yet it is probably in private practice situations, where there is a continuing therapeutic relationship between patient and doctor, that patients are most docile, least informed, and most likely to be exposed to risks for no valuable public purpose. The license to practice medicine, earned following medical school and an additional year of training, gives physicians leeway to perform almost any procedure under the rubric of therapy. A good deal of worthless and possibly dangerous "experimentation" continues to take place in ordinary medicine. An overall approach to control of human experimentation must in some way come to terms with practices outside research institutions and with the unrestricted mandate associated with a medical license. It may be reasonable to restrict physicians through licensure to those types of medical practice for which they are trained and competent, although it might be argued that such restrictions tend to have the effect of raising the costs of more specialized and restricted procedures. There is some expectation that the implementation of Professional Standards Review Organizations will have the effect of restricting the work of the ordinary practitioner, but this remains problematic.

In short, because of the way regulation has proceeded, a double ethical standard has developed. The rules are most detailed and strict for, and have greatest impact psychologically and legally on, the best-trained and accomplished researchers who are part of demanding scientific peer groups. Although administrative guidelines have been developed and elaborated for the scientist receiving public funds for research in universities, research institutes, and hospitals, the ordinary physician who engages in the use of "experimental therapies"—often with ineffective designs for research or no design at all—is left untouched. In effect, ethical researchers who have a serious purpose, potentially beneficial to society, are far more restricted in their procedures for obtaining information than are advertisers, market researchers, newspaper reporters, police investigators, credit agency investigators, and others whose intentions and ethics may be more dubious.

Let me be absolutely clear—subjects solicited for an experiment or research project must be assured protection. At minimum, subjects should have sufficiently detailed and accurate information to make a reasonable judgment about participation. Beyond that, they deserve further protection—regardless of their willingness to participate—from exposure to significant risks for which there is no scientific benefit because the study either is not worth doing or is so flawed in methodology that it is unlikely to yield useful information. Research subjects are not in a position to assess the value of an experiment or the integrity of its methodology. Although they can make a reasonable assessment of whether they wish to assume particular risks—assuming the issues are presented fairly—the worth and integrity of the investigation itself must depend on evaluation by a scientifically sophisticated peer group.

IMPROVED SOCIAL REGULATION OF EXPERIMENTATION

In recent years we have developed a cumbersome bureaucratic structure to regulate research and experimentation through federal guidelines and human subjects committees at institutions receiving federal support for research. The structure is relatively expensive in time and effort but, from all indications, is not impressive in its effectiveness.[19] No doubt regulation has limited the grossest abuses, but the issue is whether such a cumbersome bureaucratic structure is necessary for the identification of major abuses. Moreover, there is indication that at least some researchers engaging in questionable practices tend to evade the human subjects committees entirely by carrying out their efforts as part of clinical practice, by doing research using private funds, or by carrying out research in countries where the ethical requirements are more limited. If one of the consequences of ethical rules in experimentation is to shift research to areas where the people used as subjects are less likely to gain from our research than we are, we may be compounding rather than alleviating ethical problems. If pharmaceutical firms test new drugs in Africa or Asia because the Food and Drug Administration will not approve human trials in the United States, we are certainly not improving our moral stance.

The usual regulatory approach, and the one associated with recent history on the regulation of experimentation, has been to continue to elaborate the rules that institutions must follow in approving research as new problems develop. The rules are now so detailed that many researchers are probably not aware of them except in the most general way. Researchers usually know that their proposals for federal funds must be approved by a human subjects committee and that they are required to obtain informed consent, but they probably know relatively little about the precise requirements that have been developed. Those in favor of further regulation would argue that institutions have a responsibility to inform their professional staffs better. But researchers and clinicians are busy people already flooded with paper work, and such bureaucratic directives often end up in the wastebasket unread. Researchers may learn the rules when their proposals are rejected or turned back for modifications from the human subjects committee, but evidence indicates that this is more the exception than the rule.

Regulation must now cope with the danger that more and more investigators regard human subject procedures as unjustifiable restrictions reflecting a diffuse and distant bureaucratic authority. They increasingly become cynical about the procedures and regard them as barriers to get around, not as principles to agonize over in reviewing one's research plans. Speaking as an investigator myself, I can say that I regard the statement on social risk quoted earlier in this chapter as an unrealistic standard for social research which, if taken seriously, would interfere with research clearly in the public interest. The statement on social risk does not heighten my ethical sensitivities; the lack of reality, and even hypocrisy, of the statement just frustrates me. Yet the statement is sufficiently imprecise and ambiguous to cause no real problem in obtaining approval of research. It breeds cynicism, which is hardly the purpose of stating ethical rules. Many biomedical researchers I have talked with have similar reactions to some of the rules affecting patient research. As Beecher has noted:

> There is a disturbing and widespread myth that codes . . . will provide some kind of security. While there is value, doubtless, to be gained from their examination as guides to thinking of others on the subject, the reality is that any rigid adherence can produce a dangerous trap: no two situations are alike, it is impossible to spell out all contingencies in codes. . . . Most codes dealing with human experimentation start out with the bland assumption that consent is ours for the asking. This is a myth. The reality is that informed consent is often exceedingly difficult or impossible to obtain in any complete sense.[20]

It is not my contention that the view of medical researchers, the view of Beecher, or my own view on any guideline is necessarily correct. What I do maintain is that if rules are to have the respect and effect we desire, their legitimacy must be accepted and they must appear reasonable in light of the circumstances. I contend that the present difficulty is that, although we have a regulatory apparatus that scientists tolerate because they have no alternative, many rules lack legitimacy and do not have the desired effect on ethical thinking or on the work of many scientists. Achieving legitimacy is no easy matter, and dependence on the innate integrity of the scientist also is unlikely to be sufficient. What we need is a framework of regulation that is simple, that is responsive to the conflict between patient rights and societal needs, and that stimulates ethical concern—in contrast to ethical regulations—in research. This is no easy accomplishment, but in the comments below I wish to specify some of the conditions under which such a system may come about.

Traditionally in biomedical research, research participation was seen as a quid pro quo for medical care. One of the contentions in support of the ethics of heavy use of charity patients in research was that medical care on teaching and research units was demonstrably of higher technical quality, patients were monitored more carefully, and they had available the most specialized modalities. Although research on quality of care in teaching hospitals generally supports the contention that they provide better care than do hospitals unaffiliated with education and research programs,[21] the evidence remains circumstantial. The best interests of patients in research units have clearly been compromised at times for the sake of a study or of medical education. The advantages to patients in a teaching hospital may be due more to the increased availability of personnel and their competence than to the fact that being involved as a research subject results in better care. I know of no evidence to support the contention that research subjects in teaching hospitals receive more effective care than patients in the same hospitals who are not participants in research investigation, although this hypothesis remains plausible.

With the growth of health insurance and federal programs for the elderly and medically indigent, the assumption that good medical care is a quid pro quo for research participation is no longer tenable, if it ever was. Yet as we noted earlier such patients are still disproportionately used in research.[22] One possible perspective on research and teaching participation is to view those who volunteer their participation as providing benefits to others who do not. Since everyone shares in the consequences of discovery or in the successful training of excellent physicians, we should consider what such participation is worth to the society as a whole. The value of such benefits may then be transferred back in various ways to the participants.

In many ways, human experimentation fits Calabresi's categorization of "tragic choices"—"situations where there is no right decision."[23] Society requires research for its welfare, and it is impossible to eliminate risk from this research. Those who are selected or who volunteer participation assume risks that other beneficiaries do not assume. Although consent is a prerequisite for choosing those who participate, difficulties in communicating risks and in the social psychology of consent suggest that it is never fully a "free choice." Society can at least minimize the social cost of such risks by developing adequate mechanisms to provide compensation to subjects who are injured in research.[24] Such protection should extend not only to areas where researchers were at fault and are legally liable, but to those situations where dangers are unknown but where injuries nevertheless occur. Such protection should cover the needs of future health care, self-maintenance, and adequate financing for dependents. Existing insurance mechanisms provide inadequate compensation for persons who suffer injury for the sake of society. Something akin to a veteran's benefit package for subjects injured in research would not be unreasonable. Such a compensation system, of course, would not reduce requirements that researchers be prudent in research involving risks or in obtaining consent. Eliminating most research risks would probably be impossible, and would significantly retard advance of medical science even if this could be achieved. Reasonable policy on research, like any reasonable policy on traffic regulation or industrial health, makes it inevitable that occasional subjects will suffer injury, and it is irresponsible for the community to ignore this fact. There are technical problems—establishing which injuries result from experimentation and which result from the patient's condition, for example—but they are not insurmountable.

Some have argued that to insure the integrity of research and education, participation by patients should be required as a condition for obtaining medical care. While this evades the tragic choice of deciding who will be the volunteers, requiring participation for patients who wish not to be involved is contrary to law and morally unacceptable. However, although patients have a right to refuse to participate in medical research and education, they have no inherent right to receive medical care under any conditions and in any location they choose. To the extent that real treatment alternatives are available to patients, requirements to participate in educational and research programs in teaching and research contexts may be a choice situation not very different from many others we face during our lifetime. To allow such a policy requires making available to patients real alternatives to the care provided in research institutions. Although personnel in many teaching institutions presently regard participation in teaching, and even sometimes in research activities, as a condition for receiving care in these institutions, this is assumed rather than stated explicitly, and patients may be given no real choice. Legally, such institutions have no right to assume participation, and are required to obtain consent from patients for participation in each research study. Research, however, is sometimes carried out in the context of clinical care, and may not be explicitly defined as investigation.

Many people feel it is unethical to pay subjects large sums of money to assume research risks or to use as subjects prisoners or other involuntary inmates who may perceive participation as a price for better treatment by authorities. Although such practices can readily lead to abuse and subtle intimidation if not carefully monitored, the argument that research should not be allowed in these instances remains unconvincing. Much of daily living involves subtle duress and incentives for performing behaviors others desire. Risks are present not only in research, but also in many other life situations. Dangerous occupations are an example. Few people see as unethical paying people in dangerous occupations higher wages because they assume higher risks. By the same token, it is not clear why subjects who willingly and knowingly assume certain risks for valued social purposes in return for remuneration should not be allowed to do so. Similarly, prisoners have been incarcerated because in the judgment of the community, however erroneous that might be, they have violated valued social rules. It does not seem unreasonable to lighten the price such persons pay when they knowingly take risks in the public interest. We must, of course, do whatever is possible to insure that such judgments to participate are made fairly and with maximal information. But to bar the possibility for such participation on the basis of a vague ethical principle is to establish standards in this area far higher than those that prevail elsewhere in society. Prisons tend to be brutalizing and damaging to esteem. Research policies that allow prisoners to limit their "debt" to society and to engage in a "gift" to mankind do not impress me as a negative or unethical aspect of human experimentation, although there have been obvious abuses in the past.

Developing appropriate guidelines for control over experimentation is complex. As I have argued throughout this chapter, however, arbitrary guidelines that do not take account of the underlying assumptions of therapeutic interaction or the larger context of research may promote dysfunctional and ritualistic practices, and may encourage conformity with the form rather than with the substance of the guidelines themselves. If society is serious about promoting greater ethicality in research it must provide the resources to do so, rather than assume that these resources will be squeezed out of existing research budgets. It is irresponsible for policymakers to impose increased requirements on institutions and researchers for patient education and consent without providing the means to implement these goals. Serious conformity with consent principles is time consuming and costly. If administrators seriously wish to change current practices, and not just to achieve nominal conformity with bureaucratic forms, they will have to provide resources that facilitate the patient's understanding and participation and the ability of the researcher to communicate effectively.

Several systems that may truly improve the ethicality of research have been suggested. Norman Fost, for example, has been experimenting with a surrogate system of consent.[25] There are numerous circumstances in which trying to explain the details of a study to obtain consent invalidates the study, or in which subjects because of their personal stress or illnesses cannot realistically be expected to make a considered choice. Under such conditions it is possible to bring together a group of former patients who have faced similar medical problems and who therefore were once in a situation very similar to that of the proposed subjects. These surrogates are told about the project in detail and encouraged to raise issues about its appropriateness. Fost's experience is that such sessions raise important issues that the researchers have failed to consider or have taken for granted, and improve the ethicality of the researcher's procedures. Brad Gray,[26] in his book on the conduct of experimentation, illustrates a method by which subjects in experiments can be interviewed to identify consent problems and the extent to which consent is "informed." Such interviews could be carried out on a sampling basis to evaluate the procedures used in various investigations and the extent to which subjects understand their participation. The knowledge that their subjects might be interviewed would put investigators on notice that consent is a serious issue, and that the attention they pay to it will have some bearing on their careers.

The issue revolves around the extent to which the scientific peer group truly values the priority of consent. To the extent that it does not, no bureaucratic procedure will be very effective. However, when those with authority place emphasis on ethical practices in research and make it clear that promotions, salary, the ability to carry out further research in the institution, and other valued goals are, in part, dependent on how research is practiced, the potential for improving ethical research will be greatly enhanced. It is apparent that we need more empirical investigation of the real consequences of varying consent procedures. We must stop relying on intuition. Although some researchers argue that patients cannot truly understand the nature of risks involved in experimentation, this hypothesis has not been examined under conditions where special efforts are made to achieve understanding. The devices for review described above are no panacea, but they contribute a perspective closer to the process of research than is involved in the more formal reviews by human subjects committees.

In the last analysis, the right of subjects to know the risks they are assuming in an experiment is a very basic one. No researcher, however important the research, has the right to assume that the risk to the patient is worth the price. The researcher's moral responsibility and practical obligation is to communicate to the patient what the patient can contribute as a subject. This requires time and effort, and the test of the seriousness of policymakers about the value of personal choice is the extent to which they make it possible to implement the value of an informed choice by the resources they provide. The willingness to assume risks without benefits to oneself, or in the light of very remote ones, is a form of gift giving and stems from human beings' basic altruism. Like with most gift exchanges, there are satisfactions for both the receiver and the giver. The scientist as receiver has an obligation not only to protect the rights of the subject, but also to facilitate and reinforce the subject's gratification in altruistic giving.

A NOTE ON THE GROWING PROBLEM
OF MEDICAL MALPRACTICE LITIGATION

Informed consent is just one aspect of a much larger question concerning the appropriate standards for the practice of medicine. The area of medical malpractice, like the issue of informed consent, is made more intelligible by taking into account the complexities of physician-patient communication and its special social psychological features. It also poses similar policy issues concerning how best to regulate physicians' work so as to allow them to practice effectively and efficiently, but also in a way that protects patients against harm.

Although in some situations negligence may be apparent and the act speaks for itself (for example, when the surgeon leaves an instrument in the patient), it is often extraordinarily difficult to differentiate the consequences of the disease from those that result from the physician's intervention. Since we can never scientifically determine what might have occurred had the physician not followed the course chosen, some method is necessary to resolve disputes that develop between patients and physicians.

The traditional mechanism is the adversary process and the clash of experts, through which it is ascertained whether fault exists and what the proper compensation should be when fault is found. The adversary process not only provides a usable mechanism for identifying fault and awarding compensation to injured patients, but it is also believed to deter negligence and to inspire a higher level of caution and responsiveness in medical practice. The extent to which it does so is, of course, an empirical question, and the process has obvious drawbacks, but the key issue is whether we can identify alternatives that are not equally flawed for resolving such disputes. Most physicians are extremely unhappy with the law of medical malpractice. They feel that patients' litigation is often mischievous and unduly encouraged by lawyers' willingness to accept contingency fees. They blame large malpractice awards on the ability of lawyers to "inflame" juries, and feel that the concept of fault is stigmatizing and humiliating. They attribute some of the increased cost of medical care to "defensive medicine," that is, procedures carried out to protect physicians from malpractice judgments rather than to provide good medical care. They are also alarmed by increases in the rates of malpractice insurance and by the growing number of insurance companies that find it an uncertain business to insure physicians. Many physicians hope to see an alternative system developed, and in particular one involving n fault insurance,[27] but the various suggested systems also have inherent problems.

A major difficulty in considering no-fault models as an alternative to malpractice is the objective problem of defining the source of the patient's injury and suffering, and the consequent problem of determining whether and how much compensation should be awarded. Some physicians believe that a commission to adjudicate claims, such as in workman's compensation, or an ar-

bitration board would be preferable to the current system where juries sometimes award large amounts to litigants. It is worth noting that although physicians are alarmed by very large awards, partly because they lead to significant
increases in malpractice insurance costs, it does not follow that the awards are
unjustified. If a 25-year-old patient has been paralyzed and will require
continued and intensive care for life because of the clear negligence of the physician, who is to say that a very large award is not merited? Such awards may
appear to be unjust to physicians because they appreciate the great complexity
and risks involved in even the most careful use of modern medical technology,
and they know that a small oversight can have devastating effects on a patient.
Thus, the size of the judgment against the physician may seem disproportionate
relative to the extent of the negligence. There is, of course, some basis to the
physician's viewpoint. But it is also true that many of the claims made by physicians about medical malpractice are one-sided and represent their own very
special perspective.

Although settling disputes over negligence through a mechanism other than
malpractice may have advantages, it may also be more costly than the present
system. Even a cursory examination of medical practice would reveal large
numbers of transactions in which consent is violated in some fashion, or in
which there is evidence of negligence on the part of the practitioner, and which
result in some harm to the patient. Under the present system such injuries can
only be redressed if the patient makes a claim of wrongdoing, which is sustained either through informal negotiation or through the judicial process. The
cost of a no-fault system in which we attempted to compensate all patients who
are unnecessarily injured by medical treatment could be extraordinarily high.
If, in contrast, we only compensated on a no-fault basis patients who made a
claim, compensation awards would be inequitably distributed among the injured; distribution would favor the better educated and more sophisticated
patient.

If the definition of a fault is difficult for physicians to agree upon, it is even a
more problematic issue for their clients. Patients are relatively naive about both
the possibilities and dangers of medical treatment, and have no good standard
by which to assess whether they have been harmed by the physician. If a
medical transaction is to become a case of malpractice, the patient must come to
an initial determination that the physician was negligent. Most negligence is
unrecognized and undefined, while cases in which negligence played no role
may be perceived as malpractice. We have no clear idea of the relationship
between the population of transactions in which fault "objectively occurs" and
those that are brought to the stage of initial inquiry or to litigation.

Patients may believe that faults have been committed in their cases as much
because they think the physician lacks interest in them or has treated them dis-
courteously as because of the objective quality of the medical care received.

Many patients who are aware that physicians have been negligent in their care would not consider litigation because of their personal relationship to a physician whom they feel tried to do the best he or she could. Whatever the result, the intentions are viewed as good. In contrast, litigation often follows disputes about fees or an experience in which the physician is perceived as callous, unresponsive, and without humility.[28] It has been suggested that the growth of malpractice litigation in medicine reflects the growing segmentation and impersonality of doctor-patient relationships, which before their erosion insulated physicians against the threat of malpractice suits. Of course, other factors are also relevant to changing patterns—the increased opportunity to obtain medical testimony, the greater willingness of lawyers to attempt litigation now that medical testimony is more readily available, awareness among the public that physicians carry insurance against liability, and changing values more generally about litigation as a means of seeking redress. Also, while medical technology now offers more possibilities for successful outcomes, it involves greater risks and possibilities of significant injury to patients.

Once a patient has come to believe that a fault has occurred, the patient is likely to make inquiries and to discuss the experience with relatives and friends. To make a claim, he or she must contact a lawyer willing to pursue the case. To the extent that lawyers are inclined to take such cases on a contingency basis, the opportunities for pursuing grievances are enhanced. The ability to make successful contact with a lawyer probably depends on the patient's sophistication and social network and on the characteristics of the bar in the region in which he lives. The willingness to take malpractice cases, particularly on a contingency basis, will depend on the lawyer's or the firm's experience and specialization in such work, the probability of obtaining a reasonable award for damages, and the availability of convincing medical testimony.

It is difficult to obtain data on the sequence of decisions involving the establishment of a malpractice claim and such matters as the number of patients who consider malpractice claims, who make informal inquiries, who contact lawyers, who initiate a case, and the like. Some picture of the process emerges from studies carried out by the staff of the Commission on Medical Malpractice.[29] Although the Commission's data come from only 26 insurance companies providing malpractice insurance, those studied were the largest carriers; and the Commission staff estimates that their study covered close to 90 per cent of the volume of the malpractice market. The staff found that in 1970 a malpractice incident was reported or alleged for 1 out of every 158,000 patient visits. A claim was made for 1 of every 226,000 visits. Only 1 in 10 claims ever reached a court trial, and two-thirds of the payments made in response to claims were for less than $5000. The public's view of the malpractice situation is very much biased by the large but atypical jury awards that are creating considerable stress in the malpractice insurance market.

The Institute of Social Research at Temple University carried out a consumer survey of 1017 heads of households in the United States for the Malpractice Commission. About two fifths of the sample reported that within the past ten years either they, their spouses or their dependents had had a negative medical care experience. Since these are perceptions, however, they provide inadequate evidence of the actual magnitude of negligence or malpractice. What is more interesting is that only eight per cent (37 respondents) of those who reported negative experiences indicated that they considered seeking legal advice. Only 14 actually reported talking to a legal advisor, and only six made a claim of malpractice. Of the six, two later withdrew their claims without settlement, two settled before trial, and two were still in process at the time of the study.[30] The analysis adds further evidence that only few grievances lead to claims of negligence.

The National Commission, on the basis of a survey of lawyers, found that lawyers accepted approximately only one in eight claims a nong clients alleging malpractice. Half of the claims rejected by lawyers were rejected because they perceived no liability. Before lawyers accepted a malpractice case they usually required some evidence that there was a reasonable possibility of malpractice, corroborated by a physician's opinion. Attorneys felt that malpractice claims took more time than other negligence work, and thus reported that they would turn down worthy claims that involved too little money relative to the necessary work. Once a lawyer has decided to take a case, his or her ability to carry through with it is likely to depend on local norms, the lawyer's knowledge and experience in handling such cases, and the degree of cooperation he can obtain in moving the case toward a successful resolution. When conditions are less advantageous, we assume that lawyers are more willing to settle early, to get what they can with minimal investment. We can also assume that in cases where evidence of negligence is very strong, there will be considerable motivation on the part of insurers to settle early and minimize their loss. Approximately two-thirds of cases are settled, the great majority before coming to trial.

The implications of malpractice judgments for the future occurrence of faults and their deterrence is unclear. The principles developed from the selected sample that reaches the stage of adjudication may be inapplicable to the types of issues that arise in everyday practice. While the case law developed may deter some dangerous practices by defining responsibility and threatening liability, it may also encourage protective maneuvers that are expensive but that have relatively little value. For example, some physicians maintain that the growing threat of malpractice litigation induces them to overuse expensive, and sometimes risky, diagnostic procedures, to provide a record protecting them against liability should their care be at issue. This would of course unnecessarily inflate the costs of medical care, costs that in one way or another would eventually be passed on to the consumer. The problem of determining the extent and consequences of defensive medicine, as it is called, resides in the ambiguity of medical standards.

Presumably, defensive medicine occurs because physicians feel that they are vulnerable to charges of negligence when they fail to perform certain tests or procedures such as a skull X-ray following trauma. But physicians would only be vulnerable if other physicians practicing in the same specialty believed that such tests and procedures were not redundant but rather an important aspect of adequate management of the case. The complaints about inducements toward defensive medicine, thus, either imply something about the imprecisions and confusions as to what adequate standards of management are or about the deviant views of some physicians who may feel that the standards they are held to are redundant or unnecessarily high. The purpose of the standard in the first place, however, is to bring the practice of each physician to a minimal norm of acceptable practice. It should be clear, therefore, that the problems of malpractice and alleged defensive medicine are more of a medical than a legal problem. Any standard established—whether implicit as in the case of fear of malpractice if failure in performing certain procedures occurs, or explicit as in the case of those established by PSRO's or administrative guidelines—must be seen in a cost-benefit framework. When standards are established in areas where physician practice varies, disagreement on the value and relevance of the standard may exist. The effect of the standard is to induce persons to carry out certain procedures that may not be carried out in its absence. Those who agree with the standard see this as quality care; those who disagree see it as defensive medicine. In short, arguments about defensive medicine inevitably reflect disagreements and confusions about the practice of medicine itself.[31]

If defensive medicine were as large a problem as many physicians allege, one might expect certain regional variabilities in practice. For example, one would anticipate that in states or localities with high rates of litigation, physicians in specified specialties would be much more likely to use certain procedures in dealing with problematic cases than would similar physicians in low litigation areas. Although there are no large-scale studies of this question, one attempt to examine this hypothesis could find little evidence in its support, suggesting that varying patterns of physician behavior are more likely to reflect local norms and professional customs than the threat of litigation.[32] Although some physicians may order tests and procedures that they feel are unnecessary because they fear that the failure to do so may lead to their liability, the fact may be that these tests and procedures should be done. Medicine has become too complex for us to continue to accept the myth that the clinical judgment of the physician is sacrosanct. The real issue is one of standards, and in the area of standards, medicine is in a muddle.

As new Professional Standards Review Organizations become established, and as they develop standards for peer review, these new norms could serve as guideposts in locating negligence as defined by the medical peer culture. Physicians, however, would like to insulate PSROs from public scrutiny, and argue that the deliberations of such bodies should be privileged and confidential. There is no doubt that physicians will vigorously resist cooperation with such review organizations if reviews are to be open to public scrutiny, and perhaps justifiably so. But, then, how is the public to identify negligence without resorting to litigation or other means of identifying malpractice? It is hard to believe that the public would find acceptable the idea that PSROs should make these judgments without making their data available to nonphysicians as well. And if they will not, we are back to where we started.

I have some sympathy for the view of my colleague, Dr. Jacob Fine, that it would be preferable to have an independent judicial commission of impeccable credentials resolve issues of negligence on a no-fault basis. Such a system would have the potential of resolving issues more accurately from a scientific viewpoint than the adversary legal process, but it could be very expensive if an effort is made to redress all errors that resulted in harm. One aspect of the malpractice issue that is not widely appreciated—and particularly in the emotional discussions of the multimillion dollar award—is that the present system is relatively inexpensive in comparison to a system that would attempt to compensate more fairly those who suffer injury due to error. While the latter system would in all probability be fairer to a larger number of patients and physicians than the present system, its potential cost is large.

A major issue for public policy involves the question of who can best bear the cost burden of malpractice. Certainly, those least able are the patients who have been injured. Patients in the aggregate will, of course, bear the major burden since the costs of medical malpractice are likely to be passed on to the medical consumer in any case. But there is a social function in holding physicians accountable for their errors even if they transfer much of the financial burden. While there is some sense in alleviating the pressures on any subgroup of physicians, such as those in high litigation specialties, by sharing the costs of malpractice more widely among physicians, it seems reasonable to continue to impose higher liabilities on individual physicians who are especially prone to being sued. Any doctor can be sued once or even twice; but physicians who face multiple allegations of malpractice are clearly doing something wrong.

The present difficulties in the medical malpractice area are largely due to problems relating to the uncertainty of calculating risk and working out a system to pool risks among doctors in varying specialties. Although it seems clear that there are ways to deal with medical negligence in a manner that provides compensation to patients in a fairer way than at present, it is an illusion to believe that such a system would be less expensive than at present unless the burden of malpractice costs were transferred to injured patients—a consequence that clearly would be undesirable. Perhaps the greatest contribution of a no-fault system would be a more equitable distribution of compensation among patients who were injured as a result of medical practice, and growing realization among the public that errors are inevitable in the use of a powerful and complex technology. Perhaps such knowledge would encourage greater prudence among some patients in their demands for certain types of medical services.

In the final analysis, the growing debate in society concerning medical malpractice and informed consent largely reflects the erosion of authority and the breakdown of trust. A basic premise of the practice of medicine is that patients believe that physicians act in their interest and will do their best to be of assistance. As medical knowledge has become more complex, and as the institution of medicine has come to encompass varying conflicts of interest, trust is more unstable, and thus regulatory remedies are attempted. While these developments are in part inevitable in a more complex society dominated by large and powerful bureaucracies, they also reflect certain failures of medical practice, its growing focus on technical as compared with humane considerations, and its neglect of nurturing better relationships with patients. Social regulation, although necessary, is a poor substitute for mutual trust and understanding. Although we will never return to the days where medical practice was an uncomplicated, continuing relationship between patient and a single physician, medicine can do a great deal to limit the erosion of trust and in the process to protect itself from even greater assaults in the future.

NOTES

1. Professor Jay Katz of the Yale University Law School has put together an extraordinarily useful casebook on informed consent and other problems of human experimentation. This chapter uses several of the sources available in his casebook. See J. Katz (1972), *Experimentation with Human Beings: The Authority of the Investigator, Subject, Professions and State in the Human Experimentation Process* (New York: Russell Sage).

2. Department of Health, Education, and Welfare (1971), *Institutional Guide to DHEW Policy on Protection of Human Subjects,* p. 8.

3. See B. Barber et al. (1973), *Research on Human Subjects: Problems of Social Control in Medical Experimentation* (New York: Russell Sage).

4. See B. H. Gray (1975), *Human Subjects in Medical Experimentation: A Sociological Study of the Conduct and Regulation of Clinical Research* (New York: Wiley-Interscience).

5. P. Beeson (1964), "Moral Issues in Clinical Research," *Yale Journal of Biology and Medicine,* **36**:465.

6. A. Capron (1964), "The Law of Genetic Therapy," in J. Katz (1972), op. cit., p. 575.

7. H. Becker (1974), "Consciousness, Power and Drug Effects," *Journal of Psychedelic Drugs*, **6**:67–76.

8. D. Mechanic (1968), *Medical Sociology: A Selective View* (New York: Free Press), pp. 185–189.

9. B. Gray (1975), op. cit.

10. S. Milgram (1974), *Obedience to Authority: An Experimental View* (New York: Harper & Row).

11. F. Moore (1969), "Therapeutic Intervention—Ethical Boundaries in the Initial Clinical Trials of New Drugs and Surgical Procedures," in P. Freund, ed., *Experimentation with Human Subjects* (New York: Braziller), pp. 374–375.

12. H. Beecher (1966a), "Consent in Clinical Experimentation—Myth and Reality," *Journal of the American Medical Association*, **195**:124.

13. P. Beeson (1964), op. cit., p. 465.

14. H. Beecher (1966a), op. cit., p. 124.

15. H. Beecher, (1966b), "Ethics and Clinical Research," *New England Journal of Medicine*, **274**:1354–1360.

16. R. Titmuss (1971), *The Gift Relationship: From Human Blood to Social Policy* (New York: Pantheon).

17. B. Barber et al. (1973), op. cit., pp. 54–57.

18. C. H. Fellner and S. H. Schwartz (1971), "Altruism in Disrepute," *New England Journal of Medicine*, **284**:282–285.

19. See B. Barber et al. (1973), op. cit.

20. H. Beecher (1966a), op. cit., p. 124.

21. M. Goss (1970), "Organizational Goals and the Quality of Medical Care: Evidence from Comparative Research on Hospitals," *Journal of Health and Social Behavior*, **11**:255–268.

22. B. Barber et al. (1973), op. cit., pp. 54–57.

23. G. Calabresi (1974), "Commentary," in Institute of Medicine, *Ethics of Health Care* (Washington, D.C.: National Academy of Sciences), pp. 53–54.

24. C. Havighurst (1970), "Compensating Persons Injured in Human Experimentation," *Science*, **169**:153–158.

25. N. Fost (1975), "A Surrogate System for Informed Consent," *Journal of the American Medical Association*, in press.

26. B. Gray (1975), op. cit., pp. 250–251.

27. For a discussion of the application of no-fault insurance to the medical area, see C. Havighurst and L. R. Tancredi (1973), "'Medical Adversity Insurance'—A No-Fault Approach to Medical Malpractice and Quality Assurance," *Milbank Memorial Fund Quarterly*, **51**:125–168.

28. R. Blum (1960), *The Management of the Doctor-Patient Relationship* (New York: McGraw-Hill).

29. Department of Health, Education, and Welfare (1973), *Report of the Secretary's Commission on Medical Malpractice* (Washington, D.C.: DHEW), Publ. No. (OS) 73–88; (1973), *Appendix: Report of the Secretary's Commission on Medical Malpractice* (Washington, D.C.: DHEW), Publ. No. (OS) 73–89.

30. Ibid, pp. 658–694.

31. For a more detailed discussion of this and many other issues relevant to the malpractice dilemma, see D. Mechanic (1976), "Some Social Aspects of the Medical Malpractice Dilemma," *Duke Law Journal*, in press.

32. Defensive Medicine Project (1971), "The Medical Malpractice Threat: A Study of Defensive Medicine," *Duke Law Journal*, **1971**:939–993.

Chapter 14

Social Science and
Health Policy
in the United States

To this point, emphasis has been placed on the difficulties in implementing bureaucratic designs that achieve their intentions. Social scientists often feel that managers and administrators fail to utilize available behavioral knowledge that would contribute to more effective health policies and organizational designs that are responsive to needs and expectations of clients. This chapter considers how health policy is formulated and how social scientists might increase their impact on the health policy process. In the chapter that follows I focus more specifically on one area, evaluation research, where I believe that social science has a particularly important role to play.

Health policy in the United States culminates from decisions made in a vast range of public and private agencies at federal, state, and local levels. At the federal level, policies of the executive branch and its operating agencies and congressional mandate provide a framework for directing the health industries that exceed annual expenditures of $100 billion. Although all public expenditures in health care constitute less than two-fifths of the total, public investments and particularly federal expenditures have vast potential for influencing the character of the entire industry. That this influence has not been exerted in a consistent fashion toward a national health policy in no way detracts from its potential.

The character of the appropriations process and the numerous agencies involved in administering categorical programs result in a fragmentation and dispersion of administrative and regulatory power. Such agencies with their complex operating procedures and administrative guidelines frequently work at cross-purposes. This fragmentation exists not only in the separations among health activities in different spheres of government such as DHEW, Defense, and the Veteran's Administration, but is also evident within each of these agencies and their subdivisions. Although there has been no shortage of bureaucratic personnel at all levels of health operations, the organizational structure of health decision-making is a confused bureaucratic web with little focus or clear definition of responsibility.

Health care is largely delivered in the private sector, and professional associations and the health industries exert great influence. Not only do they operate as any other interest group with a stake in legislation, but some of these groups have a more direct role in the specification of standards, in regulatory and accreditation activities, and in the performance of other quasi-official functions. Professional organizations often have a disproportionate influence on policy, not only as a result of their special expertise, the availability of financial resources, and their internal cohesion, but also because of their research capabilities and their ability to monitor carefully the policy-making process.

Although a national health program could supersede significant state and local legislation in the health arena, much potential power is concentrated and exercised at these levels through the provision of financing for services and educational programs, the licensing of facilities and personnel, and the existing regulatory opportunities. Similarly, much of the daily character of the provision of services results from thousands of administrative and operational decisions, and these limited decisions in the aggregate have a profound effect on the scope, quality, and accessibility of health services available to the population.

Consideration of the role of health policy must take account of the complexity of the health sector and the multiplicity of decision points among legislators, government officials, administrators of service programs, professionals, third-party providers and suppliers, and numerous other groups having a stake in the choice of one or another policy option. Moreover, the options and the ability to influence them come about in diverse ways: some are highly visible, others hidden; some seem momentous in character, others appear commonplace; some appear to be policy with a capital P, others little more than administrative minutiae. Also, they affect the system in varying ways. A congressional decision on financial entitlement will have a dramatic impact through the entire system if the benefits are broad enough, but the implementation of a new technology or a new pattern of organization facilitating greater accessibility will have to diffuse among a vast number of professionals and other providers.

Consideration of possible roles for the social sciences must also take account of limitations of social science in both its substantive and methodological aspects. For some issues social science knowledge may be crucial; for others social science has little to contribute or is incapable of responding within the allowable time. Any framework for increasing social science involvement must be attuned to the political realities of policy formulation, the varied modes of participation of groups with interests at stake, and the extent to which particular policy solutions are outgrowths of complex compromises between rational considerations and political pressures.

Attempts to increase the relevance of social science in policy formulation must take account of its limitations, and efforts must be made to delimit carefully the appropriate range of social science participation. Work in the social sciences is relatively slow and ponderous, and it is difficult to generate relevant results in time to have impact on many policy decisions. Moreover, since results carefully acquired are often heavily qualified, and their generalizability is frequently uncertain, legislators or administrators who seek clear guidance may find them of little help. Moreover, social scientists who have only limited familiarity with the health sector will design studies or give advice that clearly reflects their lack of appreciation of the character of health services and diminishes the overall credibility of social science activities. Serious considerations of how social science can play a greater role in policy formulation must come to terms with the fact that many policymakers have no great admiration for social science research and are skeptical that it can be of much assistance to them. Most frequently, policymakers seek reliable information and projections, not elaborate theories, models, or examinations of forces not amenable to legislative manipulation.

Social science probably has its largest impact not on policy but in shaping the larger climate of opinion in society. Social science research and theory contribute to the formulation of assumptions, perspectives, and alternatives. Such thinking is transmitted through the mass media and the educational process, and contributes indirectly to the way in which issues are defined and decisions formulated. The impact of social science on policy may be most lasting through this indirect route rather than through more specific advice given on any particular issue. Recommendations made by advisors external to the relevant bureaucracy are rarely attuned to the organizational realities that decisionmakers must face in bringing an issue to its resolution. Such advice is likely to be most effective on more restricted technical matters where the scientific community has a special expertise, but as the issue broadens to one of policy, which involves political and organizational matters as well, the role of such advice, or even its utility, becomes more unclear.

A social science capacity built into policy-making organizations is likely to have a far greater impact than advice—no matter how proficient—that is offered from the outside. The disproportionate influence of lawyers, and perhaps economists among social scientists, on social policy stems in large part from their proximity to decision-making processes, although it is also related to the adaptability of their tools to the questions at issue. Both lawyers and economists are more likely than other social scientists to work as staff members within bureaucracies, and they frequently write legislation or administrative guidelines. The impact of policy may be as dependent on the nitty-gritty of administrative implementation as it is on the big policy issues.

Proximity to the policy-making process puts the analyst in a good position to react to the daily contingencies and the changing formulations of policy issues. It also leads to other advantages, since it brings the staff member into continuing interactions with higher level policymakers. Such interactions allow trust and dependence, ingredients frequently absent in external advisory arrangements, to develop. It also provides an opportunity for policymaker and staff members to become aware of one another's perspectives, to learn how to communicate with one another, and to experience the norms of the operating system. Policymakers do not live in a vacuum; they are part of a highly competitive system where their mistakes are costly and where they must jockey for position. Outside advisors are usually immune from risks or responsibility for their advice since they are not integrated into the reward structure of the bureaucracy. This gives them greater freedom but also less credibility. Within the bureaucracy able staff members soon come to understand the constraints and the organizational difficulties the policymaker can anticipate. They learn that there are ways to present issues to stimulate visibility and response to certain problems. Their suggestions often are combinations of policy and strategy. But outside advisors are rarely sufficiently attuned to the concerns of the bureaucracy to have any useful views on strategy. It may be that all of these strategic views add up to very little in reality, but the system operates on the basis of what participants believe and not on some abstract reality.

Looking at the issue in a somewhat different way, I would contend that the informal influences on policy formulation are often more profound than the formal structures that have been developed. Most persons in high policy positions lead hurried and harried lives. The daily pressures requiring immediate response push long-term considerations to the background. Policy issues develop unexpectedly and frequently require a very rapid response. Often the first response constrains future courses of action. In such circumstances there is a particular need to know whom to trust, and policymakers are rightfully reluctant to depend on outside advisors or even on the existing bureaucracy. Social scientists have limited impact on health policy in part because relatively few serve as primary staff to high government officials, congressmen and senators, state legislators, professional associations, or large providers of care.

In considering how to enlarge the role of social science, we might note the extraordinary lack of an effective analytic capability in most government agencies, particularly in state governments but also within the federal structure. In many states, legislative committees concerned with major health issues have no staff at all, and in the federal government the staff available is often at work on the continuing daily bureaucratic demands. Given both the immediacy of work demands and the short tenure of personnel, there is a failure to develop an analytic capacity to deal with complicated, long-range issues of great importance. This failure is related to the need for trust discussed earlier, since the analytic staff tends to be replaced with changing political administrations. But one result of the process is a failure to come to terms with long-range policy issues.

When policymakers lack their own analytic capacities, they are much more susceptible to the influence of special interest groups for the definition of issues and possible responses. Organizations that have a stake in health legislation—such as professional organizations and medical industries—often have excellent research capacities allowing them to follow policy developments and to influence not only decisions but even the definition of issues. When policy issues are of high interest and visibility—capturing newspaper headlines, as in the case of National Health Insurance—political factors frequently become the prime determinants of policy resolution. Most policy issues, however, are relatively invisible to the public and rarely reach the mass media. In these circumstances the sources of information on public consequences derive from whatever capability the government has to obtain relevant facts and to define issues and from the efforts of special interests who have a stake in the matter. Such special interests are not evenly matched, however, for the larger and richer groups can devote greater resources to influencing the manner in which the issues are defined and resolved; and some groups whose interests are also at stake have no resources or organization at all, do not become aware of the issue until it is already resolved, and have limited capacity to gain access to those making decisions.

An important function for social science research and analysis is to make perspectives salient that are not evident to the policymaker or practitioner. Both come to observe the development of health policy from a particular vantage point, and the perspectives they come to adopt and the images of behavior and problems they have derive from their work and its special problems and their particular location in the health care structure. Practitioners come to view the problem from their experiences and particular needs and not from a larger view of the problems as they occur in the community as a whole. Similarly, policymakers frequently come to think in administrative terms and are often unappreciative of the profound human consequences of one or another administrative solution. We all adopt stereotypes based on our own experiences that facilitate making sense of our world and coping with it, but when applied to new situations they can be faulty and maladaptive. Social science can assist in avoiding such errors which, when they occur as part of a nationwide policy, cause great suffering.

There is presently much agonizing in the health area concerning community participation and client influence. In the policymaking sphere, some alternatives are not considered, not because they would be unsuitable or even politically unacceptable, but more because there is no one available at the points where policy is formulated to present them. In the absence of viable consumer controls, social science—incorporated into the policymaking process—can be of assistance in serving as a form of community representation by proxy. Particularly in areas of policymaking with little visibility, the social scientist can attempt to put forth in the most reliable and objective way the likely repercussions of one or another policy on varying groups in the community who are not represented in policymaking discussions. Through these means, an objective and honest social science can enhance the democratic process by limiting the dominance of special interest perspectives. There is no assurance that a balanced view will prevail, but social science through its analyses can represent, or at least bring into consideration, the needs of affected groups outside the mainstream of government decision-making. I am not naive as to the political difficulties of such a role or to the danger that social science will itself become a captive of its own or other special interests. The responsibility for objectivity, openness, and accessibility to criticism and review is great indeed.

This role, I believe, is particularly important when the issues at stake are hidden from public view. The typical policymaker must make hundreds of decisions. Some of these decisions appear highly important to the policymaker, others appear more trivial; on some he or she has strong value predispositions or his constituency is involved; on others he is uninformed and apathetic. Where the policymaker stands will depend on the case made and on who makes it. If a staff member has a special interest in an issue that seems of little importance to the policymaker, the staffer may be allowed to pursue it. Or if an important constituent or interest group makes a strong case they may prevail, particularly in the absence of a competing view. Thus, proximity to the policymaking process is a condition for influence, and much of the failure of social science is the failure to achieve proximity. In government agencies, in Congress, and in legislatures, as well as in administrative agencies, supporting staff are responsible for much of the work that culminates in policy. Unless social science becomes part of this staff structure in a significant way, it will remain relatively impotent in affecting the policy-making process.

THE ROLE OF A SOCIAL SCIENCE
CAPABILITY IN POLICY-MAKING

Keeping up with the day-to-day demands in government is an energy-draining process, and the policymaker is often uncertain where the next issue will surface. A social science capability can be of considerable assistance in anticipating future issues, obtaining relevant analysis and information necessary for the formulation of alternative policy responses, and for examining the consequences of existing programs. Moreover, effective monitoring of the consequences of policy and the nature of public needs requires a sophisticated information system that is sufficiently simple and practical to provide current information relatively quickly and without prohibitive cost. The information system must be simple enough to be used readily with limited retrieval time, yet sufficiently sophisticated to deal with the true complexity of the problem.

The requirements for "intelligence," monitoring of ongoing programs, policy analysis and evaluation seem simple enough when stated blandly, but they are enormously difficult to implement effectively. Implicit in "intelligence" and long-term policy analysis is the existence of a group of analysts insulated from the daily bureaucratic pressures, but such insulation becomes difficult to sustain when immediate problems require solution. In such circumstances policymakers call on the best people they can muster, pulling them away from the longer range concerns to which they had been assigned.

If policy analysis is funded outside the governmental structure in universities, "think tanks," and consulting firms, those settings offer other obstacles. Universities usually offer the most sophisticated analytic capacities, but tend to work on a different time scale; and the disciplinary concerns of the analysts and the effects of the reward structures of which they are a part lead them to drift away from the concerns as policymakers see them. Consultant firms, vying for contracts, tend to develop a formula for policy analysis that is too frequently sterile and incompetent. While they may parade considerable talent in acquiring contracts, much of the work is done by others in an uncreative way. Policy institutes closely associated with the work of government may offer greater promise, but it is difficult to develop situations in which there is an effective balance between long-range analysis and response to more immediate need. If the distance between policy institute and policymaker is too great, the institute is unlikely to be sufficiently responsive to policy needs, but if the distance is inadequate, the policy institute may become nothing more than a fire-fighting subsidiary. A useful compromise is a policy institute funded for a range of activities involving both short-term and long-range interests. This provides possibilities for effective trade-offs. Thus, in universities, analytic talent can be attracted to work on short-range needs with the understanding that the institute would also fund some of the related interests of investigators which are more disciplinary in their character.

There is some resistance to funding institutes or program grants on the assumption that such organizations with block grants tend to support both adequate and mediocre work. It is maintained by independent scientists that a competitive individual grant program buys better research for a given expenditure. This would be correct if information useful for policy were generated in this way, but the grant system is not usually responsive to policy needs. Thus the government has moved more and more to contracts, where the quality of work is uneven. Unlike the case of competitive grants and contracts, institutes have greater incentives for developing effective interdisciplinary problem-solving groups capable of dealing with complex policy issues. Although contracting firms potentially have similar incentives, few have adequate social science capacity. University-based institutes and program project grants in the health area have little stability and have been disrupted and demoralized by changing funding policies and the lack of long-term support.

Much of what is termed "program evaluation" in government consists of self-serving data aggregation that argues for the continuance of existing programs or the termination of unpopular ones. The appropriations process includes few incentives for administrators to examine their own programs objectively or to search for indications that they are ineffective. Ideally, we would like to encourage experimentation and modification of existing programs and an empirical attitude, but administrators well know that failure to argue for the effectiveness of existing programs may bring little more than budgetary reductions.

Part of the difficulty in evaluation research, whether done internally or by outside evaluators, is the resistance among administrators toward clarifying the goals and targets of the programs they administer. To the extent that goals are ambiguously formulated, there always remain opportunities to shift one's ground. Moreover, administrators are frequently given programs that they know can never meet the aspirations that were stated when they were enacted or the goals that were used to argue for their implementation. The legislative process encourages an exaggeration of rhetoric that few programs can match, and wise and experienced administrators attempt to keep program options flexible so that they and their agencies can continue to survive. Thus, the governmental process and competition for funds among agencies encourage resistance to serious evaluation. In the case of some major programs of high cost and visibility, evaluation may be achieved through independent studies by outside contractors, but most programs never receive serious scrutiny. Therefore, success becomes the ability to maintain one's proper share of the budget and to edge slowly forward, and this may require above all that the agency's external constituency is kept active and effective.

The failure to enunciate clear goals is a general characteristic of policy in the United States. Much legislation is a compromise between competing factions and emerges from coalitions that support the program for varying and even contradictory reasons. Thus, the failure to specify goals is frequently the result of more than the protective instincts of an experienced administrator. Although the higher levels of the executive branch may impose criteria for evaluation, this too is usually part of a political process in which monies are reallocated and less favored programs, for whatever reasons, eliminated.

Social scientists involved in evaluation efforts need considerable patience and must work closely with administrators in defining reasonable criteria for study. They must anticipate exploitation by all parties whose interests they might serve, and thus it is essential to anticipate the claims of varying groups and build them into the evaluation as well. Furthermore, possible unanticipated consequences of programs must be formulated as part of the evaluation, although there are always limits to such efforts. Only naive investigators are not aware that however well they do their study, there will be attempts to discredit it by those who have something to lose if the findings are sustained. Problems of evaluation are discussed more fully in the next chapter.

THE IMPLEMENTATION OF A
SOCIAL SCIENCE CAPABILITY

There are no simple devices that will facilitate the use of social science in policy formulation and implementation if policymakers have no respect for the social science enterprise. Many policymakers believe that social scientists have too much theory and too little data, that they are excessively ideological, that they are unrealistic about possible policy options, and lack understanding of the policy-making process. While such policymakers can identify some social scientists they may trust and whose advice they find useful, they frequently feel that much of what social scientists do is irrelevant to the "real problems."

Policymakers do not have a clear idea of what social science is. They do not differentiate clearly among the activities of varying disciplines or among varying levels of activity in academic departments, consulting firms, and advisory panels. Their views may have been influenced by specific experiences involving social scientists that resulted in little of benefit to them. Part of the problem resides in the confusions within social science itself and in the educational failures of social scientists in the universities and in the society generally. No doubt some policymakers lost interest in sociological analysis after taking an introductory course in the university, and I would emphasize that the quality of our teaching is as important in shaping public policy in the future as anything we do on advisory committees. We should not minimize the extent to which initial attitudes formed during educational experiences are generalized in later life. One important way to improve the role of social science is to elevate the existing level of social science education and the quality of social science reporting in the mass media. Improvement in these spheres would go a long way toward institutionalizing social science thinking as a way of viewing problems more generally.

It is clear that social scientists—and particularly sociologists—are not being prepared to work in policy-making roles, and few are encouraged to aspire to positions on congressional and legislative staffs, in federal agencies, and in other locations in close proximity to policy-making. Yet the greatest impact on policy is likely to come from those who work with decisionmakers on a daily basis and not from the occasional advisor. As opportunities in the universities for roles in teaching and research contract, we would do well to direct students to these new roles and improve their preparation for them.

Much of the involvement of social science thus far has been in advisory roles to various government agencies. These roles generally fall into three categories: disbursement of research funds as in the peer review process of DHEW; technical advisory committees to advise government on the feasibility of certain decisions and their likely consequences; and advisory roles on the formulation and implementation of policy. Although each of these roles has its critics and defenders, it is generally agreed that the first two operate with greater effectiveness than the third.

The greatest difficulty with the policy consulting role resides in the complexity of policy itself and the processes through which it develops. Although we all know that policy is formulated in various phases and at many levels, policy advisors often become disillusioned when they see how little of the fruits of their efforts and energies is incorporated in the final decisions. If outside advisors took the role of the policymaker or legislator, they would soon appreciate that they too are in the same situation. But while the typical government official comes to accept this, many academic advisors come to resent the fact that their advice did not prevail.

It is not clear that participation in policy formulation—with its implicit inhibition of later advocacy—is necessarily a more effective role than advocacy itself. Some persons who have participated in advisory policy roles have serious reservations about their efficacy, and it is conceivable that a strong public advocacy position might in the long run contribute more to the definition of priorities. It seems apparent, however, that both roles are important and can be performed simultaneously by the social science community.

FUTURE CONTRIBUTIONS OF THE
SOCIAL SCIENCES TO POLICY

In its essentials, the difficulty of the role of social science in policy formulation is not very different from problems faced by other scientific disciplines. To the extent that the discipline has special expertise, it can be useful in rendering an opinion on the state of the art or on the technical feasibility of one or another course of action. The success of the peer review advisory committee process derived from the fact that assessments were being made by individuals who had the recognized special knowledge and technical skills to provide a reasonable judgment of the quality of the efforts proposed. Since the scientific quality of work was the only question at issue, the process worked well.

As research funds became more limited, some study sections were faced with competing objectives. Not only were they asked to indicate the technical quality of a proposed effort, but to take into account as well the extent to which such efforts were consistent with the agencies' priorities of the moment. Since the priorities of the agencies were not necessarily those of the participants, the process was painful for some scientists who saw work of superior technical quality being superseded by other efforts of lesser creativity that were more attuned to the agency's mission. But the conflicts generated by these competing values were relatively small in comparison to the conflicts implicit in the formulation of health policy.

In policy formulation it is far easier to play a negative role than to play an innovative one. As an outside participant on anything but the highest levels, it is particularly difficult to initiate new directions or approaches to problems. Initiation must frequently come from above, and if the advisor has any influence, it is more likely to be one in indicating why a particular policy course is unconstructive or ill-advised. A convincing case for why a policy under consideration will not work, particularly when there is no prior commitment to the policy, will have far greater effect than one supporting a course that will, but has not been previously considered. Policy options are usually not taken seriously unless there is already a considerable interest or consensus supporting them. The process of building such a consensus is a difficult one, particularly for an outside advisor who is not in continuing contact with the emerging policy-making discussions.

In short, elevating the role of social science in policy requires means to bring social science analysts in closer proximity to the policy-making process wherever it takes place. This can be achieved by participating in roles in government and elsewhere that allow direct input in the policy formulation process and, by organizing visible interest groups external to policy formulation, that bring social science analysis and research to bear on issues of major national concern, such as welfare reform or national health insurance. Such efforts could be much enhanced by the development of educational programs that maintain the strengths of the disciplinary perspective but are more realistically attuned to the needs of policy analysis and the larger context of policy formulation.

Chapter 15

Evaluation of Health Care Programs: Problems and Prospects

It takes none of the great virtues to proclaim the importance of evaluation and the necessity to assess the impacts of expensive social programs that compete for scarce resources. Posing questions in a fashion that allows them to be addressed effectively and that facilitates appropriate research designs requires somewhat more sophistication, but certainly these are skills that can be taught and learned without too much difficulty. The slow pace of evaluation efforts, thus, results less from failures to proclaim their importance or to initiate studies than from the political context of social programming, the vested interests of administrators and program personnel, and the perceived threat implicit in the development of evaluation efforts. These same considerations have much to do, ultimately, with the flawed quality of many evaluations. If we do not attack these issues frankly and realistically, our methodological and analytic skills will come to naught.

Increasingly, the concept of evaluation is being narrowed to describe the assessment of the effectiveness of programs targeted toward specific social goals by means of the more sophisticated social methodologies used to study such interventions.[1] I prefer to retain the wider meaning of the concept to designate the broad range of efforts that administrators and others engage in to assess what it is that they are doing and their effectiveness in reaching their goals. Evaluation thus spans a range of activities, *from* the qualitative assessment of how adequately an agency balances its commitments in respect to a variety of competing goals *to* large-scale social experiments designed to ascertain the relative impacts of differing policy interventions on a variety of critical indicators. We may be able to learn what we want to know through feedback from personnel, recipients, and other interested persons, or our questions may require formal collection of statistical information and special investigations. In this regard, Suchman's distinction between evaluation and evaluation research is pertinent:

> [Evaluation] will be used in a general way as referring to the social process of making judgments of worth. This process is basic to almost all forms of social behavior, whether that of a single individual or a complex organization. While it implies some logical or rational basis for making such judgments, it does not require any systematic procedures for marshaling and presenting objective evidence to support the judgment. Thus, we retain the term "evaluation" in its more commonsense usage as referring to the general process of assessment or appraisal of value.
>
> "Evaluation research," on the other hand, will be restricted to the utilization of scientific research methods and techniques for the purpose of making an evaluation. In this sense, "evaluative" becomes an adjective specifying a type of research. The major emphasis is upon the noun "research" and evaluative research refers to those procedures for collecting and analyzing data which increase the possibility for "proving" rather than "asserting" the worth of some social activity.[2]

I firmly believe that it is necessary to make the process of evaluation as rigorous and scientific as possible. Thus, given a choice, evaluation *research* is always preferable to other methods of evaluation. There are, however, circumstances that lead skilled administrators to resist evaluation research to protect their programs from political attack or budgetary reductions. In such cases alternative approaches to evaluation must be stimulated and incentives that achieve this must be developed. This chapter begins with some general considerations concerning evaluation and the sociopolitical context within which it takes place. This is followed by an examination of the formulation of the evaluation task and its various aspects. The discussion then focuses on particular types of evaluation, such as social experiments, monitoring, and social indicators. The discussion concludes by addressing such issues as the appropriate criteria for assessing the value and potential of evaluation research, the implementation of evaluation, evaluation as education, and possible incentives for improving efforts in the evaluation field. My conclusion, which I amplify in a variety of ways, is that the potential for evaluation is greatly enhanced when it builds on the common desire among professionals and administrators to do their jobs more effectively and when it is implemented in a manner that minimizes threat and uncertainty. In short, I maintain that evaluation is more properly viewed as part of a process of continuing education rather than as a regulatory function.

GENERAL CONSIDERATIONS

Since the goals of evaluation—as well as the resources that can be devoted to it—are so diverse, the tools of evaluation are also varied. They range from simple monitoring or self-assessment to sophisticated multivariate analysis and social experiments to measure the intended and unintended effects of particular policy interventions. Evaluation may be carried out intramurally as part of a service program where personnel wish information about how better to allocate their efforts, or it may be imposed from above and implemented by an independent research agency. The evaluation may reflect internal needs of a particular agency or requirements for self-justification, or it may be for the purpose of policy planning and budgetary allocations at a higher administrative level. There are, of course, better and poorer methods of evaluation—those that are confounded and self-serving, and those that are more rigorous and disinterested. While we strive to implement the most valid methods to fit the circumstances, we appreciate that the choice of methods and the approach to evaluation may come into conflict with personal and organizational needs, political factors, and professional pride and insecurities. If we insist on being purists, oblivious to the practicalities of existing situations, we serve the goal of evaluation badly in the long run. By stimulating evaluation efforts, even those with imperfections, we contribute to upgrading the standards applied to policy decisions. As higher standards of evidence develop, it is likely that social agencies will come to see that more serious evaluation built into programs from the beginning is important to their own survival as well as to a more effective response to social problems.

Evaluation is an inclusive concept encompassing such activities as organizational intelligence, monitoring, the use of social indicators, demonstration projects, applied social research, and the like. The concern may be with the practical and administrative problems of program implementation, as in many demonstration efforts, or with the impact of changes when successfully executed. Evaluation research is somewhat more restrictive than applied social research in that the latter concerns itself with a wider range of influences than those generally characteristic of policy formulation or social intervention. Although evaluation efforts are broad, they are concerned with variables that are believed to be within the range of control of social policy and social programs. Thus, in the health field, evaluation research is more likely to focus on the study of specific therapeutic interventions, varying forms of financial incentives, and different manpower arrangements rather than on such issues as sociocultural differences among populations, varying social values and orientations, or dominant patterns of power or influence in the community.

In considering varying social policies, the more rigorous evaluation researcher tends to focus on behavioral outcomes and, thus, assumes a relatively conservative stance. For example, it is typical for such persons to maintain that if a particular social intervention has not been proven effective, then public programs should not extend such services. In contrast, both administrators of intervention programs and the interested public may value a service—not because it has with some degree of frequency objectively altered behavior in the desired direction, but because it has been deemed valuable in the society more generally and provides a sense of security or reduces a subjective sense of discomfort. Whatever the uncertain effects of psychotherapeutic intervention, and I, for one, believe that they are uncertain, the fact that those who are more affluent value such services makes it likely that those with lesser means will aspire to more equal access. In the political context, it is not scientific demonstration that often carries the day, but rather what the public defines as the reality; and this requires the evaluator who focuses primarily on more objective behavioral outcomes to pause for thought. The public's views may reflect ignorance, as scientists have argued from time to time, but they may also reflect the fact that the indicators valued by the researcher are not identical to those valued by the public. The tenacity of chiropractic—and the recent history of its extension under various forms of social insurance—should alert us, I think, to the fact that what people seek from help sources in the community may not be the services that help providers believe they are there to give.

From the administrator's perspective, evaluation efforts have costs as well as benefits. First, they require time, manpower, and funds. Serious evaluation is frequently expensive, and when there is a failure to understand how such expenditures will result in more efficient or effective performance, or will enhance the organization in other ways, the feeling frequently emerges that such resources might better be spent more directly for organizational activities. To the extent that funds are explicitly earmarked for evaluation and cannot be converted to other uses, evaluation may still be resented but does not pose the same trade-off problems that exist when administrators have an option. Second, there are frequently pressures from evaluators to modify organizational behavior in some fashion to meet the needs for a more rigorous methodological design, or at the very least evaluation research may require efforts on the part of program personnel to provide information, to complete forms or keep special records, or to allow their work to be observed. While much research emphasizes the importance of assessing the consequences of one or another clear intervention over time, practitioners tend to be highly eclectic in their efforts, may change their practices with new information, and thus are frequently resentful of limits imposed by a research design. To the extent that the types of data demanded by the evaluation depart substantially from those routinely recorded, to the extent that the research demands that practitioners adhere to some artificial routine, and to the extent that the purposes of the research are not well understood or perceived as threatening in some fashion, resistance is likely to be encountered. Increasingly, those in evaluation research are developing approaches that are less likely to impose artificial limits on an agency and that do not demand that the agency adhere to a particular time sequence before modifying its operations.

One important source of resistance to evaluation results from the fact that organizational personnel are often professionally and psychologically committed to the interventions they promote. It is proper and desirable that they have such commitment, and fortunate that they do not remain detached and solely engaged in the bureaucratic game. Without a sense of commitment and the conviction that one's activities count, much of the enthusiasm and the possible impact of program interventions are lost. To the hard-nosed researcher, intervention effects may be merely "Hawthorne effects"; but from the point of view of the people served, "Hawthorne effects" may be as important as any others. Particularly in the human services, it is necessary to convey to clients a sense of optimism and hope;[3] and when professionals doubt their own efforts, they are likely to communicate these doubts to their clients and create a climate of despair. This commitment to one's programs creates a certain protectiveness and suspicion of evaluation research.

Beyond simple self-protection, evaluation can also be a tool used by administrators to support and enhance their own position in the competition for continued and new funding. Such data, however, are frequently not collected for the purpose of objectively and fairly appraising performance and need, but rather to make the case that the agency's programs are of vital importance and deserve priority and resources. Given the general administrative structure of programs—particularly within government—administrators who fail to buttress their claims with whatever supporting data they can muster are delinquent in their responsibilities to their goals and soon lose ground in the battle of maintaining resources. The process thus encourages cycles of exaggeration and justification that conform to few of the canons of serious assessment.[4] Evaluation becomes the chips with which various parties play political poker, but the currency is frequently counterfeit. But in a context where decision-makers have difficulty differentiating the counterfeit from the real, the incentive is to trade in bad currency.

It is commonly advocated that the more stringent methods of evaluation useful in one type of setting be applied to others. In recent years one of the most pervasive evaluation techniques—cost-benefit analysis, which was a valuable tool in military planning—was inappropriately urged on administrators who worked with problems and outcomes that were more intangible, and where it was impossible to specify in any quantitative sense the various costs and benefits.[5] Although the implementation of such analysis was farcical from one viewpoint, it was useful in directing administrators to consider more consciously the costs and benefits of various alternatives that might be appropriately applied in their areas. It fostered a useful style of thinking about social programs. Particularly in professional agencies, which have an orientation toward using whatever technology is in vogue regardless of the absorption of resources,[6] cost-benefit consideration was a valuable corrective even if it could not provide any precise answer to the conceptual issues. It is important to address ourselves to frameworks for program planning and evaluation that help make salient those issues important for administrators to consider.

In developing approaches to encourage more widespread evaluation efforts, we must do so with full understanding that social policies are the culmination of a political process in which objective information is only one of many elements—a fact often not genuinely appreciated by academic researchers. But even in the political arena, feedback from the environment is essential to shape goals and future efforts. There are issues of social intervention, such as welfare policy or national health insurance, that are highly visible in the public arena and, therefore, highly politicized. Although research is relevant to the resolution of such problems, because of their public visibility decisions are likely to be dominated by political considerations. But a good many important issues affecting administrative policy, incentives, and implementation of programs are neither visible nor of particular interest to politicians or to a very large public; and it is in such areas that good evaluation probably has its greatest potential and impact.[7]

One of the greatest difficulties in implementing evaluation efforts is inherent in the threat they pose under conditions where program support and survival are substantially part of a political process. An unfavorable evaluation can potentially threaten and weaken further claims for resources and support, particularly if the sponsoring legislature or bureaucracy is not seen as supportive of the agency's goals, or understanding of the difficulties or the problems they are trying to cope with, or sympathetic with the fragmentary state of knowledge of what works. Administrators also know that there is a political rhetoric that encompasses the slogan "evaluation," which may mean anything from "We don't care much for your kind of program," to "Provide us with some justification," to "Let's seriously evaluate the best use of our dollars to deal with these problems."

Yet all in all, although there are many bureaucratic and professional resistances to evaluation, I am firmly convinced that most agency personnel want to be effective. Their resistance stems, thus, not from lack of interest in self-improvement, but from the fear of uncertainty and the sense of threat. Introduced in a nonthreatening way, evaluation can become a positive force toward self-improvement.

Rather than bemoan the anti-intellectualism or the ignorance of the self-protective maneuvers of the administrator, the proponents of evaluation research would do well to give more attention to the environmental contexts in which serious evaluation is nurtured and to the incentives that might be developed to promote the conditions for its success in improving practice.

FORMULATING THE EVALUATION TASK

The first requirement for evaluation is that the goals and expected impact of program interventions be formulated as explicitly as possible. While seemingly simple, agreement on intended effects is frequently exceedingly difficult to achieve. Many major programs are enacted without clear specification of goals or expected impact. Indeed, the political process may require sufficiently complex and ambiguous goals, so that varying interests support the program for different reasons. Some may support methadone treatment programs because they regard them as a humane alternative to no program regardless of its objective impact; others may provide support not because they believe it will necessarily assist the addict, but because they believe it may result in a reduction of crime and lessen the possibility of social disturbances; others may believe that it improves the functioning of persons addicted to heroin and increases the probability that they will work; and still others may see it as a way of alleviating the anxieties of an aroused public opinion. Many social programs are shaped in a process of compromise among groups having different values and preferences and who may support a program for different and even contradictory reasons. Evaluating methadone treatment is relatively easy compared with many other social programs, but even here the assessment of both short-run and long-range effects on a variety of dimensions is no simple task.

To take a somewhat more difficult example, evaluators are increasingly asking what effect the extension of medical services has on health outcomes, and it has become commonplace to assert that increased use of medical services has only marginal influence on health. The broad statement, however, is frequently misleading because it begs the question of the appropriate measures of health or the functions of much of medical practice. In the case of particular interventions, one can clearly inquire about the outcomes in respect to specific conditions and populations. Similarly, one can inquire whether a particular modality is properly applied, consistent with knowledge of its effects and adverse consequences. Medical practice consists of many interventions, varying in effectiveness and in their correct application to appropriate populations. But in each case the question must be addressed in a specific sense. Much of medical practice has greater relevance to relieving pain and discomfort, minimizing disability, and providing a sense of security and relief of worry, than to modifying physical conditions. Much of ambulatory medical care is sought by persons who require support and caring services, and to measure the effect of such services by indices of mortality misses the point. This is not to assert, however, that the current conceptualization and practice of medicine maximizes those outcome measures we value, whether they be longevity, lesser disability, relief from discomfort, or whatever. But if evaluation is really to be useful, it must give attention to the entire range of functions of multipurpose organizations and must address the more intangible impacts as well as those that are readily measurable. Even if we knew that medicine and psychiatry had little impact on disease outcomes, I think we would find that the population would continue to seek assistance for problems that are frightening or with which they could not cope.

It has become fashionable in health and in other areas to inquire whether limited social programs have impact on global characteristics of persons and populations that are in reality a product of a vast number of influences. It is not difficult to demonstrate that social programs tend not to have major impact on these global indicators whether they be overall health status, academic achievement, or whatever. Using a multiple regression approach and such indicators of impact, most programs could be shown to explain only a very small amount of variation in the dependent measure. Selma Mushkin has stated this problem extremely well.

If a study attempting to determine whether diphtheria immunization makes a difference in national health were to use a familiar regression technique, a superficial finding would be "no go." Diphtheria immunization would be quantified as having little explanatory power in the variance of health status.

The reasoning behind such a finding would go something like this. Before the development of the toxoid, diphtheria had an incidence rate reaching 3 per 1,000 persons of all ages. It occurred, on the average, in 9 of each 1,000 children. Of those who suffered from the disease, some fraction had no long-range consequences, 5-10 per cent died, and impairment of varying severities continued for the remaining number of cases. At the present time, all but 2.5 per cent of children receive some diphtheria toxoid doses. In 1971, no diphtheria deaths were reported for the over 200 cases of the disease. Obviously, immunization has removed the hazard of the one specific disease, diphtheria. But in a static regression analysis limited to a single recent year, such as 1971, the difference in diphtheria immunization and incidence is small and the figures would be interpreted as having little power to explain difference in the general health status of the population.

Given a finding of little or no explanatory power of diphtheria toxoid on general health status, would we conclude that immunization doesn't matter? Would findings suggest that one could press for reallocation of resources away from diphtheria vaccination? Is it wasteful to ask the local health departments, or the states and the Congress, to finance diphtheria immunization? Should parents spend their income on things other than diphtheria immunization for their children? In brief, the analyses based on data for a single period (after diphtheria is no longer a hazard) say little about policy conclusions based on such analyses.

In a multiple regression analysis in which the dependent variable that is being explained is a fairly general factor (such as crime rates, death rates, rates of recidivism, stays in mental hospitals, or educational achievements) each of the many independent variables that may be included in an analytic model is likely to have small power to explain variation. Further, analysis of variance in regression does not methodologically produce the causal connections required to examine any hypothesis made regarding the programs. Yet the results of regression analyses are being applied as if they in fact examined those causal relationships and concluded in the negative.[8]

In evaluating a program, one attempts to specify as carefully as possible the immediate and long-term goals. One also attempts to anticipate unintended or possible adverse effects that must be taken into consideration in balancing the advantages and costs. Although every evaluation must limit its concerns to selected variables, it is prudent to begin with an extensive inventory of possible effects, then perhaps to limit the measures used on the basis of methodological and practical considerations. By reviewing relevant literature, examining the issues that were raised when the program was implemented, and by discussions with administrators and operational personnel, it is possible to obtain a fairly extensive sense of possible intended and unintended effects. Since evaluation results are usually contrary to someone's interests—and therefore likely to be attacked, however well executed—the best recourse for the evaluator is a strong offense—careful specification and measurement of as many of the dimensions of impact as is feasible. If funding constraints or other practicalities make it important to limit the study considerably—and thus only a small subset of indicators can be included—these should be selected to represent the most important contrasting views of the impact that the program might be having. This selection may be undertaken at a sacrifice, and it might be maintained that it is most prudent to assess one type of impact well through a variety of proxy measures rather than to scatter one's efforts too widely. This is a matter of judgment, but in general the usefulness of evaluating the typical multipurpose program on a single dimension is dubious.

In such areas as mental health, the problems of specifying and measuring the impact of interventions are particularly difficult. Intervention programs claim to do everything from maintaining mental health and preventing mental disorder to providing community supports and reeducating important decision-makers. Although controlled trials are a powerful methodology for considering specific interventions for particular kinds of patients, they are more difficult to apply to the overall organization of services in mental health agencies. It is particularly difficult to get therapists to define their goals, and such goals are often expressed in vague terms such as "maturity," "self-realization," and "reeducation." The problem is further compounded by the introduction of concepts such as "symptom-substitution," which tend to deprecate alleviation of specific disturbing symptoms or behavior because a more fundamental "reorganization of personality" has not been demonstrated. Thus, not infrequently, tangible measures of impact are dismissed as irrelevant or superficial, while vague and unmeasurable concepts continue to justify existing practice. The evaluator—by selecting a range of measures of outcome, including proxy measures for some of the more vague psychological terms—is in a stronger position than one who dismisses the vaguer concepts as therapist resistance and makes no effort to examine their basis. Although it is often difficult to develop adequate indicators of symptom substitution and other current psychological concepts, with some attention to the issue it is possible to develop credible measures. Thus, for example, while one cannot prove that symptom substitution does not occur, one can measure a wide range of symptoms and behavior, and demonstrate to what extent the patterning of other symptoms has undergone change. Research, after all, is a matter of plausibility and credibility. If researchers make a serious effort to understand the concepts and goals of therapists—and to include consideration of these in their studies—they carry greater credibility. Also, by including a variety of measures of both objective and subjective outcomes, researchers are in a better position not only to consider a variety of outcome dimensions, but also to examine to what extent they present a consistent pattern.

CONTROLLED TRIALS AND SOCIAL EXPERIMENTS

The evaluation of most social programs involves several different questions. First, there is the specific issue—does a particular intervention lead to intended changes in specified populations, by whatever indicators are used to measure impact? At this level, evaluation is logically the same as in the assessment of any therapeutic modality, such as particular drugs or surgical interventions. Although careful clinical observation of responses to new therapeutic agents may be extremely valuable in assessing impact, such evaluation is frequently associated with wishful thinking, the confusion of suggestion effects with effects attributable to an active therapeutic agent, and to unconscious biases introduced by the clinician. The methodology of controlled double-blind clinical trials has been well developed, and it is fully appropriate to many evaluation questions in the health services areas. There are, of course, serious resistances to the application of controlled trials to health services delivery problems; but as Cochrane has so beautifully illustrated—as much by his own example as through his advocacy—we often have opportunities for controlled clinical trials in health services research that are not inconsistent with ethical standards or the needs of practitioners.[9]

To the researcher there is nothing more elegant and convincing than an experiment, one that successfully randomizes recipients and exposes them to varying interventions or no interventions at all. A successful experiment eliminates the difficulties of selection which is a pervasive bias in much social research and which interferes with making clear inferences. The elegance of the experimental methodology has led some to the short-sighted conclusion that nothing less than an experiment is acceptable and has infrequently resulted in the arrogance expressed in one researcher's statement that "the fault lies not in the model, but in those who out of ignorance prevent the random assignment of units to programs or control groups."[10]

Whatever the advantages of randomization and experimentation—and there are many advantages—they may be significantly eroded by the real difficulties and constraints characteristic of carrying out complex experiments in uncontrolled social settings. Outside the experimental laboratory, the researcher has little control over the multitude of variables that may change the meaning of the experimental manipulations. An example occurred in the New Jersey Negative Income Tax Experiment when the state changed its welfare payment structure and disrupted the ongoing experimental manipulations.[11] In situations where we require informed consent and where there are significant resistances to particular social treatments, the problems of nonparticipation and attrition of subjects become difficult. We have not yet learned how to cope with the attrition problem in long-term experiments, except to find out that to the extent that it is large and nonrandom, we no longer have an experiment at all. Social experimentation can be extremely expensive in time and resources and, frequently for both practical and methodological reasons, quasi-experimental methods[12] or other types of evaluation approaches are more promising.

Experiments are most feasible when the issue concerns the impact of a specified intervention within a relatively narrow time period rather than a complex set of interventions directed toward a variety of goals. In the areas under consideration here, randomized controlled trials are far more useful to study approaches to treatment of specific problems than they are to an overall evaluation of government policy. Thus, an experiment is the optimum way of evaluating methadone treatment or a program that offers a community alternative to hospitalization for schizophrenic patients. However, an experiment is not a particularly good approach to evaluating the impact of such multipurpose institutions as mental health centers or to assess the impact of training programs on the mental health sector. Of course there are significant resistances to experiments that are both feasible and appropriate, but there is a growing tendency to urge very expensive experiments that are not appropriate for answering the social policy questions at issue.

SOCIAL MONITORING AND SOCIAL INDICATORS

In situations where programs have multiple goals and where the bulk of agency effort is given to no single goal, the agency requires some feedback to know how well it is dealing with its responsibilities. To obtain feedback, monitoring is a useful device. Monitoring refers to the continuing effort to assess the occurrence of various events, including unexpected changes, in the environment. Through experience we have developed a variety of social indicators such as those that assess the state of the economy. In the health field the most common indicators include birth and death rates, occurrence of morbidity and use of health care services, and disability and impairment. These indicators make administrators sensitive to emerging problems, to unanticipated changes, and to significant differences among subgroups in the population that require social action. The information is useful for the agency in carrying out its programs, but it does not clearly delineate what impact agency programs have. For example, a public health department may monitor the rate of infant mortality as one of its program responsibilities. But positive changes in such indicators may be indicative of a wide variety of possible influences and cannot be attributed to program efforts. Such information does, however, alert agency personnel to geographic areas or social groups that require special attention and perhaps special studies as well.

Public agencies frequently cannot monitor important indicators themselves, and thus depend on the availability of vital statistics from local and state authorities and from the National Center for Health Statistics. If these data are to be most useful, they must be up to date, they must be relevant to public policy issues, they must provide estimates for important subgroups in the population, and they must be compiled in a fashion that provides not only an estimate of morbidity but information as to the extent to which these problems are being dealt with or corrected. For example, a report on visual acuity in the population is more useful for public policy if it also includes information on the extent to which problems of acuity have been adequately corrected.[13] Furthermore, the data systems should be organized to facilitate obtaining further analyses than those published that are particularly important for a given program. The Committee to Evaluate the National Center for Health Statistics has made a variety of useful suggestions which, if implemented, would contribute importantly to improving health monitoring at the present time.[14]

ASSESSING THE VALUE AND
POTENTIAL OF EVALUATION RESEARCH

Because of the sociopolitical factors already discussed in this chapter, it is un-reasonable to evaluate the effectiveness of evaluation research on the basis of whether there is an immediate implementation of the research findings. An immediate response may be impossible because of political factors or because of the very long time lag between the formulation of the research conclusions and the diffusion of this information to the many decisionmakers who have responsibility for social programming. Moreover, few evaluations are sufficiently clear-cut or unequivocal to avoid criticism or conflicting interpretations of their relevance or implications. Thus, it seems that we require more modest and more realistic criteria to assess the value and significance of the evaluation process.

One important dimension for assessing the significance of evaluation research is the extent to which it contributes to growing sophistication about the appropriate questions to ask and how to evaluate information about social programs. Even when the results of evaluation efforts are not directly implemented, if done carefully and in communication with the personnel involved in carrying out these programs, evaluation affects the climate of thinking and may affect the direction of future efforts. It may contribute to an active and analytic perspective, which stimulates program personnel to be more involved in their work and thoughtful about it, and indirectly may contribute to morale and intellectual ferment. Evaluation can have adverse effects as well if it undermines commitment to goals or induces despair. But if properly done, evaluation contributes to a sense of direction and development of mastery, and becomes an important component of excellence of performance.

Perhaps the most common form of evaluation in social agencies is to monitor program efforts. Its popularity stems from the ease with which it is performed. Moreover, in the bureaucratic game it provides a device that one can always use to make claims for success. But of all of the possible forms of evaluation, program monitoring is perhaps the least effective and least informative. It might be far more valuable for social agencies to devote attention to a sample of their most important programs, using more powerful evaluation devices, than to dilute their efforts and resources in routine program monitoring.

With patience and persistence it is possible to make some progress. However, how much evaluation is carried out and how it is carried out must depend on the circumstances involved. Of course, there are many circumstances in which successful evaluation depends only on minimal cooperation of the agency being studied, as in surveys of recipients of human services. In still other circumstances, cooperation is mandated by the administrative program of which an agency may be part.[15] But I hope that our view of the evaluation process is far broader than this, and that we seek ways to make most administrators and professionals receptive and committed to seeing evaluation as an important instrument to increase their potential. However, I would not deny that the presence of a mandate assists the development of both receptivity and commitment.

THE IMPLEMENTATION OF
EVALUATION OF SOCIAL PROGRAMS

Much of this discussion has addressed the issue of whether a particular intervention significantly affects outcome. A related but somewhat different issue, which too often receives inadequate attention, concerns the effective implementation of a successful intervention. Health programs are highly decentralized and have innumerable points of decision concerning implementation. Much ineffective care results not from the lack of knowledge and experience but rather from the difficulty of diffusing experience and knowledge to the decisionmakers who administer and carry out health programs. Many interventions, appropriate in particular circumstances, are applied in a fashion that induces iatrogenic illness and disability, while others that should be used are frequently not understood or implemented. The problem of diffusion of appropriate practice patterns is enormous for even the more straightforward therapies, such as use of antibiotics and simple general surgery. As one moves to more complex intervention approaches that are more difficult to understand and apply, error is further compounded. Evaluation must not only be concerned with what effect programs have, but also with the failures to use established interventions appropriately and the misapplication of those that are used.

Many social programs are not administered and executed by a single administrative entity, but rather by a variety of programs and agencies at the local level. The actual operational units may be state and local health departments, universities, hospitals or other nonprofit corporations, profit firms, individual practitioners, or a conglomeration of individual programs. Even when the intent of a program is clearly specified at the highest administrative levels, the translations at the local units can be quite bizarre; and the operational units tend to have their own agendas and priorities and often quite diverse goals. To some extent the diversity might result from the fact that agencies and programs may solicit funds for a project as a means of sustaining other activities as well—to which there may be greater commitment. Variabilities also result from the fact that agencies deal with different populations with varying profiles of problems, and the availability of other community resources may differ substantially as well from one context to another. Also, the skills and leadership available may make concentration of effort on particular areas a reasonable and effective way of using resources. All of this is very untidy to the evaluator, but it is the reality with which evaluation must cope.

In many if not most circumstances, we do not have a developed strategy for evaluating the efforts of social agencies. Too frequently, policymakers and administrators have not explicitly thought out what might index reasonable progress and whether the efforts of the organization might be better applied in some other way. All social organizations take on a life of their own with their own particular dynamics and priorities; and without an unequivocally clear mandate, the goals and practices tend to drift toward those that are most enjoyable, comfortable, and that confer the greatest prestige. The emphasis on evaluation will have made an enormous contribution if it does nothing more than encourage administrators to think through clearly what their options are and how they are expending their effort, and if it stimulates a more active and searching perspective among those who deliver social and medical services to the population.

EVALUATION AS EDUCATION

Evaluators must always be clear about the purpose of their efforts. In many circumstances a valid study is impossible, and the concern in any case is improvement of the quality of work among relevant practitioners. Here it may be more useful to develop tools that facilitate practitioners' abilities to assess their own efforts without threat and defensiveness. If we are honest with ourselves, we know that few of us enjoy being subjected to outside evaluation, and particularly by parties we feel are not sympathetic to the problems of our work and the difficulty of our tasks. The fact that we might resist such evaluations does not mean that we are not interested in self-improvement or in developing skills to do our jobs better. How to use this commonly shared desire for self-improvement in improving performance is a major challenge.

I am impressed by the extent to which some of the medical specialty societies appreciate these concerns and by the programs they have developed that allow physicians to evaluate anonymously their strengths and weaknesses, with feedback on how to improve performance in areas requiring remedial efforts. No doubt the complaint that persons who participate in such programs are frequently those who need them the least is often true; yet it is possible to provide incentives to many professional workers for continued self-improvement without threatening them or making them defensive. Moos[16] has developed relatively simple measures of treatment environments for mental health facilities that can be applied to various treatment contexts and that can be used to measure the outcome of directed change, providing relatively simple feedback to treatment personnel. In England, the Royal College of General Practitioners has developed means to encourage practitioners to investigate their own practices so as to have a better appreciation of what they really do and how they can better organize their efforts. They have developed various materials that allow general practitioners with little research training to carry out investigations in their practices. Since the goal of evaluation is improved practice, I believe that we must give great attention to the issue of how to assist professionals and others to make their own assessments and to improve their own performance.

INCENTIVES FOR EVALUATION

In urging evaluation and critical self-awareness, we must face the dilemma noted earlier. Much of helping works because the therapist has self-confidence, and the patient has confidence in the helper. By inducing doubts and self-criticism, and making consumers aware that at least objectively the emperor has no clothes, do we produce human betterment? By making therapists skeptical of their own efforts, do we so dampen enthusiasm and commitment that we lose rather than gain ground? The physician still remains somewhat of a priest and magician, and part of the effectiveness of medicine is the mystique of medicine.

This is no easy or trivial question, and where one stands depends in part on one's values and life perspectives. Thus I provide no resolution but only some considerations relevant to the larger question. Secular values generally support demystification on the assumption that, all things considered, it is best for people to come to terms with their real options, and that the scientific aspects of helping can only be developed through a critical and searching perspective. Much of the problem is inherent in the fact that medicine, which had its early origins in religious concerns, has been translated and conceptualized in technical and scientific terms so as to make scientific effectiveness synonymous with what is worthwhile. Thus the caring function of medical practice has come to be seen as the province of the romantic or the theologian.

There are, however, things to be done because they are right and humane, regardless of their demonstrated effectiveness in altering "objective outcomes." Practitioners must come to accept that some functions of medicine are too important, too central to our sense of ethics and humanity, to judge them solely by utilitarian criteria. It is my hope that these considerations are not so romantic that evaluators cannot apply them as criteria in evaluating how helping institutions enhance the quality of life. To the extent that the caring function is accepted as an important part of medical practice, it is more possible to remain optimistic and enthusiastic in the face of discouraging evaluations on the ability to alter "objective outcomes." Also, to the extent that commitment is built around the idea of searching for the best techniques for managing patients in contrast to being developed around particular forms of treatment or schools of thought, it is more possible to maintain momentum than if egos are tied up in particular treatment philosophies or modalities. Organizations must search for ways to build commitment around tasks and goals in contrast to specific interventions. I am not naive about the professional and other barriers to achieving such changes in values and commitments, but the fact that they are difficult to achieve makes them no less important.

In examining the outcomes of health services, somewhat different criteria must be applied to techniques of caring as compared with techniques of cure. All treatment involves some balance between benefits and risks. Treatments that carry the greatest risks to life and health and those that involve the most expensive modalities must meet the most rigorous of evaluation criteria. Those that are less expensive or involve few potential adverse consequences should be judged not only by the extent to which they bring about demonstrable change in the course of illness and disability, but also by the degree to which they make patients feel more comfortable, more hopeful, and more optimistic. Evaluation must inquire not only whether things work and to what degree, but also about the possible dangers and costs of using particular treatment options relative to others that offer comparable management at less risk and less cost.

In short, evaluation is a complex and multifaceted process. Its definition and elaboration are highly influenced by social values and political processes as well as by scientific method. It can be used as a political tool or as a means of self-assessment and improvement. And depending on how the effort is organized, it can be seen as a threat or as a valuable adjunct to one's efforts. Because of this complexity and the political and professional sensitivity of evaluation, it is often talked about but less frequently implemented. In considering both the costs and benefits of evaluation as a tool for government and professional practice, I am convinced that its effects are likely to be influential if evaluation is viewed as part of a process of education and continuing education, and not as a policing or regulatory function. Evaluation methodologies can be developed to assist practitioners of all types in comprehending what they are doing, in sharpening their thinking and practice, and in using their energies and resources with greater effect.

NOTES

1. P. Rossi and W. Williams, eds. (1972), *Evaluating Social Programs: Theory, Practice, and Politics* (New York: Seminar Press).

2. E. Suchman (1967), *Evaluation Research* (New York: Russell Sage), pp. 7-8.

3. J. Frank (1974), *Persuasion and Healing*, rev. ed. (New York: Schocken Books).

4. A. Wildavsky (1964), *The Politics of the Budgetary Process* (Boston: Little, Brown).

5. I. Hoos (1972), *Systems Analysis in Public Policy: A Critique* (Berkeley: University of California Press).

6. V. Fuchs (1968), "The Growing Demand for Medical Care," *New England Journal of Medicine*, **279**:190-195.

7. D. Mechanic (1974), *Politics, Medicine, and Social Science* (New York: Wiley-Interscience).

8. S. Mushkin (1973), "Evaluations: Use with Caution," *Evaluation*, **1**:30-35.

9. A. L. Cochrane (1972), *Effectiveness and Efficiency* (London: Nuffield Provincial Hospitals Trust).

10. T. R. Houston, Jr. (1972), "The Behavioral Sciences Impact-Effectiveness Model," in P. Rossi and W. Williams, eds., op. cit. p. 63.

11. D. Kershaw (1972), "Issues in Income Maintenance Experiments," in P. Rossi and W. Williams, eds., op. cit.; D. Kershaw and J. Fair (1973), *Report on the New Jersey Negative Income Tax Experiment*, Vol. 3 (Princeton, N.J.: Mathematica), Chapter 12.

12. D. T. Campbell and J. C. Stanley (1963), *Experimental and Quasi-Experimental Designs for Research* (Chicago: Rand McNally).

13. Institute of Medicine, National Academy of Sciences (1973), *A Strategy for Evaluating Health Services* (Washington, D.C.), pp. 3-5.

14. Report of the Committee to Evaluate the National Center for Health Statistics (1973), *Health Statistics, Today and Tomorrow* (Washington, D.C.: Government Printing Office), Series 4, No. 15.

15. J. Wholey et al. (1970), *Federal Evaluation Policy: Analyzing the Effects of Public Programs* (Washington, D.C.: Urban Institute).

16. R. Moos (1974), *Evaluating Treatment Environments: A Social Ecological Approach* (New York: Wiley-Interscience).

Chapter 16

Prospects for National
Health Insurance:
Promises, Hopes,
and Cautions

Since the United States is clearly moving toward some system of national health insurance in the near future, I want to conclude this book by examining some of the hopes and promises of various proposals, the trade-offs involved in making one or another choice, and difficulties likely to be encountered in translating ideals into realities.

The proposals for National Health Insurance vary in scope of services and population coverage; in the extent to which they mandate new forms of financial arrangements and organizational modifications; and in the roles of government, employers and employees, insurance companies, and providers of service. Some of the proposals seek primarily to extend insurance coverage to segments of the population that presently have inadequate coverage; others propose to protect consumers against catastrophic costs that exceed either fixed dollar amounts or fixed proportions of their income; and still others seek universal coverage financed through the federal government and major alterations in the way medical services are planned and delivered. Much has been written about the proposals,[1] and although I will describe them to some extent, the central purpose of this chapter is to define what I believe to be the most productive course to follow, and to analyze the problems of implementation in light of the organizational issues I have raised throughout this book.

My preference is for a national health insurance system that includes the entire population, provides easy access to medical care without financial barriers, and is under greater economic control by government. Although I believe that the role medical care plays in promoting health status is often exaggerated, I share Fuchs' view that "a national health insurance plan to which all (or nearly all) Americans belonged would have considerable symbolic value as one step in an effort to forge a link between classes, regions, races and age groups."[2]

A relatively comprehensive, equitable, and economic national health program requires a reasonable level of control over the allocation of medical resources. This, in turn, requires the use of an established budget that controls the total level of expenditures. The proper point to achieve economic control, I believe, is where expensive and elaborate decision-making takes place, and not at the point of access that keeps people who are worried or upset from seeking assistance and reassurance. If we move to a system where budgetary pressures require professionals to establish priorities for medical work, it is more likely that efficient and effective use can be made of available health personnel and of existing facilities.

Most proposals for national health insurance that increase the available insurance, without altering the delivery system, tend to increase both the demand for and the costs of care.[3] An important exception are proposals for catastrophic insurance that becomes operative only after the patient has reached a specified level of expenditure. Most such proposals are highly inequitable since paying first-dollar costs are a greater hardship for persons with less income. However, a proposal by Martin Feldstein overcomes these inequities by relating the extent of obligation of the consumer for the "first-dollar" payments to their income levels. Since no person would be obligated to pay more than a fixed proportion of his or her income for medical costs, and since individuals who are below given incomes can be excused entirely from out-of-pocket payments, this approach does not necessarily place an undue burden on the poor. And, as the argument goes, consumers are more prudent in purchasing services when they must pay the "first-dollar" expenditures themselves. This proposal has had considerable appeal among participants in the national health insurance debate because it has promise for controlling expenditures, deals with the problem of inequities, and appears to be relatively simple from an administrative point of view. But as Victor Fuchs suggests, the approach has many shortcomings:

> First, since initial expenditures would be paid by the patient and only large subsequent expenditures by insurance, there would be less incentives for persons to seek early care or preventive treatment; rather, the emphasis would be on expensive tertiary care. Second, the catastrophic approach would impose a large

administrative burden on both patients and the government. Every family would have to maintain comprehensive records on all medical care expenditures in anticipation of eventually exceeding the deductible amount and becoming eligible for insurance coverage, and the government would have to establish means for checking these records. Most proposals call for the deductible to vary with the level of income of the family, so additional checking would be required to determine each family's income level in relation to its medical expenditures. The incentive to try to lump expenditures into the year when the deductible is exceeded, as well as the temptation to indulge in more flagrant forms of chicanery, would be very great.

Major-risk insurance would not deter utilization once the deductible had been satisfied, but it is the marginal expenditure over which the patient frequently has the most discretion. In hospital care, for example, the marginal decision frequently is whether to remain an extra day or so. The first several days' stay is often determined primarily by medical considerations; the last day or two are usually much more likely to be subject to patient preference. Given the size of the deductibles now proposed for major risk insurance (about 10 per cent of income, with an upper limit of about a thousand dollars), the average hospitalized patient would satisfy the deductible in the first several days and thereafter be under little or no financial pressure to cut short his stay.

Moreover, it is not clear how the provision of major-risk insurance by the federal government would prevent families from also acquiring "first-dollar" or "shallow" coverage from private insurance companies if they so desired. It should be noted that although major-risk insurance in various forms is now available from private insurance companies, the demand for it is less than overwhelming. If major-risk insurance is really what people desire in the way of medical care coverage, why don't they buy it now? And why do union leaders and representatives of other groups seek more coverage? I believe one reason is because people want an easy, convenient, systematic way of *paying* for medical care. It is a great mistake to view the purchase of health insurance as simply the result of the desire to avoid risk.

Finally, it should be noted that the major-risk approach concentrates exclusively on the patient and does nothing about organization of care, problems of access, or efficiency of delivery systems. In my view, its appeal is extremely deceptive. It seems like a cheap way of getting out of a crisis, but it offers little hope of solving the major health care problems now facing the American public.[1]

As the momentum builds for national health insurance, it is commonplace to support accessibility for the entire population within a responsive, humane, high quality, and economically efficient system of care. Agreement on these general aspects, however, shields basic disagreements about almost every aspect of medical organization and financing. The advocates are full of promises; and that, of course, is the role of the proponent. The discussion that follows suggests a greater sense of skepticism that any of the proposals—even the one I endorse—will live up to the claims made. I believe that if we are critical and cautious, and skeptical of the commonplace rhetoric without abandoning idealism, opportunities for implementing a more effective system are much enhanced. In the past decade the gap between our theories of organization and intervention and our experiences has been wide. If this has taught us anything at all, it is that there may be a wide distance between our theories and the realities of human behavior. I strongly share Fuchs' belief that national health insurance will be more likely to serve its function well if we do not expect too much and if it is not oversold.

CRITERIA FOR EVALUATING NATIONAL HEALTH INSURANCE PLANS

Despite the appearance of consensus on such goals as accessibility and quality among adherents of national health insurance proposals, various proposals contain basic and deep philosophical differences. Some proposals, such as those that would subsidize purchase of private health insurance by those with lower income, seek to maintain intact the existing system of care but with some increased access. More comprehensive approaches, such as the Health Security Plan (a plan introduced by Senator Kennedy and Congresswoman Griffiths and backed by organized labor), seek a regionally planned and centrally financed system of medical care with universal coverage. Some proposals are based on the philosophy of self-help, on the assumption that persons have a responsibility to assume directly the costs of a major part of their care. Others view access to medical care as a "right" and seek to insure it through federal law. The Health Security Program, despite provisions for diversity and freedom of choice, has incentives encouraging greater homogeneity in the way medical care is organized. Other proposals are designed to preserve the existing diversity— many say chaos—of present organizational arrangements. Most proposals attempt to contain costs through cost-sharing provisions, such as coinsurance and deductibles; but the Health Security Program eliminates almost all financial barriers to care, intending, in contrast, to contain costs through the use of a centrally planned prospective budgeting procedure. And while some plans, such as those designed to deal with "catastrophic" costs, provide incentives for physicians and for the medical system as a whole to devote disproportionate efforts to more intensive and expensive services, others seek to limit more expensive forms of care through budgetary restrictions and peer review processes, putting far greater emphasis on increased access to primary medical care and the provision of preventive and supportive services.

Financing, of course, is usually the guts of any discussion of policy alternatives. Here is where it is most difficult to sort out various claims and counterclaims. There are serious uncertainties in estimating the costs of any program, particularly those where structural changes such as new deployments of manpower, varying types of incentives and controls, and new types of organization constitute major components of the proposal. Our experience is often too limited to make even good gross estimates of the likely savings resulting from one or another change in the delivery system. Also, such estimates and the public debate tend often to confuse the total costs of the program with expenditures that come directly from public funds. The Department of Health, Education, and Welfare, in estimating expenditures under eight proposed programs for fiscal year 1975, including both the most expensive and least expensive proposals, estimated the range of total expenditures to vary only from $107 to $116 billion, with an estimate of $103 billion if things were left as they are.[5] The major difference among these proposals is the proportion of expenditures directly paid by the federal government; these estimates varied from 38 to 90 per cent.

In the final analysis, of course, the consumers pay the bills whether the funds come indirectly through taxation or directly through out-of-pocket expenditures. As Fuchs notes:

> Nor is there any secret formula that can transfer the cost of health care to "government" or "business" without the burden eventually being borne by the public through more taxes, higher prices, or lower wages. Granted, the choice of financing system can make a significant difference to families at the highest and lowest levels of income, but the average family will have to pay the same share under any system.[6]

The issue of where the funds come from is hardly trivial, since modes of financing have varying consequences for employers' willingness to hire new employees when they must assume certain health benefits, for the coordination of varying social benefit programs (particularly in dealing with the so-called "notch" problem), and in income tax implications under varying alternatives. Some examples will illustrate the possible consequences of financing decisions.

The National Health Insurance program, first developed during the Nixon era and supported by the current administration, would require employers to contribute significantly to the health insurance premiums of eligible workers. While this is unlikely to have a major effect on most large companies who already pay for a significant amount of such benefits, it can have a far more serious effect on more marginal employers. Given the requirement to contribute toward a significant proportion of the health insurance premium through a payroll tax, an incentive is created to avoid hiring additional employees, to use part-time manpower who would not be eligible for the health benefits, to use existing workers overtime in contrast to hiring additional workers, and to hire single workers or wives of workers who are likely to require smaller premium payments. Also, under the administration's Assisted Health Insurance Plan for the poor, serious "notch" problems develop. As Rashi Fein has noted:

> an increase in family income of $500 (from $4,500 to $5,000) would lead to an increase of $300 in premium costs, of $50 in per person medical deductibles, and of almost $200 in maximum liability. Though the dollar amounts differ a similar situation is found in the Medicare-replacement program. It is unlikely, but possible, depending on income levels, to find that a one dollar increase in income leads to an increase in premium and other medical care costs of over $400—an effective tax rate of over 40,000 per cent! While this is an extreme illustration, the fundamental point is clear: at low incomes, *and only at low incomes,* the Plan severely penalizes persons whose income increases sufficiently to move them from one income class into another.[7]

The key questions in respect to financing concern the total costs of a program and its distributive effects. Any plan should be carefully evaluated in terms of the extent to which it promotes equity and the degree to which it is financed by progressive or regressive taxes. Health insurance plans tend to be more equitable to the extent that they are funded from general income tax revenues which are more progressive than most sales taxes or a fixed payroll tax, such as the social security payroll tax. A program such as the one proposed by the administration that mandates employees to contribute a fixed proportion of the health insurance premium is regressive in that it requires employees with relatively lower wages to contribute a larger proportion of their income toward the required coverage than would be the case for better-paid employees.

Another issue relating to cost involves the comprehensiveness of the benefit package. Most proposals limit the availability of outpatient psychiatric services, optometry, dental and orthodontic care, and payment for drugs. Limiting the benefit package is, of course, a major way of controlling medical care costs, and those items involving costs that are most difficult to control, or where there exists a large unmet need, are most usually limited.

One of the most important issues in considering national health insurance alternatives involves the existing incentives within any proposal for correcting inefficiencies and irrationalities in the organization of medical care. Key questions are to what extent a given proposal would encourage a more adequate distribution of physicians by geographic area and type of work, more efficient use of health manpower, controls over unneeded hospital and surgical care, and greater efficiencies and responsiveness of health services more generally. From an administrative point of view, it is also necessary to consider whether the mechanisms suggested within any proposal are really operational and whether they can be implemented in a fashion that approximates the design and intentions of the proposal.

Perhaps the most pressing problem we face is the escalation of medical care costs, which now exceed 100 billion dollars and give no indication of leveling off. Most of the proposals for national health insurance offer little to control this trend other than by limiting the benefit package available. There is some hope but little evidence that the implementation of the Professional Standards Review Organizations will aid the effort to contain costs, and most of the plans that basically extend existing insurance programs offer few means to hold either prices or total costs down. The most ambitious program to contain total cost within a broad benefit package and few economic barriers to care is the Health Security Program. Since this program would be centrally financed and would depend predominantly on public funds, controls on total costs would be maintained by the ceiling imposed on expenditures by political and administrative decisions. The ceiling on the budget, so the theory argues, would require providers to make rational allocation decisions using available resources to optimal advantage. Moreover, it is maintained that incentives for unnecessary care would be limited by using capitation more extensively as a method of payment, and such payment would also encourage more effective use of less expensive paraprofessionals.

Although the theory has considerable potential, certain cautions are prudent. To the extent that the system as a whole is believed to be performing at less than an appropriate level, considerable political pressures could mount for increased investment in care. Various disease constituencies could be politically mobilized in a manner that introduces distortions in investment and service patterns. The United States, where expectations about health care tend to be very high, may find the experience of other countries using a fixed budgetary allocation less than fully applicable to its own experience. Also, we cannot assume that in requiring physicians and health units to establish priorities in care they will necessarily make the most reasonable choices. Preferences and professional socialization among physicians are very strong; although it is plausible, we must be careful in assuming that accurate assessment of need in the population will take precedence over professional habits and desired patterns of work. Data on primary care physicians in Kaiser-Permanente, seeing approximately the same patient mix, show considerable variabilities in patterns of work and the use of the laboratory.[8] This suggests that the economic and structural aspects of practice may not necessarily be as influential on practice patterns as we often believe. If such a system is to work, the fixed budgetary mechanism must be reinforced by adequate feedback devices for providing information to physicians on their performance and effective peer review.

Both the attractiveness and dangers of more comprehensive proposals, such as the Health Security Program, result from their promise to achieve a great deal within tight economic constraints. But the prior discussion in this book suggests that while the Health Security Program would eliminate economic barriers to care, it would not eliminate the rationing of health services. No system of care in the world is willing to provide as much care as people will use. All systems develop mechanisms that limit allocation of services. It is instructive that the Soviet Union, which reports average utilization rates almost three times that of the United States, continues to define increasing access to medical care as an important priority.[9] Although those wishing to replace economic rationing with other devices hope that they will encourage greater rationality in medical decision-making, this is a process to be carefully monitored and not a goal to be assumed. In noneconomic rationing, the most basic instrument is the limitation on available resources; other major means of controlling utilization are limiting the available sites of care, increasing the queue for service, providing more hurried and impersonal services, and increasing bureaucratic barriers. Although some barriers if judiciously used need not be as disadvantageous as fee barriers to service, they can affect care adversely if they are excessive. As I have emphasized, the most sensible rationing scheme is one that facilitates patients' entry into the system but limits, through controls over provider decisions, the manner in which expensive and more dangerous modalities are used.

The Health Security Program is intended to cope with the problem of increasing equity in the distribution of medical care by redistributing through a central budgeting process financial resources by geographic area. Examination of implementation of legislation by DHEW in a variety of fields including welfare and civil rights suggests, however, considerable unwillingness to be aggressive in the face of vigorous political opposition.[10] The administration of the Health Security Program, like any other, would be subject to all of the political pressures in society more generally that attempt to maintain special privilege and avoid redistribution of resources.

This process has been operative in systems such as the National Health Service of England. Logan,[11] a long-time observer of the National Health Service and a well-known health services researcher, has lamented the fact that after 20 years of nationalized medicine so little has been achieved in bringing about more equal distribution of medical resources and manpower. Although the National Health Service was to be a planned system based on rational considerations of need and appropriate redistribution of health care resources, the system has been relatively disappointing in bringing about greater equity. Equity was enhanced by a form of organization that eliminated most economic barriers to medical care and provided free general practice and hospital services, but the practitioners and facilities are unevenly distributed throughout the country; more affluent areas have an excess of providers of care. For example, the Southern and South-Eastern Regions have better facilities, more physicians relative to the population, and provide NHS patients with more amenities than those in the North and Midlands. As Logan indicates:

> There is little difference in the age distribution of the population across the fifteen hospital regions of England and Wales, and while the industrial North of the

country seems to have slightly more sickness and death, this is not sufficient to account for the wide differences in rates of inpatients in all specialties (except obstetrics and psychiatry). Rates range from 120 per thousand population in the Liverpool Region, to 86 in East Anglia, but the Manchester Region is intermediate at 103; the neighboring Sheffield, also in the North, is even lower at 85, while the Greater London area, enjoying the lowest sickness rates, admits 113. The varying rates for hospital use are not in fact related to either the need or the demand for hospital admission, but rather to the actual availability of a hospital bed. . . . As the bed has to be serviced by manpower, there is the same ranking in the distribution of hospital doctors. . . . The gradient of the supply of nurses and the supporting "hotel" staff follow the same pattern. . . . After twenty years of the National Health Service, these differences in comparable industrialized areas have not narrowed, and indeed, if anything, have widened. Faced with such evidence, even the most optimistic cannot claim that whatever planning there might have been in an organized society such as Britain, it has produced an equitable distribution of resources across such a homogeneous nation.[12]

A planned economy is not immune to the pressures and influence of those groups in the population who are more educated, aggressive, and vocal. These groups have higher expectations, demand more services, and are more likely to define their interests in a manner that induces politicians to respond. They are unlikely to tolerate reductions in services or facilities; thus, unless the system is willing to make large new investments in care, inequalities in distribution will inevitably remain. Moreover the providers, like in other countries, wish to practice in the more affluent and attractive areas, and policies that depend on voluntary behavior and weak incentives are unlikely to achieve significant changes in distribution. Although the British have used some incentives such as additional increments of remuneration for doctors who take up practice in needy areas, to achieve more effective manpower distribution, and although they have also been willing to follow a policy that closes overdoctored areas to new general practices, these measures have been applied cautiously and have not achieved equality in distribution of these public resources.[13]

The difficulties faced by government are to some extent illustrated by health center policy in England. The key feature of the National Health Service was to be the health center, in which groups of doctors and supporting professionals were to provide the basic ambulatory services in an integrated and effective way. The government soon realized, however, that the introduction of such health centers on a wide scale would be expensive, and in the face of economic pressures the implementation of the policy was neglected for a quarter of a century.[14] Instead, the government continued the traditional pattern of the lone general practitioner, operating in a relatively inefficient way and with less than full potential, a legacy that persists today. Similarly, the costs of renovating the antiquated hospital system and building new hospitals were seen as prohibitive, and the government allowed facilities—particularly those that were less visible and, therefore, of less concern to vocal publics—to decay. Such issues as hospital construction, better long-term facilities for the aged, hospital and community care facilities for the mentally ill, new ambulatory care settings, and the like were neglected until some problem made the issue more visible to a larger public. But, for the most part, the decision-making process through which budgetary allocations were made to varying sectors of the economy within the centralized financing structure was insulated from the demands of unorganized and less vocal groups who might be particularly affected by such allocations.

In the United States, many people feel that socialized medicine is a highly expensive means of organizing health services; but the reverse is more often correct. Centralized financing systems have far greater control over the expenditure of resources in any sector and the degree to which they will be rationed. It is perhaps ironic, given the typical propaganda of those who have always opposed the National Health Service, that one of the areas in which it is most criticized by knowledgeable observers is its inability to command sufficient resources in competition with other sectors of the economy. In contrast, in the United States the diverse sources of expenditure decisions make it difficult to limit investments in the health sector without significantly sacrificing equity.

Since we have no scientific standard to determine what is the most reasonable allocation of resources among the varying sectors, this remains a matter of judgment. Certainly, given the needs of the British population in housing, education, transportation, and a variety of other areas, it is difficult to challenge the wisdom of limiting escalating health expenditures. But to those who speak for the health sector, such limitation may be seen as a disadvantage of a more centralized system. Despite the lean financing of the National Health Service, it has important symbolic significance in English society and probably contributes to the social cohesion of the country. The vast majority of the population continues to support it vigorously despite its imperfections.

Returning to current proposals for national health insurance in the United States, a major issue is the role of economic barriers to service in the form of coinsurance and deductibles. Such economic barriers constrain the behavior of persons with lower incomes but have less influence on the affluent. In contrast, the types of rationing typical in systems without economic barriers have greater effect on the affluent since they are less likely to tolerate the waiting and the inconvenience that the poor accept out of necessity. However, even within these conditions, the affluent often obtain more service because they tend to be demanding and aggressive and more capable of coping with bureaucracies. The data from England, and more recently from Canada, suggest that eliminating deductibles and coinsurance has the effect of redistributing services from the most affluent to those who are of lower incomes.[15] While noneconomic rationing processes tend to maintain approximately the same level of medical services, the elimination of economic barriers results in a lower rate of utilization among the affluent and a somewhat higher rate among the poor. This is consistent with trends in physician utilization in the United States following the implementation of Medicare and Medicaid. Although the national per capita utilization rate remained approximately the same as before, the poor now consumed a larger proportion of services, eliminating the traditional inverse relationship between socioeconomic status and physician use.[16]

Coinsurance and deductibles, which are primarily instituted to control costs, are usually justified as a means of eliminating frivolous and unreasonable use of services. Unfortunately, however, such controls constrain the behavior of the poor the most—those who have a higher prevalence of illness and a greater need for medical care—and thus affect the utilization of necessary care as well as perhaps less critical services. The theory of coinsurance and deductibles implies that people "know" when they are "really sick" and when they are not. My discussion of help-seeking patterns and attribution in Chapter 8 should make clear the weaknesses of this assumption. If the issue of when people are "sick" is so clear-cut, why is it necessary for physicians to incur such large costs in making such determinations? The issue, unfortunately, is not as simple as some cost-conscious economists would like us to believe. A rational system of medical care encourages people who are worried and insecure to obtain access to care and to be reassured. Access itself is a relatively inexpensive component of the medical care process. The major costs stem from the elaboration of work by physicians in their evaluation and management of patients. It is here that we can most benefit from very careful evaluation of the medical care process and those components of appraisal and management that are valuable and those that are less necessary. And it is in this arena that controls against unnecessary costs can be applied most realistically.

Any incentive system developed must take into account the needs of doctors and other health professionals as well as patients' needs. The fee-for-service structure encourages some medical and surgical work that is of marginal value but, conversely, some types of capitation payment can eliminate important incentives for improved efforts. Certainly one of the problems seen by patients and policymakers is a shortage of physician time relative to patient load. But existing evidence, reviewed earlier in this volume, suggests that physicians working on a salaried basis devote less hours to medical practice. We should be able to devise incentives that bring forth the best efforts of physicians under varying types of capitation, but this will require experimentation with incentive plans that take into account productivity and physician responsiveness to patients. There are a variety of rewards that motivate people, and that can be activated under capitation programs. We must not naively believe, however, that a simple salary or capitation formula, without other incentives, will encourage doctors to work as hard as they do under a system where they are rewarded for each patient they see.

Also, it is inevitable that a centralized system of financing health services will contribute to the already apparent trend of the growing bureaucratization of medical care, unless vigorous measures are taken to limit unnecessary growth of medical organizations. The possibilities for economies of scale are often not as large as many assume, and we would do well to discourage very large or highly centralized delivery systems. This can be achieved under a capitation plan by weighting the capitation payment to discourage an organization from becoming too large. Intelligent organization enhances efficiency and effectiveness of services, but we should be constantly aware of the dangers of a developing attitude toward patients that is casual and impersonal and that undermines the caring function in medical service. Growing bureaucratization poses a threat of increasing dehumanization of care, and efforts will be required to insure that planning in medical organization takes account of the responsibility to enhance human dignity and choice. I believe that decentralized facilities and patient choice among providers organized in varying ways are consistent with this goal.

One of the highest ideals in the practice of medicine is to provide services to those in need that are not only technically competent but also are responsive and humane.[17] While humane care has consequences for how patients respond to treatment and thus affects the quality of care, the case for humane care can be made on its own terms. While there has been much polemics over the role of money and profit in inhibiting humane care, and while claims have been made that a national health system eliminates economic and exploitative motives, the fact remains that humanization of care and responsiveness are far more complex than such simplified contentions imply. Experience throughout the world suggests that lack of responsiveness to people is often a consequence of conflicts in priorities of work, heavy work loads, the bureaucratization of organization with its associated complexity and specialization, and inadequate selection and preparation of those who have the responsibility of dealing with people. Moreover, the incentive system in most medical bureaucracies only rarely rewards the health professional who behaves in a particularly humane way, in contrast to those who do research, who participate in technical innovation, who handle heavy work loads, or who are effective managers.

Large medical organizations in particular tend to be impersonal and unresponsive to the social and psychological needs of the patients they treat.[18] Often such behavior results from attempts to manage heavy work loads with limited resources, and under such conditions the predominant values define what constitutes the more pressing business. To some extent, impersonal care reflects the inherent competition between the time and attention necessary to provide personal care and other functions such as teaching and research. And in part it reflects the complexity of care characteristic of such institutions, the multiplicity of workers who may have some role in any patient's care, and the more elaborate division of labor in which each worker takes only responsibility for his or her special function, with an ambiguous definition of who has responsibility for the total management of the patient. Such complexity also may impede quality of care. When many physicians and hospital services play some role in the patient's treatment, difficulties in communication and coordination are common, and serious failures may result in implementing in some consistent way a management plan for the patient. This often results in redundancies in procedures, in conflicting advice to the patient, and in errors in medication.

As we attempt to increase "efficiencies" in hospitals these problems are likely to increase. Doctors and other health personnel, whatever their personal motives, are guided more by their technical interests and competence than by concern for the social and psychological comfort of patients. The extent of inhumane care within a nationalized system of care, inspired by lofty ideals, is illustrated by Ann Cartwright's study[19] of patients' reactions to their hospital experience. This study portrays how poor communication frequently was between patients and staff. The point is not that British hospitals are any worse than hospitals elsewhere; perhaps they are better. But the complexity of organization, the need for stretching resources, and the ideologies that guide professional practice all come to shape behavior. Ideals without an incentive system to reinforce desired behaviors are too often empty rhetoric.

In the implementation of any new incentive system, it would be unwise to neglect the importance of professional patterns and the extent to which they can thwart desired organizational approaches. It is one thing to design a rational system of work among departments and varying types of personnel; it is quite another to have it operate as anticipated. This general point can be illustrated by examining the relationship between British general practitioners and consultants in British hospitals. Although, in theory, the general practitioner is expected to manage the patient in the community, home, and office unless the patient requires more intensive and specialized care, there are no clear and agreed-upon standards for what problems are best managed in different contexts. The unfortunate fact is that many consultants regard GPs as inferior doctors, and have little confidence in their judgment. General practitioners, in turn, are often resentful of consultants, are sensitive to their relatively lower status, and complain frequently of the poor communication that follows the hospitalization and release of their patients. Although in theory the hospital outpatient department is to return the patient promptly to the GP so that the GP can resume management of the problem, a British study found that almost a third of new referrals were still attending the outpatient clinic six months after their first visit instead of being returned to their family doctor.[20]

Specialists commonly complain that doctors refer trivial patients to specialty clinics without evidence of adequate prior evaluation. They suggest, as do many GPs, that the absence of an economic incentive to evaluate the patient carefully within a busy general practice, organized on a capitation basis, encourages GPs to shunt off to the hospitals patients that they should evaluate and manage themselves. In turn, GPs often feel that consultants repeat such evaluations because of their own bias toward GPs, making the latter's work redundant. Having no confidence that their work will be treated as valuable, they are more likely to prepare only a perfunctory referral note addressed to the outpatient department. The lack of coordination between GPs and specialists predates the National Health Service by many years, and has been linked to the competition between them for patients prior to the enactment of the National Health Insurance Act of 1911.[21] For many years GPs in Britain were regarded as the residual group of medical graduates who lacked the ability or stamina to pursue a satisfactory specialty place. Perhaps the split was best exemplified by the remark of Lord Moran, appearing before the Pilkington Commission, when asked about the suggestion that generalists and consultants were equal. Emphatically denying this, Lord Moran asked: "Could anything be more absurd? . . . How can you say that the people who get to the top of the ladder are the same people who fall off it? It seems to me so ludicrous."[22]

The pattern of health services, like other institutions in society, has been shaped by a particular history, social structure, and sociocultural environment. Patterns that have been ingrained in professional training and the personal perspective of the physician are not easily modified. I have already suggested some of the problems resulting from status differentials among doctors in the British context; similar problems exist between doctors and other health professionals, paraprofessionals, and local government. In some circumstances status differentials are perceived as fair and legitimate. But, increasingly, nonphysicians are viewing such differentials in power and rewards as discriminatory, and are demanding more voice and rewards in the medical context. Status differentials, particularly when they are perceived as unfair or when they are under challenge, hamper effective communication. This in turn retards coordination, dampens the commitment and enthusiasm of personnel, and very much limits the care that is theoretically possible with the resources at hand. In the case of such differences among doctors, a variety of adaptations may develop that are not conducive to good care and consultation. General practitioners, often sensitive and insecure in their relationships with specialists, may cope by limiting their referral arrangements to a few doctors with whom they feel comfortable. In Britain many practitioners do not accompany consultants on domiciliary visits, although the purpose of such visits is consultation, and they can serve as a useful source of continuing education of the GP. Similarly, although general practitioners have no official role in the care of their patients in the hospital, it is desirable for patients to have a supportive visit from a doctor whom they know and who is familiar with their problems. General practitioners tend not to make such visits, complaining that when they do they can have no input into care and that they are sometimes treated with less than full courtesy. Thus, attempts to protect oneself from embarrassment or insecurity resulting from invidious status comparisons result in a pattern of care in which parallel rather than team services are provided.

In the United States, rivalries among varying specialties and subspecialties are common. These differences of perspective and struggles over control may become dysfunctional to care by disrupting orderly communication and coordination. As attempts are made to rationalize and systematize relationships through health planning, it will be foolish to assume that such human problems will not persist. They may even become more severe. Competition and rivalry are likely to become more bitter when resources are more limited and when struggles take place over beds, space, equipment, and funds. Similarly, although we can only speculate about the possible impact of the Professional Standards Review Organizations, it seems possible that such review can become the chips in a "game" quite different from the one intended—departments and specialties faced with contracting resources and a new set of incentives may battle over control of the medical domain and the distribution of resources through this process.

The existing organization of health services in the United States is in disarray. Most of the proposals for national health insurance will perpetuate and exacerbate existing problems. They will do little to change or rationalize the organization of health care, and they will contribute to inflation rather than to control over spiraling medical care costs. Only two alternatives provide a reasonable opportunity to deal with the economic consequences of increasing access to health care and to increased demand resulting from more comprehensive insurance. One approach is through catastrophic insurance, but this approach does not come to terms with many of the basic criticisms of current practices and patterns of organization. The only real alternative approach presently advocated is the approach typified by the Health Security Program.

In endorsing the Health Security approach, I do not necessarily approve of all its details. Throughout this chapter I have emphasized the many problems we can anticipate in moving from the poorly defined administrative structure presently embodied in the idea to its implementation. The idea provides a possible framework for substantially improved performance in the delivery of health services, but much effort and attention must be given to defining more clearly the administrative mechanisms and incentive systems that will achieve desired results. As I have argued, we need considerable experimentation, and thus I would favor a loosely organized administrative structure, encouragement for a decentralized pattern of services, incentives for competition within the framework among competing delivery patterns, and a clear plan and associated incentives to promote increased emphasis on humane and responsive care and on caring as a central aspect of performance. Although it would not be wise to expect such a system to improve vastly the nation's health or to solve all problems of access immediately, these goals provide some sense of new priorities such as health promotion, patient education, and an emphasis on using the self-help resources of the community as part of the overall pattern of delivery of services. To avoid unfulfilled expectations, we must be realistic. But we must also have aspirations that stimulate the involvement and participation of both providers and patients. Utopia is not around the corner, but having goals toward which we aspire is an important facet of any organizational effort.

In short, it should be apparent that the designs of new systems of behavior and coordination are more difficult in practice than they are in theory. They must cope not only with theoretical conceptions of systems design but also with the sociocultural context and behavioral aspects of human organization. For doctors and patients are simply not pawns for policymakers to manipulate in line with current social theories, but active participants who are aware of attempts to design their behavior and capable of manipulating these designs in light of their own needs and goals. The area is complex and innumerable questions remain unanswered, but it seems likely that approaches to design that recognize the difficulties and that provide opportunities for experimenting with varying alternatives have greater potential for success.

NOTES

1. Social Security Administration (1974), *National Health Insurance Proposals: Provisions of Bills Introduced in the 93rd Congress as of February 1974* (Washington, D.C.: DHEW), Publication No. (SSA) 11920; R. Eilers and S. Moyerman, eds. (1971), *National Health Insurance* (Homewood, Ill.: Richard Irwin); "National Health Insurance: Which Way to Go?" *Consumer Reports*, February 1975, pp. 118–124.

2. V. R. Fuchs (1974), *Who Shall Live: Health, Economics and Social Choice* (New York: Basic Books), p. 150.

3. J. P. Newhouse, C. E. Phelps, and W. B. Schwartz (1974), "Policy Options and the Impact of National Health Insurance," *New England Journal of Medicine*, 290:1345–1359.

4. V. R. Fuchs (1974), op. cit., pp. 135–136.

5. Department of Health, Education and Welfare (1974), *Estimated Health Expenditures Under Selected National Health Insurance Bills: A Report to the Congress.*

6. V. R. Fuchs (1974), op. cit., p. 128.

7. R. Fein (1974), "The President's Health Insurance Program—Is It the Best Way?" *Health Care Policy Discussion Paper No. 14*, Center for Community Health and Medical Care, Harvard University.

8. M. Greenlick and D. Freeborn (1971), "Determinants of Medical Care Utilization: On Choosing Appropriate Measures of Utilization," Keynote Address, Engineering Foundation Conference on Qualitative Decision Making for the Delivery of Ambulatory Care, Henniker, N.H.

9. O. Anderson (1973), "Health Services in the USSR," *Selected Papers No. 42* (Chicago: University of Chicago Graduate School of Business).

10. See, for example, J. Handler (1972), *Reforming the Poor: Welfare Policy, Federalism and Morality* (New York: Basic Books).

11. R. Logan (1971), "National Health Planning—An Appraisal of the State of the Art," *International Journal of Health Services,* 1:6–17.

12. Ibid., pp. 11–12.

13. R. Stevens (1966), *Medical Practice in Modern England* (New Haven: Yale University Press).

14. D. Mechanic (1972), *Public Expectations and Health Care* (New York: Wiley-Interscience), pp. 130–134.

15. A. Cartwright (1967), *Patients and Their Doctors: A Study of General Practice* (London: Routledge and Kegan Paul); P. E. Enterline et al. (1973), "The Distribution of Medical Services Before and After 'Free' Medical Care—The Quebec Experience," *New England Journal of Medicine,* 289:1174–1178; and A. D. McDonald et al. (1974), "Effect of Quebec Medicare on Physician Consultation for Selected Symptoms," *New England Journal of Medicine,* 291:649–652.

16. T. Bice et al. (1972), "Socioeconomic Status and Use of Physician Services: A Reconsideration," *Medical Care,* 10:261–271.

17. See J. Howard and A. Strauss, eds. (1975), *Humanizing Health Care* (New York: Wiley-Interscience).

18. R. S. Duff and A. B. Hollingshead (1968), *Sickness and Society* (New York: Harpers).

19. A. Cartwright (1964), *Human Relations and Hospital Care* (Boston: Routledge and Kegan Paul); R. Logan (1971), op. cit., p. 14.

20. R. Logan (1971), op. cit., p. 14.

21. B. Abel-Smith (1964), *The Hospitals: 1800–1948* (London: Heinemann).

22. Quoted in P. Ferris (1965), *The Doctors* (London: Gollancz).

Index